Paul Wenzel Geissler, Richard Rottenburg, Julia Zenker (eds.)
Rethinking Biomedicine and Governance in Africa

MatteRealities/VerKörperungen
Perspectives from Empirical Science Studies

Volume 15

Editorial

Since the late 1970s, *empirical science studies* have developed into a key field of research at the intersection of science, technology and society. This field merges a repertoire of theories and methods stemming primarily from cultural anthropology, sociology, linguistics and history. Its main characteristic is the detailed analysis of scientific practices and epistemic cultures and how these become entangled with public discourses and everyday life. This focus tries to reveal specific, local configurations and their epistemological as well as social consequences. Beyond a mere deconstruction, science studies are constantly looking to engage with the fields in which they do their work. The goal of this book series is to offer to scholars a German and English speaking Forum that

- develops inter- and trans-disciplinary bodies of knowledge in the areas of medicine and the life sciences and makes these nationally and internationally available;
- supports young scientists through opening up a new field of work which runs across existing disciplinary structures;
- encourages the formation of *tandems* through co-authorship. In particular, it supports, evaluates and comments on collaborative projects with colleagues from the natural and engineering sciences.

The series is directed towards scholars and students from both the empirical science/social studies and the natural sciences and medicine.

Paul Wenzel Geissler, Richard Rottenburg, Julia Zenker (eds.)

Rethinking Biomedicine and Governance in Africa

Contributions from Anthropology

[transcript]

This volume emerged from the work of the research group »Law, Organization, Science and Technology« directed by Richard Rottenburg, financed by the Max Planck Society and located at the Max Planck Institute for Social Anthropology, Halle, Germany.

Bibliographic information published by the Deutsche Nationalbibliothek
The Deutsche Nationalbibliothek lists this publication in the Deutsche Nationalbibliografie; detailed bibliographic data are available in the Internet at http://dnb.d-nb.de

Cover layout: Kordula Röckenhaus, Bielefeld
Cover illustration: Collaborative medical research fieldwork in the city. 2009. Drawing from a series of illustrations of scientific research work by Johnson A. Ondiek, staff member of KEMRI, Kenya.
Typeset by Michael Rauscher, Bielefeld
Printed by Majuskel Medienproduktion GmbH, Wetzlar
ISBN 978-3-8376-2028-3

Content

Missing the Nation State

Longing for Citizenship

21st century African biopolitics: fuzzy fringes, cracks and undersides, neglected backwaters, and returning politics

P. Wenzel Geissler, Richard Rottenburg, Julia Zenker

Introduction

This volume, based on a workshop organised by the research group Law Organisation Science and Technology (LOST), and held at the Max Planck Institute of Social Anthropology, Halle, Germany, in June 2009, is about biomedicine and governance in Africa. Biomedicine was introduced to the continent in line with its own evolution as 19th century scientific endeavour, and its engagement with African maladies—new germs, new modes of transmission, and new measures of experimentation and control—has in turn profoundly shaped the universal forms of "modern" biomedicine (see e.g. Vaughan 1991; Baronov 2008; Tilley 2011). The intimate entanglement between medical endeavours and government—notably the nation-state and its colonial precursors—has been particularly marked in Africa given the limited availability of private biomedical practice during most of the 20th century, and due to the contrast to the much more prevalent *non*-biomedical ideas, organisations, and practices of healing which until fairly recently, and with few exceptions were distinctly non-government in the sense of not being endorsed by state institutions and not pursuing a governmental, population-wide perspective (see e.g. Last 2012). Biomedicine in Africa affords thus a privileged perspective on the relationship between government—in a wide sense comprising direct state policies and practices, as well as other forms of control ranging from subjects' own self-making within wider power relations, to population-wide efforts of categorisation and discipline—and its evolution across the tides of history.

Changing times

Our motivation for the workshop, and for this volume, was twofold: On an empirical level, all participants share the impression that the African present, the early 21st-century, constitutes a departure as compared to an earlier period, half a century or so ago (e.g. Ferguson 2006; with respect to bioscience see e.g. Rottenburg 2009). While few of us propose tidy, tidal shift type, historical periodisations, we all observe, with varying emphasis, contrasts and changes. Between the 1970s and the present, scientific-technical shifts occurred, for example the growing importance of first immunology and later genomics, and the attendant shift to an increasingly costly, high maintenance diagnostic and therapeutic apparatus. This shift was accompanied, across most of Africa, by epidemiological changes; first and foremost the HIV/AIDS epidemic—which brought exceptionalist policies, obscured the continued prevalence of equally dramatic diseases, and called for interventions on an unprecedented scale—as well as the gradual emergence of non-communicable health problems such as cancer and diabetes (Livingstone 2012; Whyte 2012).

During the same period, funding mechanisms and institutional frames for biomedicine and science in Africa changed, broadly shifting the emphasis from national institutions to collaborative transnational endeavours, and from nation-state government funding to various forms of private-public partnerships (see e.g. Geissler 2012). This change in the organisation and financing of medical science was paralleled by radical changes in government financing, reducing state expenditure and control, largely through outside pressure, and, in consequence, privatisation of health care as part of larger economic and political privatisation. These large-scale medical-technical and political-economic changes where accompanied by the proliferation of new conceptual frames and social forms: Non-governmental organisations and private public partnerships filled some of the gaps left by crumbling states; and 20th century "public health" with its strong ties to the nation-state and citizenship, was replaced, on the one hand, by "humanitarian" imaginaries and modes of intervention, driven by the logic of emergency and exception and targeting "humans" rather than citizens (e.g. Fassin & Pandolfi 2007; Redfield 2012); and, on the other hand, "global health" focusing on health problems with global impact and promoting policies on a global, rather than merely national scale.

These larger contrasts arise from comparison between the early postcolonial period in Africa, 1960s-70s, and the present in the early 21st century. Something happened between these two points in time, and although few of us would subscribe wholesale to one neat description of periodisation and historical shift–such as "neoliberalisation"—and the concomitant implication of economic determinism, something did happen during the period of the long 1980s, from somewhere in the mid-70s to the mid-1990s, which has produced a constellation of medical governmentality that is different from what we were used to, and different from much that has been described in the history of biomedicine in Africa (e.g. Packard 1990; Lyons 1992; Feierman 1992; Iliffe 1998). Our task in this volume is not the historians' pursuit, relative to the early postcolonial period, nor historical comparison, but to capture the emergent present. There can be little doubt that biomedicine and governance—in the broad sense alluded to above—remain as closely intertwined as ever, but how and to what effect is less clear; and from this empirical question arises a political question that underlies many of our contributions: how can one politically engage with governmental medicine and medical governance that (maybe, in some parts) no longer follows the rules of 20th-century nation-state politics?

21st CENTURY AFRICAN BIOPOLITICS

The sense of an empirical change, emergent and partially articulated, posits a challenge, then, to our theoretical tools, which is the second motivation for our conversation and for the essays below. For all of us thinking about the relationship between governance and biomedicine, state and science, is inevitably framed by Michel Foucault's now classic work. The key texts pertaining to biomedicine were published in the 1970s, and radically changed thinking about medicine and knowledge, and governance and power during the "modern" era since the late 18th century. It provided a creative framework for countless innovative studies of medicine, and not least the study of medicine and colonialism, and triggered theoretical and methodological moves that changed the entirety of social science, notably through concepts derived from Foucault's "biopower", mutating into "biosociality", "biological citizenship" etc. (see below).

Yet, parallel to the creativity unleashed by Foucault's works, there is also a risk of ideas and arguments atrophying. Five decades after these groundbreaking texts about biology and medicine, some of Foucault's ideas have become formulaic, much like the reduction of Marx' subtle and sophisticated analyses to the historical-materialist determinism of 1980s student essays. Today there is a risk of Foucault's open (sometimes contradictory) invitations to profound social inquiry to be eroded to simple narratives about the relations between medicine and governance, according to which biomedical knowledge practices are key tools in modern biopolitical regimes of power. If this narrative is pushed to the extreme, childhood vaccines become disciplining tools, dysfunctional hospitals emanate power, refugee camps become indistinguishable from concentration camps, and every randomized drug trial evokes the specter of Tuskegee (Jones 1981), which does little justice to the analytical potential of such objects, nor to the lives and struggles of those involved in such phenomena—as patients and subjects, or indeed as doctors and planners.

Such reductionist narratives about "disciplining" bioscience have their own historical context of (neo)liberal ideas about the supposed separateness between state and citizen, in combination with an antimodernist thrust (which finds its expression e.g. in James Scott's work). Above all, this interpretation of biomedical governmentality has become so taken-for-granted and instinct-like that it can obscure, rather than elucidate the analytical and political challenges posed by bioscience in Africa today. It becomes particularly problematic if it is applied to contemporary political-cum-scientific constellations, without taking into account the dramatic empirical changes, flagged out above, that state and other modes of government, and scientific and technological regimes, have undergone during the past 30 years.

Our point is not to discard the biopolitical narrative; it remains foundational to our analyses as the papers in this volume will show. It is not our aim to "move beyond Foucault" in a familiar academic move—we cannot and do not want to offer a new narrative. Instead, we hope to interrogate the above simplified narrative, as well as more sophisticated derivatives of Foucault's lexicon in the light of diverse ethnographies of medical science across Africa, so as to open it up again; we aim to get at it from different, and not always commensurate angles, *not* proposing an alternative argument—anti-biopolitics vs. biopolitics—that would only push the old scholarly pendulum, but inviting new questions and routes of investigation stemming from these now classic ideas about government, body and knowledge.

MAIN LINES OF ARGUMENT

The contributors to this volume are of a post-Foucauldian generation. The oldest of us read Foucault, which then had replaced the Marxist analysts of the previous generation, since the first days of their graduate studies in the late 1970s; the youngest of us studied in an environment saturated by the profound Foucauldian impact across all social sciences and notably in those concerned with medicine and body, as well as among anthropologists and historians of former empires. By then, the extension of Foucauldian terminology and thought, filtered through the different adaptations of German, French, and especially US academia, had become taken for granted, and not rarely reduced and simplified, and began to invite—with due respect to the profound influence of the original texts—critical reflections.

The chapters below take much of their orientation from post-Foucauldian scholarship, in particular the fruitful elaborations about the theme of biopolitics in the works of anthropologists like Rabinow (e.g. 1996), or sociologists like Rose (2007), who moved issues of biopolitical discipline towards the concept of "biosociality" and "biological citizenship". With few exceptions, the texts below understand themselves as contributions to the study of biosociality, and many reflect over, and critique, the notion of biological citizenship. They are, then, "post-Foucauldian" both in the sense of a profound debt to the social science scholarship inspired by Foucault, and seeking for academic pursuits, and political practice, for an age beyond the classic modernist compound that his work arose from.

At the same time, most of the authors below engage with the political critique of late capitalism, or neoliberalisation, theoretically drawing on readings of Marx' political-economy through anthropologists like the Comaroffs (e.g. 2000) and geographers like Harvey (e.g. 2006) or Massey (e.g. 1999). While the degree of identification with this scholarship varies between the authors, all of them relate to the notion of neoliberalism and its impact on politics and well-being. In as far as they try to move beyond the simple description of the present as neoliberal, the authors display post-neoliberal sensitivities, some explicitly using this term.

Limits of Biopolitics

Many of the authors below take issue with the apparent seamlessness of the biopolitical disciplining project, with the idea that medical practices and interventions simply produce disciplined subjects, simply *work*. Against this imaginary of subjectification, some of the authors point at moments of *resistance and creativity*, even of supposedly disciplined new selves (e.g. Gerrets, Hardon). Other authors underline the inevitable *incompleteness* of any disciplining project especially in Africa, notably under conditions of post-neoliberal state attrition (Kelly, Park, Peterson, Prince, Redfield), or point even at the outright failure that is built into the biopolitical endeavour (Lachenal)

Some authors reflect further about the usefulness and limits of the now widespread use of the concept of *citizenship* in relation to disease control and public health intervention, notably in regions where direct governmental control over territory has become or remained weak. Several authors recognise that biopolitical interventions, such as large-scale treatment programs, have the potential to engender social relations and produce collectives as well as attachments to larger wholes. Some of them contrast biological disease-related "citizenships" with the standards of the older, more comprehensive project of "rights bearing citizens" that provided possibilities for political articulation and durable attachments well beyond the sort of unstable associations produced by deterritorialised, time-space limited, single disease treatment programs (e.g. Redfield, Geissler).

Moreover, several contributors raise the question whether citizenship, as well as public health, might not simply require the existence of a functioning whole, and/or a vision of its existence, such as the nation or an equivalent polity—while alternatives to the nation seeming to be difficult to identify (e.g. Park, Kelly, Redfield, Geissler).

A further qualification of the concept of biological citizenship arises from the comparison between different disease-specific interventions. While much of the writing on biological citizenship in Africa focuses on interventions to prevent or treat HIV/AIDS, several of the authors below suggest that this, rather than providing the model case for emergent biopolitical regimes, might just be one specific case among many, and rather different from, say, interventions against malaria or sleeping sickness (e.g. Redfield, Gerrets, Kelly). Far from simple disease-parochial one-upmanship, these observations regarding the specific effects of different diseases, and their diverse entanglements with social and political projects, serve as a useful caveat against generalisations based on HIV-focused studies, and point towards fruitful areas of future scholarship.

As a logical complement to reflections about overly structural representations of disciplining regimes—and the attendant tendency to overlook failures, gaps, contradictions, creativity and struggle—many of the chapters pursue, sometimes as a subtext, a search for remains and revivals of politics proper, as in spaces of struggle for rights and interests, and for alternative trajectories to that of a progressively neoliberal, and medical-technical repressive, "regime". Such new political moments and propositions emerge from very different quarters: several authors recognise the lasting purchase of the nation-state both as legitimising agency (e.g. Park, Klein, Prince) and as territorial-cum-meliorist project (Kelly, Redfield, Gerrets), as a contested future, and as a reference in the past. For others, politics emerge on the level of bodily practices of self-formation interpreted as "resistance" (Klein), in relation to mundane everyday struggles with hunger (Prince), or out of the moral dilemmas that especially medical practitioners in HIV treatment experience as a result of the incomplete and unstable order of pharmaceutical governance that they are part of (Park). Politics also raise their head in the form of desires and utopias, such as in medical research participants' longing for attachment to large, trustworthy and reliable wholes (Geissler), or in medical doctors' utopian visions of public health as government (Lachenal).

At the very bottom of biopolitical regimes, in their cracks and crevices, at their fuzzy margins, and even in their abysmal failure, the contributions to this volume recognise the potential for something other than subjectification understood as subjection. In various guises they suggest the possibility of re-emerging political subjectivity, the beginning of new positionings, contradictions, spaces, struggles. Importantly, in several accounts the search for alternative directions brings the figure of the nation back to the fore as both, state and territory, which variously appears as absent, as prerequisite, as condition of citizenship and as desire and project. Thus, while for classic post-Foucauldian sensitivities both medical science and the nation-state were intertwined dimensions of the high modern biopolitical apparatus, suspect on account of its repressive and subjectificating capacity, for many of the contributors below, and presumably even more so for the people that they engaged with in their field work in African settings, the absence of the nation-state as collective, territory and shared history, is experienced as a lack. Biopolitics, including national medical government, calls here forth not threat and loathing, but nostalgia and desire.

OVERVIEW OF THE VOLUME

Not quite disciplined

The themes above feature, in various proportions, in all the texts below. We begin with two chapters that, based on very different empirical material—one from transnational malaria experiments conducted upon discreet African territories, the other from national politics of sex and gender—suggest that apparently disciplining regimes such as disease control and surveillance and the legislation of gendered bodies, do not necessarily produce new subjects, but retain resilience, unpredictability and are shaped by effects of local and biological specifics.

Gerrets takes issue with two linked common assumptions about African biopolitics, namely the idea that public health interventions necessarily produce discipline, new subjectivities, and self-fashioning; and secondly, that specific contemporary, "public-private" biopolitical formations necessarily engender a paradigm shift from nation-state order to a neoliberal regime antithetical to nation-state government and citizenship.

Situating contemporary malaria control public-private-partnerships in Tanzania in the context of a larger historical trajectory, Gerrets shows how the shifting fates of malaria control in Tanzania have created a "changing (in) visibility of malaria", rather than one coherent regime. Intense efforts to control malaria and educate people did not simply discipline populations, but instead created unstable patchworks of specific local understandings, interlaced with older cultural meanings, and selectively appropriated health messages often contradicting fundamental biomedical tenets. Thus, although malaria has orientated governmental interventions for more than a century, the outcomes—including those of current non-governmental interventions—are less than predictable and did not bring forth a clearly defined biological citizenship. This leads Gerrets to the conclusion that, unlike AIDS, malaria does not seem to produce novel collectives or subjectivities, and that, accordingly, the social study of "global health" must take heed of the variation between the relative social productivity of different disease entities instead of extending lessons learned from AIDS to a generalised biopolitical regime (see also the contribution by Redfield on sleeping sickness, below).

Klein's ethnography of legal and medical struggles about transsexuality in post-apartheid South Africa reflects about the relation between the nation-state and the embodied subject around gender defining practices. While Klein recognises the power of the law and of medical concepts to normalise and discipline subjects, her interest is "not the passive subject of governmental, legal or medical intervention" but "subjects themselves", as agents involved in struggles about their bodies. Klein interprets what she calls "somatechnics of self-formation"– notably surgical and pharmaceutical interventions, but also legal innovations such as the introduction of a 3rd sex, or linguistic artefacts as ungendered pronouns—as forms of resistance that challenge the hegemonic supposition of an unambiguous binary sex model.

Klein's material leads on to examine the interaction between transgender activism and the post-apartheid South African diversity fetishism; these are particularly pertinent in the context of this volume, because South Africa is one of the few African states which at the beginning of the 21st-century combines neoliberal state privatisation with a strongly developed nation state ideology.

Reading Klein's ethnography one is, moreover, struck by the resonance between the body-focused, pharmaceutically and surgically enhanced vision of sexual rights, and neoliberal discourse on personal ownership in bodies, and the rejection of nation-states' interference with bodily concerns. Millennial South African transsexual politics emerge then at the intersection of a particular dominant hegemonic discourse of "diversity" and "freedom", combined with a particular South African tradition and expertise in highly invasive surgical technologies, from which arise, at this particular point in time, exuberant hybrid forms. The recognition of the particular historical juncture at which this is possible would lead to further reflection and investigation about the fate of these creations under the impact of more recent political and ideological terms.

Politics again

The next two chapters, both dealing with HIV activism and interventions in Eastern Africa, pursue this line of argument further, looking for the interplay between political discipline and its anti-political effects as well as for the re-emergence of struggle and contradiction beyond it.

Hardon takes issue with the familiar post-Foucauldian associations between biomedicine and discipline, and the idea that disease-focused biomedical projects, such as HIV activism produce predictable patterns of biopolitical subject formation. She traces the evolution of HIV activism from its origins in the US American gay community to Africa and shows how the transfer of the activist model did indeed entail the production of disciplined selves, even docile subjects; but, she argues, similar to the work of e.g. Nguyen (2010), the new social forms that arise from this governmental process might, in turn, enable new forms of agency, resistance and "potential for change". In an interesting aside, nodding towards science and technology studies, and towards the arguments by other authors below, such as Kelly or Park, Hardon suggests that unpredictability and resilience are exacerbated, beyond human agency, by nonhuman contributions, such as drug resistance or the breakdown of technology.

Prince studies HIV care and treatment programmes funded by the US government's PEPFAR, touching upon millions of Western Kenyans' lives. Drawing on funds that dwarf the National Ministry of health's budget, these programs have during the past decade produced a "medicalised economy of care and welfare" which provides much of the resources circulating in the local economy, which otherwise is marked by an exacerbating economic crisis, rising food prices, massive corruption and stark class differences. In her ethnography Prince shows how HIV interventions open up pathways of opportunity for some—employment, workshops and training, part-aid volunteering etc.—creating what is locally referred to as a new middle class. For HIV-positive people, however, these opportunities are highly volatile, and access depends upon one's visibility and legibility to NGOs. This leads to the proliferation of new social forms aiming at producing precisely this: self-help groups that make "community" and particular HIV groupings visible; projects and proposals that express needs in the terminology and budget frames of overseas funders and NGOs. Prince concludes, that while one might be inclined to describe HIV programmes as anti-political forms of governmentality, one should recognise the fact that hunger and poverty are nevertheless brought to the fore by patients, "puncturing" the "expert discourse", as Li has it (2007). And one should continue to explore the fuzzy edges of seemingly clear biopolitical forms, attending to smaller politics of life, rather than reifying their hegemonic order. Like the previous chapters, Prince's encourages the reader to refocus attention at the margins of the biopolitical regime, not to deny its potency, but to attend to the struggles, situated under particular local conditions, that it is engaged in.

Inherent failure and contradiction

The next two chapters move beyond this by pointing at the fact that contradictions, and even outright failure, are not just effects external to a biopolitical regime, but part and parcel of it.

Lachenal's history of a distinctly utopian mid-20th-century biopolitical experiment in French-occupied Cameroon—literally turning the government of a territory over to medical doctors—takes him beyond familiar discussions about African biopolitics. He takes issue with analyses of biopolitical projects that take their effectiveness for granted and critique their allegedly disciplining and subjecting consequences; yet at the same time he shows that it is insufficient merely to point at failures and complexities to counter such interpretations.

Instead, Lachenal convinces us of the productivity of failure, moving us away from the question as to whether biopolitical interventions and experiments really succeeded or failed, and suggesting that failure always is at the heart of such experiments and indeed adds to the heroic connotations of utopian social projects. As he shows in the Cameroonian example, the experimenters did not delude themselves about the failure of their pursuit, and yet, this did little to discourage or discredit them among peers. On the contrary, the persistent gap between discourse and reality was part of their performance, underlining the grandeur of the mission. Delusion, irrationality, and delirious aesthetics, appear here not so much in contrast to governmentality—as the pursuit of discipline and melioration—but as an integral part of it. Adding forces beyond rationality to our interpretations of medical science and public health, Lachenal enriches our critical engagement with biopolitics, not merely as a more or less effective regime, but always also as performance and illusion.

Peterson's reflections about the attempts to implement global intellectual property agreements under the 1995 TRIPS framework in Nigeria pursues a very different path by showing not only that the biopolitical order of pharmaceutical property regimes reaches its limits when it is confronted with local cultural notions of ownership—and interesting but relative conventional argument—but also, more importantly that it is limited by the inherent contradictions within the global system of neoliberal governance. While TRIPS aims to impose strict patent law and intellectual property protection, this would require a legal and control apparatus that does not exist in Nigeria, partly because of the persistent privatisation and downsizing of state institutions during neoliberal structural adjustment programmes, which incapacitated juridical and executive institutions. Peterson sees thus a "full-scale contradiction between structural adjustment results and TRIPS demands". The result is, then, a regime of intellectual property that is inefficient at best.

Missing the nation state

The next two chapters pursue further the figure of *the absent state*, the gap left by the transformation and reduction of state functioning over the past decades.

Kelly moves ahead, theoretically and empirically, of the preoccupation with neoliberalisation as a paradigm shift away from the nation-state and its attendant forms of territorial sovereignty and citizenship. Her case is about the *end* of a transnational scientific malaria experiment in Tanzania, funded by large-scale ex-corporate charitable organisations outside nation-state government. The problem faced here is not privatisation (or public-private partnerships), but "re-publicisation", or "municipalisation": the transfer of an experimental order inscribed upon the territory of the capital city, by global scientists through "community owned resource persons" or CORPS (locally sourced but paid by overseas charity), to the government of that city. This scaling up of an experimental order, Kelly shows, raises more than just questions of size and sustainability.

The transfer is fraught with difficulty—accentuated by the technical, logistical, cognitive and political requirements of malaria control. Kelly traces the contemporary challenges of recreating *public* health out of an experimental form back to the collapse of national malaria control after the 1980s (a national programme that had been remarkably successful; see also Gerrets) and the subsequent revival of interest in malaria at the behest of external donors who, faced with the lack of public infrastructure and resources, emphasised the need to rely upon community. Community became here shorthand for the civic, substituting for notions of nation, society and citizenship, which had been cornerstones of the successful post-independence malaria control. One question which the end of the experimental regime described by Kelly brings to the fore is whether this substitute can exist without the stabilising role, and resources, of outside experts and donors. In the current absence of a comprehensive municipality—including experts, bureaucrats, technicians and citizens contained in a larger entity—community, including supposed "community owned persons", might simply not exist, leave alone provide the foundation for a complex, labour-intensive and resource demanding public-health endeavour like malaria control.

Park's sensitive ethnography of HIV treatment programmes in Uganda casts fresh light upon the inter-animation of transnational and national forms of government. Life-sustaining HIV treatment for millions of people takes here neither the form of classic nation-state biopolitics, nor of neoliberal, privatised and extraterritorial interventions. Instead, Park discerns the outlines of a novel formation of pharmaceutical governance centred on supply chain management, and as such is technical or "infrapolitical". While the earlier pharmaceutical politics of the 1990s (see e.g. Hardon; Redfield) were struggles about HIV sufferers' rights, the subsequent forms of pharmaceutical governance are outside the political, because of their technical and de-territorialised nature.

As Park shows around the moment of "stock-outs", when drugs run out in the facilities that should distribute them to patients, the key to effective supply chain management is data and information—indicators—and considerable attention is directed within the programs at producing such numbers, which nevertheless remain flawed, making stock-outs a persistent feature of this system. Moreover, HIV drug supplies in Uganda (similar to other PEPFAR funded HIV treatment programs in Africa) are not situated within the public healthcare system—which is deemed too unstable—but in projects managed by NGOs, and in an entirely separate drug distribution system, bypassing nation-state structures. This projectification—relying upon shifting donors and policies—adds different forms of instability to the "complex and unstable entanglements" of this governance. As an important contribution of Parks's ethnography, he leads our attention to the fact that the instability of this order, and notably stock-outs, engender moral dilemmas for patients and staff, who have to reconcile clinical and ethical standards with scarce resources, take clinically wrong decisions in order to serve patients, or give contradictory messages to patients. Experienced contradictions like this might, as Clair Wendland (2010) recently discussed, revitalise political visions and engagements within the remit of seemingly technocratic pharmaceutical governance.

Longing for citizenship

The last two chapters both engage with the inchoate social projects and longings that we might find among the diverse constituencies of contemporary biopolitical constellations: *the longing for citizenship*.

Geissler's chapter on participation in HIV clinical trials conducted by US government organisations in collaboration with Kenyan institutions focuses on "experimental citizenship" as a variant of biological citizenship arising from biomedical experimentation. The term draws simultaneously attention to the inherent limitation of this subspecies of citizenship—if this is the appropriate term, still—namely the tentative, temporary and circumscribed characteristics of the experiment, by contrast to the comprehensive, enduring and territorially encompassing (national) citizenship of the rights bearing citizen. Geissler examines a particularly trivial material aspect of clinical trials, small payments of money, and highlights the emergent collectives and aimed-for social relations into which these material transfers are embedded. Rather then being simple "payments", he argues, they function as tokens of attachment, and as markers of belonging to a larger whole, such as a potent transnational medical research organisation. This desire for experimental citizenship reveals for him a lasting longing for larger social collectives and enduring attachments, ideally beyond the ephemeral order of a trial. This form of citizenship falls certainly short of the larger project which the nation-state here is no longer able to provide, but it retains its older shape as a project, and, Geissler suggests, this experimental citizenship might harbour the germs for a re-emergence of political subjectivity.

In the volume's final chapter, Redfield, using the vantage point of sleeping sickness as a neglected disease, takes issue with the increasingly liberal use of the term citizenship—such as in "experimental citizenship", above—in the literature on biopolitics in Africa and elsewhere. In general terms, he notes, the claims and attachments issued by global health interventions are qualitatively different from citizenship understood as the quality of a rights bearing subject; as such, novel concepts like "biological" or "therapeutic citizenship" in equal measure elucidate the social forms arising from interventions such as HIV programmes, as they highlight important differences in regard to such broader, classic understandings of the citizen. Upon such critical reflection, "global health engenders at best a distant form of citizenship, constructed out of humanitarian concern rather than territorial projects".

More specifically, Redfield observes, echoing similar remarks by Gerrets (this volume), the particularities of different diseases make a difference when thinking about intersections between politics and life; in other words insights won from studies of HIV programmes might not be transferable to sleeping sickness interventions (or, in Gerrets' case, malaria). From this arises Redfield's guiding question, as to whether one can be a biological citizen of a marginal medical concern. Exploring the departure of MSF as the driver of sleeping sickness work in Uganda, and the uncertain transfer of monitoring and control activities to the national government (reminiscent of Kelly's problematic), Redfield observes that although Uganda is not a "failed state", its institutional and budgetary weaknesses make it "far less biopolitical than any contemporary European polity, in the sense of actively fostering life". And thus, its effects in terms of eliciting citizenship remain limited.

Not quite disciplined

Governing Malaria: How an old scourge troubles precepts in social theory

RENE GERRETS

In November, 2003, Tanzanian parliamentarians gathered for an unprecedented event: 204 out of 295 legislators crossed the street to the recently-established Centre for the Enhancement of Effective Malaria Interventions (CEEMI). A day-long seminar aimed at gaining their support for plans to halve deaths and sickness from the mosquito-borne illness by 2010. Headed by Dr. Ali Mohamed Shein, the Tanzanian Vice-President, the seminar featured dozens of domestic and foreign experts who detailed the public health and socioeconomic consequences of malaria, the principle cause of mortality and morbidity in Tanzania as in most sub-Saharan countries. Underscoring this message, a theatre group staged a performance showing legislators the enormous suffering that malaria causes in society, especially among impoverished children and pregnant women in rural areas.

After reviewing the problems, experts turned to solutions. Representatives from various public sector institutions, non-governmental organizations, philanthropies and—a novelty—commercial enterprises informed law-makers about the latest developments in malaria research and control. Massive international funding increases, and intensified cooperation with the private sector, spurred the development of new tools—e.g., vaccines, antimalarials, insecticide-treated nets (ITNs)—that made a renewed attack on the seemingly invincible disease conceivable, for the first time in decades.
This first-of-a-kind seminar was a roaring success: Legislators promptly declared the long-neglected disease a priority topic. In the following months, they issued a range of measures aimed at facilitating malaria research and control efforts; streamlined conflicting laws and directives; eliminated obstructive taxes on necessary drugs and insecticides; and debated creating 'malaria focal persons' to coordinate and monitor affairs at the district level. Applauding these shifts, international actors followed suit. In February 2009 the Global Fund to fight AIDS, Tuberculosis and Malaria (GFATM) awarded Tanzania US$680 million to expand malaria treatment and prevention, a sum three times the annual budget of the Ministry of Health (MoH). After years of neglect, malaria was once again a priority issue in Tanzania.

Rare a decade ago, events such as the above-described malaria seminar for Tanzanian parliamentarians have become commonplace in resource-constrained countries, where they profoundly shape infectious disease research and control priorities. The apparent diversity of these events (for instance, in terms of their focus—e.g., AIDS, pneumonia, maternal mortality) obscures the fact that they share a principle that in recent years has become orthodoxy in international health: the notion of 'partnership.'

The rise to dominance of this idea in international health is exemplified by the explosive growth of public-private partnerships during the last decade. A novelty in this domain until the late-1990s, partnerships[1] were embraced as the way forward by key players such as the World Health Organization and—crucially important—the Gates Foundation (Shiffman 2006), paving the way for expanding the role of private sector institutions and corporate models in international health. Soaring development assistance to the health sector, which rose from US$ 5.6 billion in 1990 to US$ 21.8 billion in 2007 (Ravishankar 2009), further fuelled the proliferation of PPPs. Today, well over half of donor funding for malaria research and control efforts—US$ 800 million in 2007, a 20-fold increase in 15 years—is directed through partnership-like endeavours (Ravishankar 2009). Similar patterns can be observed for other diseases. Unsurprisingly, partnerships are nowadays regarded as an "unavoidable necessity" (Richter 2004).

For social theorists, the rapid proliferation of partnerships in international health raises various salient questions. These entities are currently affecting the lives and livelihoods of millions—if not billions—of people, for instance by transforming the development, testing and distribution of drugs and vaccines for a steadily growing range of neglected diseases (Nwaka 2005; Serdobova/Kieny 2006). Even ardent critics acknowledge their impressive public health achievements, so far (Buse/Harmer 2007). Yet partnerships also exert effects beyond the domain of health. As neoliberal "tools" for privatizing state functions and for governing at a distance (Colman 1989; Brinkerhoff 2002; Bovaird 2004), these entities propagate forms of governmentality centred on self-disciplining human subjects (Rose/Miller 1992). Moreover, entanglement of subjects into biomedical knowledge practices gives rise to new normative claims, expectations and subjectivities (captured by notions such as "biological citizenship" (Rose/Novas 2005) and "therapeutic citizenship" (Nguyen 2004). Following these theoretical lineages, one could plausibly reason that the PPPs boom in international health advances neoliberal agendas by fostering self-governing subjects.

1 | In this paper, the terms partnership, public-private partnership and PPP(s) are used interchangeably.

Through a historically-grounded ethnographic focus on malaria, a disease largely overlooked in contemporary social theorizing, the following paper calls into question such a line of reasoning. By examining a paradoxical feature of malaria, its concomitant visibility and invisibility, it explores shortcomings in contemporary theorizing on the relation between biomedicine, governance, and subjectivity formation, especially in African settings. The paper begins by ethnohistorically charting malaria's (in-)visibility in Tanzania, its shifting manifestations across various domains of practice (e.g., among health experts) in relation to changing domestic and international priorities. Then I draw on fieldwork conducted among a large-scale malaria intervention in southern Tanzania to discuss how decades of biomedical health education and interventions largely failed to generate intended subjectivities and practices. To conclude, I discuss theoretical implications of these findings, particularly concerning Foucauldian approaches to explore the relationship between biomedicine and governance in African settings.

THE WAXING AND WANING (IN-)VISIBILITY OF MALARIA: A SOCIO-HISTORICAL GLIMPSE

The disease Europeans call malaria[2] has 'always' been among the most common ailments in Tanzania, nowadays and during the colonial era (Clyde 1967). As in other parts of sub-Saharan Africa, most populations devised names, explanations and treatments for the affliction (Evans-Pritchard 1937; Whyte 1997). These names, explanations and treatments reflect the considerable cultural and linguistic diversity of the continent, and are grounded in cosmological principles that are similarly varied.

In some cases, there exists considerable congruity between the biomedical definition of malaria and local terms for the affliction. A striking example is the notion of *asra*, used by Ga-Adangbe farmers in Ghana, which encompasses signs such as "headache, a rise in body temperature, chills, bitterness of the mouth, yellow eyes, deeply coloured urine, loss of appetite, bodily aches and pains, weakness and easy fatigability, vomiting, pallor of the palms and soles, and cold sores around the mouth" (Agyepong 1992). However, such a high degree of correspondence between biomedical and local illness categories is

2 | In this paper, I use the term malaria in accordance with its biomedical definition unless otherwise indicated. Following this definition, malaria is an infection caused by parasites of the Plasmodium genus though even in (clinical) practice these are rarely distinguished. Reflecting this discursive practice, I use malaria here to signify any type of infection with plasmodia.

atypical in sub-Saharan Africa, and partial overlaps between these notions are far more common.

In Tanzania, local terminologies generally differentiate between symptoms associated with uncomplicated malaria—e.g., fever, chills and headaches—and severe malaria—e.g., convulsions, anaemia, and coma. This breakdown reflects prevailing cosmological principles according to which actors sort afflictions based on their symptoms and their perceived cause, which is either 'natural'—diseases that 'just happen'—or 'personalistic'—diseases 'sent' by humans (Foster 1976). This classificatory distinction between diseases of natural or personalistic aetiology is fundamental in many African societies and profoundly influences treatment decisions along with experience, available health care options and financial means (Janzen/Feierman 1992).

Among Swahili-speaking people of coastal Tanzania, this dichotomy manifests as two local illness terms: *homa* (Swahili for fever) and *degedege* (a Swahili word for a spirit in the form of a bird—*ndege*—that makes children sick by casting its shadow on them). Together, the *homa-degedege* pair denotes symptoms associated with malaria, the first uncomplicated manifestations, the latter life-threatening signs, mainly convulsions (Makemba et al 1996; Kamat 2006).[3] However, unlike their biomedical counterpart malaria, *homa* and *degedege* are considered distinct, unrelated illnesses. Herbs and pharmaceuticals are deemed appropriate treatments for *homa* but not for *degedege* since only *waganga*, traditional healers, can treat the underlying spirit-cause.

Frequently used in Swahili speech, the term *homa* illustrates the ubiquity of fever in daily life. A very common first sign of malaria, *homa* rarely worries patients if effective treatment is within reach, which has been the case since the 1950s when chloroquine became the first widely used antimalarial (Clyde et al 1964, Kamat 2006). *Homa* usually resolves with antimalarials or antipyretics, while adults in endemic areas, who develop high levels of immunity,[4] often heal without any treatment. In comparison, *degedege* is not only much rarer than *homa*; it can kill quickly. Epidemiologists have observed that although malaria is the leading cause of death in Tanzania and other countries, relatively few patients with mild disease progress to develop potentially fatal symptoms (de

3 | Further southwards, Langwick presents an excellent paper about the co-construction of malaria and degedege among inhabitants of the Makonde plateau of southern Tanzania (2007), where Swahili has become increasingly prevalent in recent decades. Reporting on classification of fevers in the Swahili-speaking town of Mombasa, Kenya, Beckerleg reports the centrality humoral understandings attributed to Arabic influences (1994).

4 | A unique feature of malaria is that immunity takes years to develop, requires continues boosting (through bites of infected mosquitoes), and is strain specific—questions that confounded and preoccupied colonial scientists for decades (see e.g., Clyde 1962).

Savigny et al. 2004). Unsurprisingly, most Tanzanians regard neither *homa* nor mild malaria as particularly worrying illnesses.

For Europeans, malaria constituted a rather different phenomenon in German East Africa and (British-ruled) Tanganyika, the colonies that gave rise to Tanzania in 1961. Many were highly susceptible to the deadly disease which—along with yellow fever—gave (West) Africa its reputation as "The White Man's Grave" (Rankin 1836; Curtin 1961).[5] Hence colonial authorities were preoccupied with malaria, which remained a major hazard to Europeans despite quinine therapy (Curtin 1985) and was moreover considered a major obstacle to African economic and social development and population growth (Cooper/Packard 1997; Bruchhausen 2003). Soon after Ross established that anopheline mosquitoes transmitted malaria (Ross 1898), scientists and health authorities initiated efforts to combat the disease using strategies targeting points in the life cycle—the parasite, the mosquito vector and the human host. Often successful in temperate zones, these strategies usually yielded disappointing results in tropical Africa.

Colonial powers tested different malaria control strategies that often reflect national and personal scientific rivalries. While British colonies embraced mosquito elimination, the "Ross method", German colonies adopted the strategy advocated by Robert Koch, targeting malarial parasites through mass-treatment of urban residents with quinine. However, the "Koch method" barely dented the burden of malaria in towns such as Dar-es-Salaam and Tanga (Ollwig 1903; Clyde 1962). After the British conquered the colony during WWI, health authorities switched to the Ross method and began targeting mosquitoes instead. These efforts suppressed malaria in urban areas such as Dar-es-Salaam and Tanga yet in rural areas they failed and were abandoned in the late 1950s. Until the end of the colonial era, malaria control in rural areas consisted primarily of providing curative services through the small but growing network of health centres (Clyde 1967).

After independence in 1961, malaria became a priority topic for the new government. Julius Nyerere, the first president, declared disease control central to his plans to develop Tanganyika (renamed Tanzania in 1963) into a self-reliant socialist state based on "African" communitarian principles, a vision captured by the ideology of *Ujamaa* or extended family (Nyerere 1962 [1975]). Since 95% of the population lived outside towns, Nyerere made "villagization" the cornerstone of his plans for developing the countryside (Beck 1981). Thus millions of rural dwellers were (forcibly) relocated into newly-constructed nucleated villages during the 1970s, where they got access to basic services such

5 | Coined by Rankin, the notion "White Man's Grave" subsequently gained widespread circulation in the popular, scientific and governmental imagination (I thank Maureen Malowany for pointing out this fact).

as schooling, piped water and allopathic health care (Freyhold 1979). Nyerere's goal to produce a healthy Tanzanian nation and citizenry rested on two legs: a massive expansion of the primary health care infrastructure, and promotion of desirable health-related behaviour.

To instil healthier behaviour among Tanzanians, a team comprised of government agencies, the ruling party TANU and the Institute of Adult Education of the University of Dar-es-Salaam developed a series of health campaigns during the 1970s and 1980s. Sporting catchy names such as *Mtu ni Afya* (literally, Man is Health) or *Chakula ni Uhai* (Food is Life), these campaigns infused public health messages with the dominant ideology of communalism and self-reliance. While aimed at all Tanzanians, they focused on *ujamaa* villagers, who were at greater risk for "malaria, hookworms, dysentery, bilharzias, tuberculosis and [unclean] water" than dispersed rural populations (Hall 1974). Thus millions of villagers were educated about biomedical disease principles through these campaigns, which not only made extensive use of radio broadcasting and printed materials but also involved thousands of community instructors and (mandatory) group activities for villagers to put newly-acquired knowledge into practice (Hall 1974). In conjunction with expanded treatment, these health education efforts helped to lower the burden of malaria dramatically. By 1973, it caused "10% of hospital admissions and 7 percent of deaths," a historical low (Beck 1981: 46).[6]

Tanzanian authorities kept malaria in check until the late 1970s, when the mismanaged economy entered the doldrums. Hampered by spiralling shortages, the health system became increasingly dysfunctional while mass health campaigns dwindled steadily in number and eventually ceased completely. With bankruptcy looming and donors loosing interest in bankrolling his increasingly authoritarian regime, Nyerere had to abandon plans to modernize his country and citizens according to his African socialist vision, eventually stepping down in 1985 (Hodd 1988). His successor Mwinyi requested aid from the International Monetary Fund which in exchange called for shrinking and decentralizing the state, privatizing service provision, and promoting 'cost-sharing' for health and education services (Lugalla 1995; Tripp 1997; Turshen 1999). As happened across the developing world, these 'structural adjustments'

6 | As with any other malaria-related figures, these are estimates that are best taken as an indication given two interrelated factors: first, the paucity and inaccuracy of health data and; second, the bias of this data. Countless studies have reported that across Africa, patients suffering from severe malaria typically seek treatment outside of the formal health system. Most deaths are not reported to health authorities while causality is rarely determined and usually attributed to other causes than the mosquito-borne disease, and for this reason official figures tend to underestimate morbidity and mortality rates while presenting a skewed, health sector-centered picture (Kengeya-Kayondo 1994; Foster 1995; McCombie 1996, Mwenesi 2005).

boosted NGO and commercial sector involvement in the health sector at the expense of state institutions, which faced mounting difficulties executing core responsibilities such as oversight and policy making (Edwards/Hulme 1995; Semboja/Therkildsen 1995; Shivji 2004). Some branches of government such as the National Malaria Control Programme essentially ceased to function during this period.

Meanwhile the global infectious disease landscape was changing rapidly (Barrett et al 1998). The media, donors, health experts, and social scientists were obsessed with outbreaks of frightening 'new' diseases such as AIDS and Ebola. By comparison, the resurgence of 'old' menaces such as malaria or tuberculosis attracted little attention. Repeated warnings by a small group of experts that spreading drug resistance and crumbling public health infrastructures were fuelling a malaria "catastrophe" fell on deaf ears (Kidson 1992). The failure of the 1955 Global Malaria Eradication Programme had given malaria a reputation as an intractable health problem that outwitted technological solutions (Packard 1998; Najera 2001) and was impossible to eradicate in African settings (Bruce-Chwatt 1969). Containment therefore came to be seen as the best feasible option in sub-Saharan Africa. However, this required costly long-term control efforts, a goal few donors and governments of rich countries and poor countries were willing to finance. Hence apathy predominated until the late 1990s, when it gradually gave way to a historically unprecedented commitment to fighting diseases of the poor (Annan 2001).

By this time, however, the scourge was re-establishing itself as the leading cause of mortality and morbidity in sub-Saharan Africa (except in countries where AIDS was inflicting an even larger toll, such as Zambia or Botswana (Trigg/Kondrachine 1998)). Alarmed by this resurgence, established organizations in the health arena (e.g., the World Health Organization, WHO) forged alliances with new players (e.g., the Roll Back Malaria Partnership, RBM; the Global Fund; the Gates Foundation) to boost material and human resources for malaria research and control efforts. These efforts were enormously successful: worldwide annual funding for the disease reached US$1 billion in 2009, a 20-fold increase in less than a decade (Ravishankar et al. 2009). Crucially, most of this money is channelled through collaborative undertakings that pivot on two tacit assumptions: First, a (long-standing) faith in the superiority of biomedical tenets. Second, the (newfound) belief that complex health problems cannot possibly be tackled by institutions working in isolation, but only by broad-based alliances that share resources and skills, benefits and burdens to pursue mutually-agreed goals (Gerrets 2010). Such 'partnerships' proved highly appealing notwithstanding criticism that the concept was ill-defined, fluid, and ambiguous (Buse/Walt 2000; Brinkerhoff 2004). Enthusiastically embraced by donors and recipients of aid, by organizations small and large, and by novel and well-established players, 'partnerships' quickly became central to contemporary thinking and practices in the domain of international health (Richter 2004).

The centrality of 'partnerships' in the contemporary international health landscape is illustrated by the proliferation and influence of novel, multibillion dollar entities such as the Global Fund or the Global Alliance for Vaccines and Immunizations, GAVI. Generally working in concert with influential donors such as the Gates Foundation, these partnerships are propelling the current expansion of malaria research and control activities in low-income countries (Ooms et al. 2010). Obviously, as the preceding historical section illustrated, these interventions take place in context-specific institutional, conceptual and semantic landscapes that influence their unfolding in particular ways. The following section takes a closer look at this context in Tanzania in order to show how, over several decades, malaria-centred health communication was appropriated in patterned ways that point toward gaps in current theorizing on the relation between biomedicine and governance.

THE CHANGING (IN)VISIBILITY OF MALARIA ACROSS TANZANIAN SETTINGS

As described in the preceding section, Tanzanian malaria research and control efforts had been very limited in scope for about two decades when international funding for the disease started to soar in 2001 (Trouiller et al 2001; Louet 2003; Moran 2005). Profoundly affected by the 1980s economic crisis and the subsequent period of neoliberal restructuring, government institutions had drastically diminished their involvement in malaria research and control efforts. The National Malaria Control Program (NMCP), the branch of the Ministry of Health responsible for developing and supervising malaria-related policies and control efforts across Tanzania, merely had six core staff members and very limited resources in 2001, posing huge hurdles to implementation of its mandate. Non-governmental organizations did not exactly rush in to fill this gap; whereas thousands of NGOs became active in HIV/AIDS or reproductive health, only a handful took up malaria-related issues (Hartwig et al. 2005; Brouwers 2011). Likewise, private sector involvement was minimal and essentially confined to manufacturing and distribution of medicines and bed nets.

Moreover, Tanzanian malaria research and control activities were not just limited in scope during the 1980s and 1990s; they were concentrated in two parts of the country, in areas surrounding two leading research institutions—the National Institute for Medical Research (NIMR) based in north-eastern Tanzania, and the Ifakara Health Research and Development Centre (IHRDC) located in southern Tanzania. Aided by strong ties with foreign institutions, NIMR and IHRDC were able to sustain research and control activities in their catchment areas while in other parts of the country such activities dwindled or ground to a halt. The remainder of this chapter focuses on the catchment area of IHRDC, the Kilombero Valley. Unlike most Tanzanians, inhabitants of the Kilombero Valley were exposed to a virtually uninterrupted chain of malaria-related activities (e.g., research, control, education).[7] Drawing on fieldwork and secondary sources, the following section explores how decades of exposure to biomedical ideas and activities influenced malaria-related beliefs and practices among Kilombero residents. This did not necessarily unfold as health experts intended.

The spread of 'maleria' in Southern and Eastern Tanzania

To understand contemporary ideas and practices involving malaria in Kilombero, adoption of a historical perspective enables deeper analysis of the processes that shape context-specific appropriation. As discussed earlier, malaria is a foreign concept that does not have an equivalent term in Swahili-speaking areas of Tanzania. Rather, as discussed at the beginning of the chapter, in keeping with local nosological principles symptoms associated with malaria are divided into two clusters. Each corresponds with a discrete, and conceptually unrelated, illness—*homa* and *degedege*. Although these terms appear in early colonial reports, little is known about the ways inhabitants of the Kilombero Valley treated *homa* and *degedege* before European missionaries and German colonial authorities introduced modern Western medicine and biomedical ideas into the area. Colonial-era documents feature recurrent complaints that patients with *degedege* usually shunned allopathic health facilities and sought treatment with 'traditional healers' (Clyde 1962). In contrast, Western pharmaceuticals quickly gained popularity as a cure for *homa* during the colonial period. Over time, these drugs were incorporated into local belief systems as culturally appropriate treatments for *homa*, a process described across the continent (Comaroff 1981; Whyte 1992).

Echoing the paucity of information about *homa* and *degedege*, it is difficult to ascertain from colonial-era documents how the notion malaria was taken up in Kilombero (as in Tanzania more generally). Since Swahili was the lingua franca of medical services dealing with native Tanzanians (Beck 1977; Iliffe 1998), it is entirely plausible that staff often used Swahili illness terms in dealings with the local population, more so than in interactions with foreigners (e.g., German or British colonizers). Commonsensical as such an assertion may seem, backing it up is challenging for colonial-era historical sources offer little concrete evidence. To examine how the notion malaria were appropriated in Tanzanian settings, I

7 | The only other site with a comparable density and continuity of malaria research and control activities is the area surrounding NIMR-Muheza in northeastern Tanzania.

therefore turn to another, more recent source—studies exploring local malaria-related knowledge, attitudes and practices and illness terms. Although these KAP-studies have serious limitations—the oldest date back to the 1980s, most are epidemiological in orientation and anthropologically shallow (Good 1994)—they reveal useful clues as to how the term malaria 'travelled' on the ground in particular contexts. When juxtaposing these accounts with in-depth ethnographic investigations, it becomes apparent how people changed the meanings of the term malaria during its appropriation into locally relevant practices and webs of signification.

A pertinent illustration of such appropriation is the use of malaria as a qualifier for *homa*, yielding the contraction *homa ya malaria* (literally, malaria-related fever or malaise). Reports from the 1990s show that lay people and health workers commonly distinguished *homa ya malaria* from other kinds of *homa* such as *homa kali* (harsh or violent fever) or *homa ya vidonda* (fever from boils) (Winch 1996). Significantly, the meaning of *homa* remains stable across these permutations whereas the meaning of *malaria* no longer corresponds with the original biomedical definition. In Swahili usage, *malaria* refers only to symptoms typical of a mild malarial infection (e.g. headache, fever), not to those characteristic of severe disease (e.g., convulsions, coma). In practice, *homa* and *malaria* are often used interchangeably and, along with *homa ya malaria,* these terms refer to a set of similar symptoms. In sharp contrast, symptoms characteristic of severe malaria are interpreted as signs of *degedege*, also called *ugonjwa wa kitoto* (disease of little children). Crucially, health professionals as well as lay people routinely use the *homa (ya) malaria/degedege* binary when talking about malarial symptoms, not just at home but also in formal health care settings (Oberlander/Elverdan 2000; Tarimo et al 2000). Through these quotidian semantic practices, they reproduce and validate the conceptual distinction between *homa (ya) malaria* and *degedege*, providing an apt illustration as to how public health messages that incorporate local illness terminologies cannot only reinforce local nosological principles but also fuel 'misinterpretation' of biomedical notions such as malaria.

When experts realized during the 1980s that the *homa (ya malaria)/degedege* dichotomy featured prominently in healing practices on the ground, they typically framed this as a serious problem that needed correcting. The *homa (ya malaria)/ degedege* binary, so reasoned many experts, hindered both 'correct' (biomedically-defined) diagnosis and 'appropriate' treatment of patients displaying signs of severe malaria, who typically were treated by *waganga (*traditional healers) for spirits they regard as the underlying cause of *degedege*. Since *waganga* do not treat *degedege* with antimalarials—such drugs are for *malaria* and *homa,* to treat spirits other medicines are used—most patients opting for traditional healers supposedly died due to ineffective treatment.[8] While such reasoning, which guided health interventions for decades, makes sense in light of local nosological principles and prevailing treatment practices, data supporting such claims are scant. In fact, despite abundant anecdotal evidence that patients with severe malaria often skirt formal health facilities, it remains largely a matter of conjecture what they actually do for their treatment trajectories are seldom examined (Gessler et al. 1995; Makundi et al. 2006; Kamat 2006). If anything, available studies suggest that many malaria patients resort to multiple treatment modalities, combining, for instance, home treatment with herbal medicine, modern pharmaceuticals, hospital medicine, or traditional healers, and evaluating each approach in terms of their therapeutic efficacy (Guyatt/Snow 2004; Kamat 2006; Nsungwa-Sabiiti et al. 2007).

In the 1980s, IHRDC experts did not fully consider these complex and dynamic aspects of therapeutic pluralism when designing interventions aimed at containing the rapidly rising malaria morbidity and mortality rates in the Kilombero Valley. Generally sticking to public health conventions, their interventions usually included a health communication campaign instructing patients with (uncomplicated and severe) malaria to seek allopathic care at formal health facilities (Degremont et al. 1987; Tanner et al. 1987). Kilombero Valley residents were therefore exposed to a fairly continuous stream of malaria-related health campaigns throughout the 1980s and 1990s, (Tanner et al. 1994), unlike Tanzanians living in most other parts of the country where such interventions became increasingly rare in the decades after the socialist era ended. These malaria campaigns in the Kilombero Valley were always premised on biomedical tenets although they regularly adopted local terminology, for example by instructing people to treat *homa (ya malaria)* or *degedege* at health facilities. On top of these public health campaigns, inhabitants of the Kilombero Valley were also exposed to years of social marketing for products such as insecticide-treated nets and malarial drugs. Involving diverse activities such as "face-to-face interactions...product launching parties, local drama groups, singing and dancing, roadside billboards and soccer tournaments," these social marketing campaigns were designed to attract and entertain large crowds while conveying public health messages about malaria transmission and treatment (Minja et al. 2001). Further adding to this health communication avalanche, radio and (less frequently) television broadcasted a steady stream of malaria-related health messages. This stream is continuing to date.

Spanning several decades, this intensive exposure of Kilombero residents to malaria-centred health communication elicited diverse effects, some

8 | The search for culturalist explanations over other factors shaping health behavior such as perceived quality of care, financial considerations, and so forth pervades international health, cf. Good (1994).

intended, others unintended. Two aspects will be discussed in greater detail with an eye on the principal aim of this paper, (re)theorizing the relationship between biomedicine and governance. Social scientific research has shown that health communication successfully heightened the 'visibility' of malaria as a major public health problem among Kilombero inhabitants and raised awareness that mosquitoes cause *maleria*—the local vernacular term for the disease. While these dimensions of public health messages about malaria were taken up as experts intended, other aspects were not. Minja et al. report that many informants dismissed the proposition that *maleria* causes fever. Rather, Kilombero residents claimed the opposite: fever causes *maleria* (2001). This notion of causality upends a foundational biomedical tenet which posits a unidirectional causal relationship between agents (such as malaria parasites) and symptoms: an agent causes a symptom (or symptoms). Reversal of this relationship—a symptom engenders a causative agent—is impossible according to biomedical epistemology. Hence, both in biomedicine and in public health such causal reasoning is not just deemed incorrect but almost "inconceivable".

Such accounts of *maleria*-generating fevers illustrate the resilience of local African nosologies which offer modes of explanation (such as a bidirectional relationship between cause and symptom) that biomedicine precludes (Feierman 1981; Langwick 2007). Still more disconcerting to public health experts, Kilombero residents also rejected the (biomedical) claim that mosquitoes cause *degedege*. Minja's informants dismissed this idea as incredible, citing two reasons. First, invoking local nosological principles, they explained that *maleria* could not possibly cause *degedege*—only spirits could cause this affliction. Second, their observations and experiences confirmed that mosquitoes could not possibly cause *degedege*. Minja et al quote an informant to illustrate this reasoning:

> "[...] if these mosquitoes were causing such serious *maleria*, everyone would be dead in the village because people have lived with mosquitoes since they were born and they are still surviving, getting bitten by mosquitoes every day during the rainy season when mosquitoes bite all the time [...]" (2001: 616)

Empirically irrefutable, this interpretation rejects and disrupts core biomedical tenets inscribed in malaria health communication. We now turn to a study by colleagues of Minja to take a closer look at how these biomedical notions were altered during their appropriation by residents in the Kilombero Valley.

Working in the same area shortly after Minja et al., Hausmann-Muela et al. investigate how peoples' empirically-grounded assessments and appropriation of malaria education and treatment practices disrupt and transform embedded biomedical messages (2002). The authors take on a vexing problem in health communication—public health messages often do not achieve desired results (le Grand et al. 1999; Airhihenbuwa/Obregon 2000; Dutta-Bergman 2005).

They investigate how people actually incorporate new information into their illness models and practices so as to identify which intended and unintended ideas and practices attend these processes of appropriation. Hausmann-Muela et al. show that although "scientific terminology, clearly reflecting the wording of health communication programs and school lessons, has been incorporated into the local discourse", residents infuse these notions with local beliefs and practices, a process they call medical syncretism (2002: 406). For instance, Kilombero residents imposed a local "logic of illness transformation" wherein *homa* merely constitutes the "first stage of illness that eventually progresses into *homa kali* (harsh fever) out of which malaria and, if it is persistent or gets worse, *degedege* (convulsions) can develop" (2002: 407). They view malaria as an illness which "emerges, disappears and reappears in different form, and progresses over years," an interpretation that blurs boundaries between illness episodes, considered separate events from a biomedical perspective (2002: 408). This view of malaria (or rather *maleria)* as an unending illness that waxes and wanes but never disappears completely makes perfect sense in areas such as Kilombero where transmission occurs perennially and is subject to sharp fluctuations (e.g., seasonal). However this view also challenges biomedical understandings of malarial infections as discrete episodes comprising successive illnesses, cures and re-infections.

Lay peoples' experientially grounded (re)interpretations of public health discourses not only upend biomedical tenets by challenging temporal understandings of malaria (and illness more generally); they furthermore call into question basic etiological concepts. Affirming Minja's findings, Hausmann-Muela et al. report that Kilombero residents viewed *homa* as the principal manifestation of an ongoing battle between malaria parasites and blood cells, their explanations often drawing on the immunological imageries that permeate health communication messages (2002). Instructed to visit health facilities when suffering from *homa,* informants noted that antimalarial treatment did not always alleviate symptoms. If the condition of patients undergoing antimalarial treatment worsened, and especially when they suddenly developed seizures, lethargy or suffered a miscarriage—all symptoms associated with severe malaria—people began suspecting that another force might be involved: witchcraft. This form of witchcraft invades and sickens its victims either by imitating malaria or by "'hiding' the parasites so as to make them invisible in the blood and thus undetectable in the hospital" (Hausmann-Muela et al. 2002). Disguised as 'fake malaria,' witchcraft outwits biomedical practitioners' knowledge and skills by sickening and killing patients who adhere to health communication messages, calling into question expert truth claims.

Empirically unassailable and socioculturally persuasive, witchcraft discourses explained invisible events such treatment failures and recurrent infections in a setting where poor quality pharmaceuticals, sub-dosage drug treatment, high transmission rates, poor living conditions and inadequate health services conspirer with rising levels of antimicrobial resistance to make malaria increasingly tenacious and difficult to treat.

Unlike these witchcraft discourses, public health messages—crafted to be simple and clear—seldom address peoples' complex, continually shifting illness experiences or their ongoing efforts to stave off unpredictable malarial infections. Paradoxically, especially in situations of pervasive uncertainty, "beliefs in biomedicine and witchcraft, rather than being contradictory concepts, not only complement but actually reinforce each other" (Hausmann-Muela et al. 2002).

Summing up, this ethnohistorical account has shown that decades of health education ensured that the term malaria was taken up in Kilombero Valley and became widely used, entering local parlance as *maleria*. However, core biomedical meanings were altered or lost in the course of this appropriation—*maleria* differs substantially from malaria. Crucially, this slippage was not the result of mistranslations or other 'errors' but arose from Kilombero residents' critical engagement with public health messages which regularly conflicted with their own empirically grounded observation and experiences. For problems such as recurrent malaria or drug treatment failure, explanations anchored in local meaning systems such as witchcraft discourses or conceptions of unending illness were more persuasive to Kilombero residents than public health messages, whose underlying biomedical knowledge claims they dismissed as unbelievable (to some degree). Decades of exposure to public health messages and their embedded biomedical principles did not marginalize local conceptual frameworks and modes of reasoning such as the distinction between afflictions of natural and spiritual causation, encountered across African societies. Rather, it was biomedical malaria that was transformed and refracted through two locally meaningful logics—the natural-supernatural dyad, yielding *maleria* and *degedege*, and witchcraft discourses, yielding 'fake' malaria—illustrating the partial and superficial penetration of public health messages among Kilombero residents.

MALARIA AND CONTEMPORARY THEORIZING OF BIOMEDICINE AND GOVERNANCE

By examining historically the waxing and waning visibility of malaria and interventions targeting the scourge, both in the international sphere and in an Tanzanian location, I aimed to think through a baffling paradox that malaria presents: On the one hand malaria is a ubiquitous problem in tropical Africa where it has long been an object of interventions that seek to boost interest in and the visibility of the disease. Yet despite the buzz these activities generate, it remains a taken-for-granted, almost invisible fact of life that generally arouses apathy rather than excitement or concern. This (in)visibility—at once visible and invisible—was clearly palpable across social groups in Tanzania, yet also in international circles. Scientists I studied and worked with often commented with considerable frustration that high-level government officials expressed little interest in malaria compared with diseases such as AIDS or filariasis.[9] Health facility staff in rural southern Tanzania often complained that if the government really cared about malaria, it would make sure that antimalarials would not run out repeatedly for weeks or months at a time (Hetzel et al. 2007). Among its key victims, poor women, the (in)visibility of malaria took yet another form; they rarely had much to say about the disease even when they said it was the biggest health problem they faced. Indeed, researchers I worked with regularly noted with dismay that malaria was not a topic that people talked about in elaborate detail (Gerrets 2010).

When juxtaposing the (in)visibility of malaria with the preceding ethnohistoric exploration of the spread of *maleria* in the Kilombero Valley, stimulating questions emerge for theorizing the relationship between biomedicine and governance, particularly in African settings. Quite surprisingly given its historical significance as a force of change in (current and erstwhile) endemic societies and on the international plane, malaria featured only peripherally in social scientific debates during the past twenty years. The disease inspired several compelling accounts from perspectives such as political economy e.g., (Packard 1984), cognitive anthropology (Packard/Brown 1997), political ecology (Brown 1986), modernization theory (Cooper/Packard 1997; Sufian 2007) and science studies (Langwick 2007). Yet in the sizeable scholarship inspired by Foucault, whose writings have been crucial for theorizing the relationship between disease, biomedicine and governance, malaria is strikingly underrepresented.[10] What makes this lacuna so peculiar is that malaria has long been a subject of government interventions. Historically, attempts to control the disease were oftentimes deeply intertwined with states' efforts to assert credibility and authority and to produce healthy, modern citizens (Cooper/Packard 1997; Mitchell 2002; Sufian 2007), as illustrated by the preceding ethnohistoric accounts of Tanganyika and post-independence Tanzania. While coercive state-centred malaria control campaigns are less prevalent this day and age, this does not mean that contemporary interventions are any less concerned with shaping and disciplining subjects in accordance with biomedical principles and ideals.

---

9 | Filariasis, also called elephantiasis, is a well-known trigger for sterilization rumors that have brought down vaccination campaigns across the continent, c.f. Feldman-Savelsberg et al. 2000.

10 | For exceptions, see e.g. Silva 1997; Mitchell 2002; Carter 2008.

To give one example, interventions aimed at improving treatment adherence—an unremitting concern since sub-optimal doses can adversely affect cure rates and spur the emergence and spread of antimicrobial resistance—seek to transform peoples' behaviour in order to align these with biomedical principles as part of achieving public health objectives. This idea is shared by many (if not most) health development interventions. Similarly, the malaria treatment regimes I observed in the field aimed to 'discipline' patients into appropriate drug use,[11] for instance by combining verbal instructions with packaging technologies.[12] However, a sizeable minority of patients, seemingly unfazed by health workers' instructions and public health messages, took medicines as they saw fit—a problem described by health workers around the world for a wide range of diseases and treatment regimes (Souares et al. 2008; Khantikul et al. 2009; Gerstl et al. 2010). In southern Tanzania, I regularly witnessed patients throwing away pills upon leaving the health clinic where they had taken (under direct observed therapy, DOTs) the first dose of a three-day antimalarial regimen and been instructed to take the remaining pills for two more days, usually punctuated with a warning that their illness might resurface if they fail to do so. These observational data dovetail with a study which reported that 75% of patients completed the remaining two days of treatment, considered a high adherence rate compared with other antimalarial drugs in Tanzania, while the remaining 25% of patients deviated from treatment guidelines (Kachur et al. 2004). Another example of the limited impact by efforts to instil desired biomedical knowledge and behaviour derived from CONTACT researchers. They repeatedly complained that many regular users of the antimalarial they were testing failed to recall its name or purpose, despite extensive social marketing of the product. What stuck better in peoples' minds was the number of pills they were supposed to take (*vidonge saba,* seven pills) or their size (*vidonge vidogo,* little pills), cues researchers often deployed to solicit information about the drug or about malaria more generally. Telling a similar story in different locations, countless reports describe the difficulty of making recipients of insecticide-treated nets (ITNs) adhere to (biomedically) appropriate treatment and usage instructions, even with intensive communication efforts (Schellenberg et al. 1999; Alaii et al. 2003; Kinung'hi et al. 2007; Ordinioha 2007).

To begin weaving together the different strands presented in this paper, I now turn to the question informing the title of this essay: what can malaria contribute

11 | Defined as completing a 3-day treatment regime and determined through interviews with patients and counting of left-over pills (Kachur et al. 2004).

12 | A growing number of antimalarials is made available through prepackaged strips that apportion specific dosages per time interval using a combination of color codes (e.g., to differentiate day 1, 2, 3 of treatment), symbols (e.g., the moon or the sun, signaling dosages for different daily time points) and text.

to contemporary social theorizing, particularly the explorations of the relationship between biomedicine and technologies of the self? A key contribution of this literature is to show how subjects' participation in biomedical management of diseases such as AIDS or conditions such as infertility (inadvertently) fosters the production of self-governing subjectivities (Biehl 2002; Gremillion 2003; Fassin 2007; Gooldin 2008). Applying this theoretical perspective to malaria, various questions emerge. Do malaria education and treatment practices foster new subjectivities? If so, which kinds of selves might malaria interventions create? If not, what does this tell us about malaria as an object of analysis? By extension, what does this say about theories positing particular relations between subjects and biomedical practices? Finally, how do contextual specificities refract these theories and shape our analyses?

Although I wish I could answer each of these questions, I do not (yet) have sufficient evidence to make authoritative claims. Nonetheless, I would like to offer some tentative suggestions in the remaining paragraphs of this paper by drawing on the themes raised by this malaria-centred analysis raised so far—its (in)visibility in African societies and on the international plane; the literature lamenting the enormous hurdles associated with advancing biomedically appropriate understandings and practices in rural African settings; and the rise of notions such as *maleria* in Kilombero that evince the resilience of 'traditional' African nosologies.

To determine if and how malaria interventions shape subjectivities, existing scholarship is extremely limited and largely restricted to historical inquiries (Carter 2008; Sufian 2007; Stapleton 2009). Unable to locate studies examining this relationship in the present, I draw on fieldwork data obtained in southern Tanzania to sketch relevant issues to consider. Just as malaria health messages or treatment practices did not seem particularly effective at promoting self-disciplining subjects, so identity issues manifested themselves in rather superficial ways. For example, health workers and government officials often made value statements about malaria patients, praising *wagonjwa wazuri*—'good patients' who took up biomedical ideas or adhered to official treatment guidelines—and complaining about *wagonjwa wabaja*—'bad patients' who failed to change their ways, supposedly because they were "backward," "uneducated" or stuck in "tradition" (c.f. Stambach 2000; Montgomery et al. 2006). During nearly two years of fieldwork, I witnessed such (derogatory) ascriptions almost daily, yet only once did I observe anything that might be considered an identity claim. It occurred in 2006 while studying the ramifications of a district-wide stock-out of malaria medicines. I drove with my motorbike into a hamlet where I had not been before and asked a male in his thirties for directions to the local government office. After pointing me in the right direction, he asked me spontaneously: "Why have all (malaria) drugs run out in the dispensary? Does the (Tanzanian) government think that this village is inhabited by Mozambicans?"

Angry that the dispensary had run out of drugs including antimalarials, this man accused government officials of ineptness, a common reaction to all kinds of mishaps and grievances in southern Tanzania. By suggesting that he and his fellow villagers were Mozambicans, he insinuated that the government did not treat them as Tanzanian citizens entitled to functioning health care. However, this reaction was unique. At no other time did I observe that malaria research and control interventions had much impact on self-making or identity politics, let alone give rise to something like biological, therapeutic or pharmaceutical 'citizenship' (Rose/Novas 2005; Ecks 2005; Nguyen 2004).

Scholars have shown persuasively that diseases such as AIDS spurred influential social movements, debates about subjects' rights and duties, and massive changes across society (Farmer 1992; Robins 2006; Fassin 2007). Once again, malaria presents a rather different story. At the time I conducted fieldwork in Tanzania, from 2004-2006, malaria sickened millions and killed over 100,000 people per year yet despite its enormous societal impact, few interest groups, NGOs or social movements were calling attention to the affliction. Compared with the massive NGO industry dedicated to fighting AIDS—its signs and offices are visible across Dar-es-Salaam—malaria attracted at most a dozen NGOs, some Tanzanian upstarts though most were offshoots from international NGOs. There exists no clearly defined division of labour between these NGOs. For example, Oxfam, Population Services International and Merlin conduct tasks such as providing emergency antimalarials to refugees or distributing insecticide treated nets among the general population whereas a handful of Tanzanian NGOs offer various malaria-related health services. Importantly, and this is my key point, none of these NGOs display features of a social movement such as a grass-roots base or actors who self-organize around a socially salient issue (Epstein 1996; Edelman 2001; Robins 2006). These entities conduct a steadily growing assortment of tasks, but their growth is fuelled more by surging international funding for malaria than by grass-roots pressure to tackle the disease.

Likewise, Tanzanian citizens were scarcely organizing themselves to clamour for better, more effective, and cheaper antimalarial treatments and prevention technologies. Nowadays, malaria inspires little social activism, unlike during the heydays of Nyerere's regime. This is surprising given that social organizing and 'shell NGOs' awaiting funders are plentiful in Tanzania. In fact, not far from the house where I resided in southern Tanzania there stood a crumbling building that served a shell NGO dedicated to AIDS orphans in the area, or so suggested the fading script on the wall. Mzee Mkongo, who owned the building and headed the NGO-in-waiting, regularly told me of his fruitless efforts to acquire funding for his mission. One day, en route to the market, I greeted Mzee Mkongo, who was chatting with other elders outside his dilapidated building, and complained that he still had not found a donor. Half-seriously, I said: "Nowadays there is a lot of money for malaria. Why don't you set up an NGO that is dedicated to fighting this disease?" Mzee Mkongo and the elders first looked a bit puzzled and then laughed heartily. As I wished the elders a pleasant day, Mzee Mkongo uttered, smiling of course: "Only a *mzungu* (a white person) can come up with such a silly idea!"

Mzee Mkongo's incredulous reaction sits uncomfortably with theoretical notions such as biopolitics and therapeutic or pharmaceutical 'citizenship,' especially when considered in conjunction with the other malaria-related issues raised in this paper. Since I observed few if any signs that malaria interventions spurred particular kinds of subjectivities, social groups, rights claims, or exerted noteworthy 'disciplining' effects in Tanzania, I am curious how the old scourge might breathe new life and directions into Foucauldian theorizing and analyses. Indeed, malaria's poor fit with this framework raises salient questions. For instance, to what extent is contemporary theorizing on the relationship between biomedicine and (self)disciplining subjects shaped by the kinds of objects (e.g., diseases, biological processes, technologies, organizational interventions) that scholars study? How might current theoretical paradigms shift if scholars were to base their analyses more on objects (such as malaria) that do not appear to be particularly productive in terms of fostering (self)discipline, new subjectivities or novel modes of sociality?

To conclude this essay, I would like to extend the questions posed above by returning to the opening vignette of this paper, which offered a glimpse of how the rise of partnership in international health is overhauling malaria-related policy setting and intervention activities in Tanzania. Events such as the CEEMI seminar exemplify an increasingly prominent mode of governance wherein infectious disease-related decision-making and policy setting involve teams of stakeholders from the public and private sectors and civil society. Such partnerships are also deemed essential for implementing infectious disease research and control interventions in poor countries. Collectively, these PPPs are assuming a growing set of tasks 'traditionally' deemed a prerogative of national governments and multilateral institutions, infusing these with private-sector notions of efficiency, market principles and accounting technologies, all hallmarks of neoliberalism (Rose/Miller 1992). Since partnerships are further seen as a

> "new modality of government that works by creating mechanisms that work 'all by themselves' to bring about governmental results through the devolution of risk onto the 'enterprise' or the individual...and the 'responsibilization' of subjects who are increasingly 'empowered' to discipline themselves" (Ferguson and Gupta 2002: 989)

then malaria elicits yet more interesting vexing questions. How does the inscribed neoliberal thrust of partnerships aimed at producing empowered, self-governing subjects play out for diseases such as malaria which, certainly in the Tanzanian context, show little evidence of fostering self-disciplining and subjectivity-formation? How does this compare with partnerships dealing with afflictions such as AIDS which appear to be better 'hooks' for the neoliberal project of fostering self-governing subjects? More generally, how might theoretical debates about the relationship between biomedicine and governance benefit by paying greater attention to contextual variation (such as the Tanzanian particularities examined in this paper)?

Obviously, answers to these and other questions necessitate empirical evidence which, so far, is in short supply. Given the ability of malaria to call into question old and new assumptions in public health, it might very well challenge and reinvigorate precepts held dear by social scientists. However, to avail ourselves of such a possibility, it is necessary to start taking objects such as this old scourge seriously as subjects of inquiry.

Configuring Trans* Citizens in South Africa: Somatechnics, Self-Formation and Governmentality

Thamar Klein

Introduction

Imagine your country being able to decide on the removal of your reproductive organs or to deny you the legal recognition of your gender. In fact, this is the situation trans* citizens face in most countries worldwide. Affirming the rights of citizens, philosopher John Locke stated in 1689 in *The Second Treatise on Government* that: "Though the earth, and all inferior creatures, be common to all men, yet every man has a property in his own person: this no body has any right to but himself" (Locke 1689: V, Sect. 27). In an analogous manner, trans* citizens have the impression that they need to safeguard the right to their own bodies against their respective states: "[...] it really is ridiculous to have to wait that long—and have to see so many people—to start hormones. People's bodies are their own property, not the State's!" (Jacques 2010).

In this chapter, I reflect on the shifting relations between state and its subjects in the gender-defining process of its citizens. I investigate the influence of biopolitically standardizing bodies on the definition of gender as well as the shifts in a society's power-diagram that enable progressive transformations in dominant truth discourses. A central aspect of transformations and social change is technology. Therefore, I will examine the Embodied Self as a social product in a technological age that connects individuals through new communication technologies on a global level, facilitating access to new discourses and somatechnics[1].

1 | Somatechnics are technologies of the body. The term connotes the inextricability of body and technology as the body incarnates in time and place situated transformative practices.

My main focus therefore lies on the relation between biomedicine and governance with regard to the configuration of trans* citizens through technologies of the self. I discuss legal, administrative and medical aspects, within the broader space of governance, shaping trans* citizens' identities and bodies in contemporary South Africa. The paper investigates how new technologies alter views on an individual and social level concerning how trans* citizens' bodies are, ought to be or could be.

Excursus: trans*

The term trans* refers in this text to citizens whose gender identity differs from their assigned sex at birth and/or challenges male-female dichotomies. I have found myself struggling with a linguistic dilemma when searching for non-discriminatory terminology. Usually, this problem is circumvented in social anthropology by using local terminology; however, South Africa has eleven official languages and recognizes quite a number of other non-official local languages. Thus there is no single local terminology.

In addition, local terms contain different meanings and often have no equivalent in English (e.g. intersexed persons, trans* people and individuals who engage in same-sex practices might not be distinguished and may be called *istabane* in Zulu). Aside from this, all of the local terminology I encountered during the eleven months of fieldwork between 2007 and 2008 (e.g. *moffie, italasi, istabane,* and *skesana*) was considered hurtful, derogatory and discriminatory by the interviewees. This is also true for pathologizing medical terminology. It can only be used by individuals to describe themselves in an act of counter-discourse or what Foucault called "reverse discourse": the reclaiming of internalized, oppressive terminology through marginalized people while insisting that their legitimacy be acknowledged through the same vocabulary by which they are ostracized (Foucault 1990: 101).

In an effort to resolve this dilemma, I use the term trans* as employed by Gender DynamiX (GDX) for people described as transsexual or transgendered. GDX is the first and only South African organization that offers services exclusively to trans* people. I would like to point out however, that many people subsumed under this terminology do not identify with it.

Keeping the diversity of South African trans* citizens in mind, I concentrate on the questions of how trans* citizens as users of gendering/sexing technologies are defined and configured—using some of Foucault's concepts such as governmentality, techniques of the self and his power-diagram. Assuming that individuals are both subjects and objects of power—as power in Foucault's sense is a transformative capacity and "needs to be considered as a productive network which runs through the whole social body, much more than a negative instance whose function is repression" (Foucault 1980: 119)—I examine allocated and usurped sex/gender-altering technologies.

For the purpose of this paper, technology is understood in the broad sense of the word; not only as material objects and techniques (e.g. medical technologies), but also as methods of organization (e.g. the (re-)categorization of gender). I will also deal in this text with technologies of the self. These have been defined by Foucault as techniques and practices that

> "[...] permit individuals to effect by their own means or with the help of others a certain number of operations on their own bodies and souls, thoughts, conduct, and way of being, so as to transform themselves in order to attain a certain state of happiness, purity, wisdom, perfection, or immortality" (Foucault 1988: 18).

These technologies of the self are situated within power relations (the power-diagram) and are inextricably connected to Foucault's notion of governmentality that encompasses the organized practices (mentalities, rationalities, and techniques) which are designed to regulate the conduct of individuals and populations not only at the administrative or political level. Accordingly, technologies of the self have a productive as well as a constraining side and build on both canonical and unorthodox individual knowledge. Thus "technologies of domination of individuals over one another have recourse to processes by which the individual acts upon himself. And, conversely, [...] where the techniques of the self are integrated into structures of coercion or domination" (Atkins 2005: 214).

Therefore, I consider the practices of classifying, standardizing and embodying sex/gender and query how power structures are mediated in and through biomedical knowledge. However, my focus is not primarily on biopower's processes of normalization (the establishing of norms) or the disciplinary processes of bringing subjects into conformity with a predetermined norm (what Foucault referred to as "normation"), but on the subjects themselves. Even though medical classifications are instruments of normalization and medico-legal technologies configure very specific citizens, South African trans* citizen are not passive subjects of governmental, legal or medical intervention. As Foucault has pointed out: "Where there is power, there is resistance" (Foucault 200: 341). Indeed, "[...] power and resistance are no more than two different names Foucault gives to the same capacity, the capacity to create social change" (Heller 1996: 99).

On the one hand, medical ideas of normality and the practices through which they are generated shape individuals' experiences of the body. On the other hand, some citizens resist or modify the processes of configuration and claim their gender and their right to adapt their bodies in opposition to hegemonic discourses and state policies. Therefore, I will examine what Foucault termed the 'power-diagram'; the net-like organization, "which permits one to act upon the actions of others" (Foucault 1982: 792) and in which mechanisms are continually transformed through the exercise of power within itself. When critical masses are reached through new communication technologies, it may lead to the employment of new somatechnics and, in turn, to the alteration of hegemonic discourses.

I will explore which specific technologies are envisaged by policy makers to be used by what kind of trans* citizen users as well as which citizens use the available technologies in unforeseen and unintended ways, or do not use them at all. Are these technologies in fact (sufficiently or at all) available to the citizens they were intended for? What are new uses for technologies that were originally invented or intended for a different cause? The last question is also relevant when studying the situation of citizens whose identities are located beyond the binary of male and female and who undermine contemporary regimes of truth regarding sex and gender. Some citizens, identifying as neither male nor female, actively experiment with biomedicine in order to modify their bodies as well as to alter discourses on maleness and femaleness, thereby departing from discursive practices around binary models of gender. One has to ask: How is the 'power-diagram' transformed through the (dis)use of certain technologies? Does the (dis)use of certain technologies lead to shifts in power relations and in the possibility of new subjectivities? These questions become important as for Foucault,

"[...] power relations are conditions of possibility for subjectivities. [...] 'Power produces; it produces reality, it produces domains of objects and rituals of truth.' It also produces people [...] Power in its positive sense is enabling, constituting subjects, even though the forms of subjectivity constituted may not be desirable" (Simons 2006: 191).

Thus gendering technologies as objects of identity projects may stabilize or destabilize hegemonic representations of gender. Even processes of normalization do not necessarily lead to the production of docile, disciplined citizens. Indeed, unexpected and unruly subjectivities arise that disrupt biomedical and legal taxonomies: new identities and social relations emerge around biomedical classifications and normalizations that have consequences beyond the field of health and that can be studied from a genealogical perspective: "[...] genealogy is, for Foucault, synonymous with the analysis of counter-hegemonic conflict [...]" (Heller 1996: 95). "Genealogy examines how subjects are constituted by others and how we participate in constituting ourselves as subjects" (Simons 2006: 191).

The present study explores some aspects of the 'power-diagram' encompassing trans* related issues, especially with regard to trans* citizens' local and global agency within the realms of supranational citizenship, citizen science and medical tourism. This draws on Aihwa Ong's observation that "in theory, citizenship as protected entitlements depends on membership of a nation-state. But increasingly in practice, entitlements and benefits are realized through specific mobilizations and claims in milieus of globalized contingency" (Ong 2005: 697).

I start with a brief outline of the methodological approach of my research project. This section will be followed by a discussion of the role of technology in the configuration of trans* citizens and the practices of classifying and standardizing sex and gender through legislative, executive and judicial organs. I then move on to the usage of medical technologies (as technologies of the self) as well as to the local and global agency of trans* citizens within the realms of supranational citizenship, citizen science and medical tourism.

Methodology

The research for this article was carried out as part of the project "Biomedicine in Africa", of the Fellow Group "Law, Organisation, Science and Technology" at the Max Planck Institute for Social Anthropology in Halle/Saale (Germany). My research project, Que(e)rying Body Perceptions in South Africa, examines medico-legal practices and discourses around queer sexes/genders in South Africa. As part of my current work on medical, legal, and political discourses concerning gender and globalization, I explore the relationships between law, medicine and queer bodies in South Africa.

This chapter draws mainly on data from 65 semi-structured interviews, of between 30 and 150 minutes in length, conducted over an eleven month period of fieldwork taking place between 2007 and 2008 in Cape Town, Pretoria, Johannesburg (and Soweto) with trans* and intersexed persons, surgeons, endocrinologists, clinical social workers, sexologists, psychologists, and legal specialists, as well as trans* and intersex activists. Besides innumerable hours of participant observation at social gatherings with trans* and intersexed people, the research involves many more informal interviews, private e-mails and excerpts from chats in internet forums from as early as 2005, when I first became interested in the topic.

Governing Sex and Gender: Whose Body is it?

Feminist scholars and those contributing to sexual, queer or intimate citizenship studies, for example Ruth Lister or Ken Plummer, have pointed out repeatedly that citizenship rights are intimately connected with the sex and gender of a citizen. Accordingly and unsurprisingly, the situation faced by trans* citizens differs from those who are cisgendered[2]. Naturally trans* citizens are not a homogenous group and the term trans* is a complex and contested umbrella term encompassing miscellaneous subjectivities. Due to limited space, it is not possible to delve into discourses pertaining to concepts of difference and sameness, universal claims to equal rights and differentiated rights claims, the balancing of the needs of special sub-groups against the good of the whole, and so on. However, the term trans* citizen is useful in distinguishing from traditional notions of citizenship which portray the citizen as being white, male, cisgendered, heterosexual and able-bodied. These models have been challenged by feminist and sexual citizenship theorists (e.g. Lister 1997 and 2008, Richardson 1998) as well as theorists on queer and intimate citizenship (e.g. Plummer 2001). Already in the early 1990s, Young and Yeatman analyzed the exclusion of the 'other' and the 'different' from citizenship (Young 1990; Yeatman 1990).

One of the main problems of trans* citizens worldwide is that states rely profoundly on a bi-sexed or -gendered system; laws are developed along a binary sex or gender model without defining exactly which attributes define a person as male or female. Legislation addressing sex (e.g. for purposes of marriage, inheritance, military service, etc.) more often than not falls short of defining the terms. It goes without saying that non-binary sexes and genders are hardly recognized as legal sexes and genders at all. As an important first step, Australia in September 2011 introduced new passport rules that allow people to select their official gender as either male, female or indeterminate.

LET'S TALK ABOUT SEX

Sex, in the scope of a medical as well as a heteronormative and binary model, refers to the male and female duality of biology and reproduction. From a medical point of view, the sex of an individual is defined by its chromosomal, gonadal, hormonal, psychological, social, internal and external genital differentiation (Pschyrembel 1994). Nonetheless, these ascribed sex-dichotomous differences[3]

2 | The Latin prefix cis stands for "on the same side", whereas the prefix trans stands for "on the opposite side". "Cisgendered" or "cissexual" describes people whose gender identity matches their perinatally assigned sex. The term was coined in the 1990s in order to distinguish a majority group (cisgender) from a minority group (trans* gender) without the use of negative prefixes (e.g. non-trans*gender) while at the same time avoiding terminology such as ,"normal" or "genetic" women and men' which would imply deviance or defect on the part of the minority group.

3 | Sex-dichotomous differences refer to aspects, which are wholly characteristic of one sex only.

are not absolute in the human population, and there are individuals who are biologically or behaviourally 'in-between' (e.g. intersexed[4] and trans* persons). Thus, a first intricacy is already posed by the birth of intersexed children and the fact that some children cannot (or not easily) be placed within the binary model. Other legal complications may occur later in life when the sex assigned at birth does not match a person's gender identity or when it becomes apparent that the outer genitalia of the infant may have looked male or female but that other sex characteristics do not match the assigned sex. In other cases, such as 5-Alpha-reductase deficiency, infants appear phenotypically female at birth until puberty when secondary male sex characteristics develop with the descent of the testes, deepening of the voice, and growth of what had been identified as a clitoris into a functional penis. There exists a huge variety of biological and psychosocial conditions due to the complex interlocking of sex-dichotomous differences. A significant fraction of the human population simply does not correspond exclusively to either female or male with regard to every level of definition.

In cases of ambiguity, the definition of legal sex relies on biomedical definitions. However, as stated above, the medical definition is not unambiguous in itself. The psychological make-up of a person (the gender identity) is already part of the medical definition (chromosomal, gonadal, hormonal, *psychological, social*, internal and external genital differentiation). Thus the conventional division of sex (biological) and gender (psychological, social) is already intermeshed. However, Hines sees an advantage in the divide and argues therefore for an understanding of gender as separate from sex.

"An understanding of gender as separate from sex thus holds the potential for a greater diversity of masculinities and femininities. From this perspective, rights can be articulated and protected on the basis of subjectivity. Such a move would represent a radical departure from medical understanding of (trans) gender, which continue to influence rights discourse and law. Accounting for subjective gender difference in this way would signpost a genuine utopian model of human rights, which foregrounds the very concept of diversity" (Hines 2009: 96).

I strongly agree with Hines that it would be a significant step to base rights on an individual's gender identity; I am, however, doubtful that a legal division

4 | Intersex is a general biomedical term for a huge variety of physical conditions in which a person is born with chromosomal, gonadal, hormonal, internal and/or external genital features, which do not fit with conventional definitions of male or female (e.g. external sex organs that seem to be ambiguous in a binary model; simultaneous presence of both testicular and ovarian tissue in one individual; chromosome combinations other than XX or XY etc.). Approximately 1.7% of all humans are born intersexed (Fausto-Sterling 2000; Samelius/Wagberg 2005: 13).

of sex and gender would lead to the desired results. Instead, such a division would imply that sex is an objective medical entity unaffected by temporal and local discourses and would be regarded as something inherently free of psychological or social factors, whereas Butler has already argued that "[...] sex, by definition, will be shown to have been gender all along" (Butler 1990: 8). Scientific knowledge is always inseparably linked to power relations and is co-produced by them. Foucault's power/knowledge thesis is reflected in the concept of "co-production" from Science and Technology Studies. "Knowledge and its material embodiments are at once products of social work and constitutive of forms of social life" (Jasanoff 2004: 2). Both sex and gender are socially constructed. An understanding of gender as separate from sex will again take up the outdated idea that sex is exclusively a matter of biology with no psychological or social dimension and it will imply that biomedical definitions are objective and inherently free of socio-historical aspects. Indeed, I am convinced that such a division will lead to a considerable backwards move, which creates the danger of having legal sex based on a biological sex (defined as inherently free of psychological and social factors). In fact, court rulings, though very inconsistent in their definitions of legal sex, are already often relying on an individual's chromosomal sex as a last resort (for an extensive review of legal decisions see Hucker 1985; Green 1992; Eskridge/Hunter 1997; Greenberg 1999 and 2000; Dunson 2001; Frye/Meiselman 2001; Walker 2001; Hong 2002; Bilharz 2005; and Sabatello 2009). I fear that the already achieved rapprochement of biomedical to formerly non-medical gender concepts and the paradigm shift by scientific and trans-communities (as described by Bornstein 1994; Hubbard 1998 and Boswell 1998) from traditional understandings of sex and gender identity towards fluidity and free expression will be undermined. My opinion is also informed by the South African status quo where, despite a legal definition of sex entailing both biological and social aspects, the latter are ignored by executive organs in favour of the former (as I will show below).

The supposed unambiguity of sex as well as its binarity are both questionable from a medical, historical and cultural comparative perspective. Sex is discursively constructed as natural through interactive performative practices by different human and non-human actors on a local, national and international level. Sex-classifications and (re)categorizations are negotiated at specific sites such as the World Health Organization's International Classification of Diseases (ICD) or the Diagnostic and Statistical Manual of Mental Disorders published by the American Psychiatric Association (DSM) and implemented on a local level such as the South African Department of Home Affairs. Currently the term "gender identity disorder" (the label assigned to trans* people) is being renegotiated as both the ICD and DSM are under review. The definition of "gender identity disorder" is part of an ongoing and controversial public debate in which not only trans* activists and medical experts take part, but also other stakeholders such as the European Parliament. In the European Parliament's Resolution of 28 September 2011 on Human Rights, Sexual Orientation and Gender Identity at the United Nations (authored by South Africa) it

"11. Regrets that the rights of [...] transgender people are not yet always fully upheld in the European Union, including the right to bodily integrity [...] 13. Roundly condemns the fact that homosexuality, bisexuality and transsexuality are still regarded as mental illnesses by some countries, including within the EU, and calls on states to combat this; calls in particular for the depsychiatrisation of the transsexual, transgender, journey, for free choice of care providers, for changing identity to be simplified, and for costs to be met by social security schemes; [...] 16. Calls on the Commission and the World Health Organisation to withdraw gender identity disorders from the list of mental and behavioural disorders, and to ensure a non-pathologising reclassification in the negotiations on the 11th version of the International Classification of Diseases (ICD-11)" (European Parliament 2011).

The European Parliament calls for the protection of trans* citizens' rights to both bodily integrity and reproductive rights. At the same time, it appeals to the WHO to remove gender identity disorders from the ICD's list of mental and behavioural disorders while simultaneously safeguarding a non-pathologizing reclassification. The ensuing public discourses resemble the debates which occurred in 1990 when the ICD's classification of homosexuality as a mental illness came to an end.

In South Africa, official locations of specific sex-identification practices and techniques are, for example, legislative, administrative and judicial bodies. These practices are dynamic and mutable while neither linear nor identical.

Legislature

South Africa has an exceptional legislature with regard to the recognition of non-binary sexes. However, even though sex, gender, and sexual orientation were included in the 1996 Constitutions Equality Clause, this mere inclusion was not sufficient enough to enshrine the rights of trans* persons, as the *Birth and Deaths Registration Act* stated that only persons who had commenced sex reassignment, or differently put, gender confirmation, prior to 1992 could apply to have their sex status adjusted in their documents. Accordingly, only ongoing transitions could be finalized but none could be initiated. As a consequence, no one could legally start transitioning after 1992.

Due to modern communication technologies this situation changed in 2004. Activists learned through the internet about the pending alteration of the *Sex Description and Sex Status Bill.* During this time, e-mail communication enabled them to communicate at high speed within a very limited time-frame and to formulate their objections and suggestions for improvement. Owing to their[5] written and oral submissions, improvements and corrections were inserted into *The Preliminary Alteration of Sex Description and Sex Status Bill* compiled by the South African Law Commission, so that the Act succeeding the Bill now conforms to the Constitution. One of these improvements was that people could legally start transitioning again due to *The Alteration of Sex Description and Sex Status Act, No.* 49 of 2003 (in the following referred to as Act 49). With it came another important legal change: genital surgery was no longer required for the alteration of one's sex description. This was an important step with regard to the bodily integrity and reproductive rights of trans* citizens. The preceding Bill stated that only persons "whose sex *organs* have been altered" [italics mine] could apply. Instead, a report from a medical practitioner stating that *sexual characteristics* have been altered has become mandatory for the alteration of one's sex description. Opportunely, the term medical practitioner was defined in such a broad way that it can include biomedical therapists as well as so-called traditional health practitioners[6]. Theoretically, any treatment by traditional health practitioners that has led to changes in the ways in which a person expresses his or her social identity as a member of a particular sex (e.g. style of dressing) must be recognized as sufficient for the alteration of the sex description on his or her birth register. However this is not legal practice and I will elaborate on this further in the section on the configuration of trans* citizens through South Africa's administration.

The rights of intersexed people were only secured in January 2006 through an amendment of Section 1, Act 4 of the Equality Act: *Promotion of Equality and Prevention of Unfair Discrimination Act* (PEPUDA), created in 2000. After the successful intervention of activist Sally Gross, founder of Intersex South Africa (ISSA), the definition of intersex was inserted through this amendment. Most importantly however, it was stated that the term 'sex' in the Equality Clause includes intersex. This is important as there was a court case in the US (Wood v. C.G. Studio) where an intersexed plaintiff brought about legal action claiming discrimination when the company with which the plaintiff was employed terminated employment after having learned that the employee was intersexed.

5 | These were activists such as Estian Smit and Simone Heradien involved with the Cape Town Transsexual/Transgender Support Group. Activist Sally Gross advocated on behalf of intersexed people. Further input was given by the Human Rights Commission and the Lesbian and Gay Equality Project.

6 | The term traditional is highly and rightly contested within medical anthropology as it indicates a static or ahistoric practice. I am nevertheless using the term in this context as it is the official term used in the Traditional Health Practitioners Act of 2004.

"The court determined that 'sex' under the provisions of the PHRA included men discriminated against because of their sex and women discriminated against because of their sex, but excluded intersexed individuals. Relying upon Webster's Dictionary for its definition rather than medical evidence, the court ruled that there were only two sexes and Wood [the plaintiff] wasn't one of them" (Bilharz 2005: 271).

Intervention by Gross and the insertion of the term intersexed into the Equality Act thus prevented the possibility of citizens' bodies becoming quintessentially outlawed. Even though they weren't formally denied citizenship, this ruling reduced their lives from 'bios' (life of a community / life brought under law) to 'zoe' (biological life of individuals; also called "naked life" by Agamben). "Zoe [...] expressed the simple fact of living common to all living beings (animals, men, or gods), and bios [...] indicated the form or way of living proper to an individual or a group" (Agamben 1998: 1). Schinkel argues

"[...] that in today's forms of population control a distinction between zoepolitics and biopolitics is relevant. Zoepolitics is primarily externally directed towards persons outside the state, as becomes visible, for instance, in the reduction to bare life of those detained in Guantánamo Bay and in the administrative detention of 'illegal aliens'" (Schinkel 2010: 156).

Through the formal inclusion of intersex into the term 'sex' in the Equality Clause, intersexed citizens were thus prevented from becoming targets of zoepolitics. Even though the South African Constitution has afforded guaranteed protection in law to intersexed people, it has to be noted that unlike to Australia, no certificates or legal documents are issued stating that intersex is the legal sex of a person. It signifies how state legislatures struggle to acknowledge more than two sexes.

The histories of the adjustment made to Act 49 and the Equality Act illustrate the medical impact on laws. The negotiation of legal sex classifications involved discussions on medical categorizations as well as the necessities of surgeries. As Foucault stated: "Power and knowledge directly imply one another; [...] there is no power relation without the correlative constitution of a field of knowledge, nor any knowledge that does not presuppose and constitute at the same time power relations" (Foucault 1977: 27).

And even though Act 49 is a progressive step in that it permits intersexed and trans* citizens to adjust their legal identities, it still inscribes medical definitions of sex into the law that will standardize citizens' gendered identities. These medico-legal taxonomies ensure specific rights to citizens but simultaneously try to restrict them to these identities. Moreover, the taxonomies are not impartial; they are never purely descriptive but are always accompanied by normative elements indicating what is 'normal'. In the case of sex and gender, normality is easily equated with health (physical and mental as set out above in the example of the ICD and DSM).

"[...] si tu n'es pas comme tout le monde, c'est que tu es anormal, si tu es anormal, c'est que tu es malade. Ces trois catégories : n'être pas comme tout le monde, n'être pas normal et être malade, sont tout de même très différentes et se sont trouvées assimilées les unes aux autres" (Foucault 1975).
["[...] if you are not like everybody else, then you are abnormal, if you are abnormal, then you are sick. These three categories, not being like everybody else, not being normal and being sick are in fact very different but have been reduced to the same thing."]

The quote above by Foucault nicely summarizes the experiences of many trans* people I have met. To not be like everybody else often brought the experience of dislodgement in the sense of not belonging, caused by a cisgender-oriented environment treating them as abnormal and ill, while dictating psychiatric treatment in order to receive legal recognition. For some trans* people, it instilled a desire for integration into normality as defined by their cisgendered surroundings. It resulted in the respective normalization and adjustment procedures of their bodies. In other cases (as citizens are neither wholly subjected nor entirely self-defining) it gave rise to a counter-hegemonic discourse containing a redefinition of normality, which allowed for a broadening of the available scope of identity repertoires. Still others were caught in the middle; even though oriented within the hegemonic binary gender discourse, they were unable, for various reasons explained below, to access the necessary gender confirming technologies. In any case, all of them had to deal with the perceived normality of a binary sex and the accompanying medico-legally ascribed physical norms.

ADMINISTRATION

What is interesting with regard to the South African administration is that it enforces its own rules. The Department of Home Affairs, where the appeals for Sex Description Application are handled, still only issues documents after completed genital surgery and demands letters from the surgeon who performed the surgery, even though Act 49 states that:

"2.(1) Any persons whose sexual characteristics have been altered by surgical *or medical treatment or by evolvement through natural development* resulting in gender reassignment, or any person who is intersexed may apply to the Director-General of the National Department of Home Affairs for the alteration of the sex description on his or her birth register" (Government Gazette 2004: 30, emphasis is mine).

Sexual characteristics are defined by the Act as "primary or secondary characteristics or gender characteristics" whereas gender characteristics "means the ways in which a person expresses his or her social identity as a member of a particular sex by using style of dressing, the wearing of prostheses or other means" (Government Gazette 2004: 30). According to Act 49, the Department of Home Affairs may not reject applications from persons who choose surgery that does not involve primary sex characteristics or who choose hormone therapy without surgery. Theoretically, any treatment by traditional health practitioners that has led to changes in the ways in which a person expresses his or her social identity as a member of a particular sex (e.g. style of dressing) must be recognized as sufficient for the alteration of the sex description on his or her birth register. However this legal practice is not executed. Not only have I met frustrated interviewees during my research who have had to cope with the absurd situation of legislative and executive organs making contradictory demands, but the inconsistency of the situation has even made media headlines, for example on the award winning South African TV-show *Special Assignment* on 24 November 2007. Nevertheless, to my knowledge this media coverage has produced no significant change.

A major shift in the exercise of power becomes observable when applying Foucault's power diagram to the South African situation. As long as the Department of Home Affairs is not stopped by court order, its conventions have a binding effect on the general public. It is here where citizens receive their legal documents; thus the Department of Home Affair as an administrative agency creates and enforces its own legal rules in opposition to the Constitution.

The South African situation is an example of the insoluble tension described by Foucault between a system based on law and a system based on medical notions of 'normality' in contemporary society. By law, South African trans* citizens have a right to the legal recognition of their gender identity without genital surgery; however, in practice, this right is denied to them through the Department of Home Affairs.

Two different official discourses prevail in South Africa concerning the configuration of trans* citizens through the state:

The legislative discourse concerns the Equality Clause in the Bill of Rights and Act 49, both secure trans* citizens' rights to marriage, parenthood and protect them from discrimination. Legally, South Africa subscribes to the Yogyakarta Principles[7].

7 | The Yogyakarta Principles are a set of international principles that clarify the nature, scope and implementation of States' human rights obligations under existing human rights treaties and law, in relation to sexual orientation and gender identity.

No one shall be forced to undergo medical procedures, including sex reassignment surgery, sterilisation or hormonal therapy, as a requirement for legal recognition of their gender identity. [...] No status, such as marriage or parenthood, may be invoked as such to prevent the legal recognition of a person's gender identity (Jurisprudential Annotations to the Yogyakarta Principles 2007: 11).

The administrative discourse entails The Department of Home Affairs insistence on a binary sex/gendered system that is able to clearly distinguish between male and female trans* citizens by means of genital surgery. An often cited reason has been the prevention of fraud. Why and how the removal of reproductive organs, which are usually hidden from the public eye, prevents fraud has never been convincingly argued. Nevertheless, trans* citizen (whether happy to comply or not) are coerced by the Department to engage in gender confirmation surgeries that entail sterilization and the use of specific (albeit very difficult to access) medical technologies, if they want to be legally recognized in their lived gender.

The Department of Home Affairs is caught in a rather awkward position; by upholding mandatory sterilization[8] it violates both the Equality Clause in the Bill of Rights and Act 49. Unfortunately, judicial interference has yet to overcome the contradicting definitions. This is partly due to the fact that the Department of Home Affairs has given in, in some cases, only after extended periods of time and when seriously threatened with a court case as well as, to some extent, to the willingness of surgeons to write rather vague reports about the surgeries[9] that have been carried out (personal communication, trans* activist 9 May 2009). Additionally, many trans* citizens are not willing to go public with a court case because the exposure makes them more vulnerable than they already are to countless forms of violence and discrimination despite Act 49 and the Equality Clause.

Excursus: international situation

South Africa is, however, not the only country dealing with ambivalent agendas and discourses. Sharpe has dealt with a similar situation in Great Britain, where the Gender Recognition Act of 2004 does not require surgery either, but where

8 | The term sterilization is an umbrella term encompassing all surgical techniques leaving a person unable to reproduce. In the South African case it refers however to the complete removal of all reproductive organs.

9 | Reassignment surgeries may entail any of a variety of non-genital surgical procedures such as mastectomy, chest reconstruction, breast augmentation, facial feminizing surgery, buttock and hips augmentation, liposuction, Adam's apple contouring, etc..

> it is clearly the expectation of the government that surgery will occur. [...] in the case of an applicant who has not undertaken surgery, the possibility remains [...] that this fact may hinder a diagnosis of gender dysphoria [which is essential for the legal adjustment of one's sex] (Sharpe 2007: 71-72).

Trans* people's existence and behaviour are defined in relation to medical concepts of the 'normal' (it is presumed that 'normal' trans* persons desire surgery in order to become even more 'normal') rather than in relation to whether or not they adhere to the law. The establishing of norms (biopower's processes of normalization here: a 'normal' trans* person will undertake genital surgery) is enforced through the disciplinary processes of bringing subjects into conformity with a pre-determined norm ('normation' here: the legal adjustment of one's sex is only, or at least more easily, achieved after genital surgery). As already stated above, one of the major arguments made by Foucault is that contemporary Western societies function fundamentally according to a medical rather than a legal model (O'Farrell 2010). Failure to comply with medical expectations can mean, in this setting, that one will be regarded not only as different but in some sense, 'abnormal' or even (mentally) 'sick'. Thus the already unprivileged become not ostracized but are disciplined as 'abnormally abnormal' and are regarded as in need of 'healing'. As Catlaw has pointed out: "Rather than being subject to strict exclusion, social antagonisms are internalized and subjected to disciplinary control" (Catlaw 2008: 465).

Currently, the UK (since 2004) and Spain (since 2007) are still the only European countries where genital surgery is not a prerequisite for a new birth certificate in the lived gender; first steps have also been made by Germany and Austria. Though legislative organs haven't reacted yet, the Austrian Administrative High Court declared in a judgment on 27 February 2009 that mandatory genital surgery for transgendered people is unlawful. A similar ruling was made by the German Federal Constitutional Court on 11 January 2011. Permanent sterility remains a requirement for a new birth certificate in the lived gender—or at least the entry of the lived gender into the old birth certificate (a highly contested procedure since it fails to protect a person's privacy)—by Belgium, Denmark, Finland, France and the Netherlands. Genital surgery is required in Lithuania and secondary sex characteristics surgery is compulsory in the Czech Republic and Greece. The birth certificate cannot be changed at all in Ireland, Italy, Portugal, and Sweden (compare Whittle et al. 2008: 22-23). This excursion into legal practice of other countries will become of interest again in the section on supranational citizenship.

So far I have dealt with those citizens who do not wish for genital surgery. For those South African citizens who desire genital surgery, it is complicated by very restricted access to medical technologies.

ACCESS TO REASSIGNMENT SURGERIES: TODAY AND DURING APARTHEID

Those trans* citizens who desire (or are happy to comply with) genital surgery face a difficult situation. Only two South African hospitals of the 16 provincial tertiary hospitals and national central hospitals that provide Level III care also provide gender confirmation surgery; these are *Groote Schuur Hospital* in Cape Town and *Pretoria Academic Hospital*. In addition, there are budget restrictions which limit the number of patients that can be seen at these two locations. At *Groote Schuur Hospital*, it was stated that they can only provide surgery for one Female to Male (FtM) and one Male to Female (MtF) per year. At *Pretoria Academic Hospital*, one interviewee stated that they "can only do one full profile per quarter" (Anonymous, 28 November 2007). Thus, waiting lists grow extremely long. According to Vincent and Camminga (2009: 695), waiting lists are up to 30 to 40 times the number of actually performed surgeries.

With regard to shifting relations between regimes of governance and healing, it is interesting to note that there had been quite a peak in gender confirmation surgeries and newly issued birth certificates in the 1980s, even though gender confirmation surgeries had already been carried out previously with regularity. According to the South African Law Commission, 150 trans* citizens were treated between 1969 and 1984 at *Groote Schuur Hospital* in Cape Town alone (South African Law Commission 1995: 8). Crichton (1993: 347) states that he carried out 58 surgeries at the University of Natal Hospital in Durban between 1969 and 1993. Additionally, it was estimated by forensic psychiatrist Robert Kaplan that as many as 900 forced "sexual reassignment" operations may have been performed between 1971 and 1989 at military hospitals.

"Recurrent allegations have been made that between 1969 and 1987 approximately 900 men and women had gender reassignment surgery, [...]. They were given new identity documents, discharged from the military, and told to cut themselves off from family and friends" (Kaplan 2004: 1415).

The number of gender confirmation surgeries was much higher during apartheid than it is today. It is important to note that they were not only 'available', but forced on hundreds of citizens as the military screened all conscripts for signs of homosexuality. "[...] the military approached homosexuality as a disease, which it attempted to 'treat'" (Vincent/Camminga 2009: 685) through electro-shock therapy and, in 'incurable cases', with genital reassignment surgery.

"The rationale for giving homosexuals reassignment surgery, in complete ignorance of the scientific literature on transsexualism, can only be described as repulsive. It was based on the simplistic belief that male homosexuals were sissies, female homosexuals were tomboys, and *surgery would end their preference for the same sex by allowing them to fulfil their projected role in the opposite sex*" (Kaplan 2004: 1415-1416, emphasis mine).

It is probably no coincidence that homosexual conscripts were institutionalized at *One Military Hospital Voortrekkerhoogte* together with conscripts who dissented with apartheid ideology; both being regarded as representatives of unruly and deviant citizens in need of 'normation' (compare also Foucault's work on prisons as a medico-judicial remedy; e.g. Foucault 1977).

"While biopolitical government largely works through self-governing participants (a governmentality which 'solves' the liberal challenge), it also permits the illiberal management of unruly individuals or groups by appealing to the notion of a 'society' that is internally complex and that may periodically require intervention by the state for its maintenance and security" (Raman/Tutton 2010: 715).

The regime of truth concerning the heteronormative gender binary produced the ludicrous notion that a man desiring another man must be a woman and vice versa. However, it constitutes an excellent sample of 'normation' through disciplinary power.

Returning to the post-apartheid situation of trans* citizens, it can be stated that surgery can be obtained in the private medical sector, at least theoretically. Persons who are willing and able to pay for the much more expensive private care can visit any private clinic in or outside the country. The few services offered in the public sector are, however, of crucial importance to the vast majority of people. Since income is still intimately connected with gender and skin colour, the situation is especially difficult for persons who did not grow up categorized as white males; regardless, private care is much too expensive even for many who have been categorized in this way. Two of my interviewees who were fortunate enough to be house owners sold their houses in order to finance their surgeries.

Besides the extremely limited numbers of patients who can be seen, the budget constraints in the public sector produce further restrictions for both patients and medical specialists. The latter have to work with limited theatre time and there is only a small team of medical experts available. Every patient at the gender clinic needs to be declared fit for surgery by a psychiatrist. However, there is only one psychiatrist available for the gender clinic at Pretoria Academic Hospital, and this psychiatrist only does private sector work, despite working for a public hospital. This is problematic; especially since the significantly higher fees for the services of the psychiatrist have to be paid by the clients. As most clients come from various parts of the country and do not live in the direct vicinity of the psychiatrist, the travel time and money needed complicate regular visits and makes them unfeasible for many.

SOMATECHNICS OF SELF-FORMATION: USERS AND SCRIPT-CHANGERS OF TECHNOLOGIES

The interaction of society, body, self and other becomes especially interesting in a technological age where individuals have increasing ability to modify their own bodies. This is particularly true as the technological age coincides with an information age, where new information technologies permit fast communication of heretofore unfamiliar discourses and somatechnics which ease identity work and self-normation. Communication technologies such as magazines, newspapers, TV and especially the internet with its social networks play an important role in the dissemination of information and new available identities.

"[I came across the word 'transsexual'] in the eighties a little bit, in reading some of the articles in some magazines, and then in the nineties when I got hold of the internet more. And I found that certain people started transitioning and they actually went forward and had surgery and [...] then I realized, that is me!" (MtF, 53 years, 15 March 2008).
"And I think when I was eighteen years old [...] I was at an internet café. [...] I've always been a fan of Oprah's, so I just kind of happened to [...] stumble across a small little article about a show she'd done on transgender kids. Um, and that was actually the first time, that I actually realized that, that it was something one could actually do. [...] My whole childhood, my teenage years, I knew that it was something I wanted. It was, it was something I wished for, but I didn't actually realize that it was something that was possible" (FtM, 21, 07 May 2008).

The evolution of social gender scripts[10] from 'a sex change' to 'a transgendered individual', can be illustrated through what Foucault called the genealogy of epistemes. The way in which the public press labels trans* citizens, associated identities and biographies of thirty years ago have undergone significant change through the internet. The internet facilitated the breaking up of a rigid pathologizing medical framework by pooling a critical mass of trans* people with counter-discourses. Genealogy in Foucault's sense includes "power relations in the ordered procedures that make true discourses possible" (Simons 2006: 189). The power relations with regard to the definition of trans*

10 | These are defined by Shapiro as "blueprints for [gendered] behaviour, belief, and identity" (2010: 9). Gender scripts are shaped not only by technologies but also by social norms, hierarchies, and power relations—and are situated in time and space.

were significantly changed through the internet's capacity for networking. It dramatically enhanced the collective impact of activists (see Shapiro 2010: 112ff and 128ff as well as my example in the section on legislature).

In the following quote one of my interviewees recalls how he stumbled for the first time in his life across an article about 'sex change' which led him to expect a dreadful biography:

"I was probably in primary school. And there was an article in [...] the Sunday newspaper, where a guy had gender reassignment surgery and [was] transforming into a woman and it made the front news by then. And that's where the first time I heard about that, yes you can change your sex. I was eight/nine years old—it was many years ago. Well, I was reading the article, and I was very young. I knew I wanted to do that route but it was also shocking. That was how the article was written. This person was rejected by society and this person lost um, her family and lost her friends, lost her job. And um, so that also kept you, you know in the back of your mind that: are you willing to do that? Um, is it worthwhile? And at a young age like that... I was brought up in a very Afrikaner house [...] very strict and very religious and um, that was not things that were talked about... [...] so I kept it for myself. I can just remember [...] that my father read that article and he just said 'shun, this person will be an outcast for the rest of her life' and I knew, well, I don't want to be an outcast. I want to be accepted for who I am. [...] It [the internet] made a major difference. Um, the internet is a valuable source of information. And there are a lot of things I wouldn't know [...] how to go about if it wasn't for the internet" (FtM, 40 years, 27 April 2008).

Besides communication technologies, other technologies like new somatechnics are constantly altering gender scripts. Moreover, technologies also carry "scripts". "Madeleine Akrich (1992) observed that assumptions about users are 'inscribed' into technologies, in the form of a 'script', by the innovators that develop them" (Rose/Blum 2003: 108).

In the same way that trans* citizens are not passive subjects and can resist or actively modify their configuration, they can also, as users of technologies, resist, modify or interpret differently the "scripts" of certain technologies. In fact, "to resist the configuring, and disciplining effects of [...] technologies may be to protest the social policies implicated by the technologies themselves" (Rose/Blum 2003: 106).

Due to the fact that trans* users are not a homogenous group, but heterogeneous along gender, ability status, ethnicity, religion, class, sexual orientation, and socio-economic possibility lines, there are innumerable options in the ways they accept, resist, modify and interpret the scripts of technologies. Access to and choice of somatechnics and information technologies for trans* citizens is likewise influenced by this diverse set of factors. Keeping the diversity of South African trans* citizens in mind, I will address the following questions:

How do trans* citizen users experiment with technologies? More specifically, what are new uses for technologies that were originally invented and/or intended for a different cause?

In the following section, I will present two examples: first, the example of the birth control pill and hormone replacement therapy as technologies originally invented for cisgendered women and appropriated by trans* women as a substitute for female hormones; second, the experimentation with technologies other than the pill or hormone replacement therapy by citizens who define their identity outside of a binary sex or gender system (e.g. breast implants in a gender queer citizen or the re-categorization of gender with regard to the corporeality of pregnant trans*men).

BIRTH CONTROL PILL AND HORMONE REPLACEMENT THERAPY

Experimentation and formulating new usages for technologies such as the birth control pill are excellent examples of citizen science. Knowledge concerning its usage is gained through acquaintances, researching the internet and self-experimentation.

"[...] because everybody think that you're a little moffie[11], they start telling you stories and whatsoever, and then this one girl said like something like...her, she's got a moffie friend and she takes birth control and it actually makes her tits big. You could never tell that to me! So there I was like looking for birth control everywhere—even telling my friend to get me some. So I like had a whole packet, like swallow it, yeah, like I went to school and I actually like fainted [laughs]. [...] I've learned then [...] it doesn't work like that. So that is when I first heard about the pill" (22 years old, self-identifies as "chick with a dick", 24 Sept. 2007).

The contraceptive pill is especially popular with trans* women as it is said to cause a greater increase in breast size than the hormones available at GPs and endocrinologists. Another reason for its popularity is that access to biomedical care and body-altering products depends to a great extent on financial resources. Many of the female-identified trans* interviewees with low or no income stated that they had tried to gain access to birth control pills instead of, or after unsuccessfully seeking admittance to, biomedical supervised hormone treatment. Contraceptive pills are available free of charge at public sector family planning clinics. However they are only given to cisgendered and not to trans* women. Thus the interviewees were dependent on cisgendered women (and

11 | Moffie is a derogatory South African term for (feminine) gay men. It also connotes trans* and intersexuality.

sometimes male-identified trans* persons who could still pass as women) for help.

"I'm actually starting to run out of the pill now, so, I have to like look for nice friends again, to say 'go fetch me the pill at the clinic'. But then most of my friends are on the injection. [...]
Th.K.: Can't you go yourself?
[...] I don't know, I haven't tried it, but I'm scared [pause] because if you go to a clinic, you have to open a folder. [...] they are obviously going to see I'm male. Who gives birth control to males if it's not condoms? So...yeah, I can't go hey? They'll probably tell me that the mental institute is that side" (22 years old, self-identifies as "chick with a dick", 24 Sept. 2007).

Trans* citizens are not only resourceful in finding access to hormones but also in increasing dosages. An 82 year old trans* woman related to me how she accesses the dosage she finds agreeable.

"I get them from the chemist down the road. [...] Some of them I get from the day hospital [...] I got a prescription from the doctor at the corner. [...] And he gave me the prescription without any query at all. [...] At the hospital of course I don't pay [and do not need a prescription] but I have to pay for them here [at the chemist with the prescription from the doctor] [...] I get both things. So I get a higher dosage [Premarin]. You see, I get 2.5, [laughs] just what I want. 1.25 is not enough!" (82 years old, MtF, 17 March 2008).

In the cited case she does not refer to birth control pills but to Premarin, which is a form of hormone-replacement therapy. Premarin pills were developed for post-menopausal women but are used for trans* and intersexed persons as well.

Citizens with (Un)Accommodated Gender Identities

I have outlined above how the executive organs of the South African state configure the trans* citizen user of sexing/gendering technologies as a person whose gender identity does not match the assigned sex at birth, but who is willing to adjust his or her body in a way that reflects the binary of the sex/gender system. Nevertheless, technologies are also used by trans* citizens that identify differently.

"[...] choosing an identity is a difficult one because I change and shift and move around. [pause] I am...South African. Hmm, I am, I identify myself as male mostly, uh, but that is not a strict definition. [...] I have a BA, an LLB and a Masters in Social Science from UCT and uh, I'm a non practicing attorney and I am currently doing my PhD in sexuality studies. [...] I'm not particularly attached to whether I'm identified as male or female because I don't really think that there's that much of a difference between them anyway. [...] So I identify myself as male because I was brought up as one and that's fine—but there's certain elements within my sexuality and within my self-identity which don't really fit that male mould, hmm, and are more on the feminine side for want of a better term. [...] as a result I've shifted my own [...] physicality to reflect that in certain ways. I've had breast implants, hmm, and sometimes play with hormones [...] but that's a reflection of an internal sense of self in terms of accessing my more feminine side. Now identifying, identifying what 'feminine' is, for me is very difficult because to me it's a human experience, and [...] identifying masculine and feminine traits is not necessarily a very helpful way of looking at things because if you could use all of those old stereotypes of hmm, kind of dominant versus submissive as male versus female and active versus passive, none of that really worked because everybody's got all of that, every human being has got all of that inherent or implicit in them" (35 years old, 07 Feb. 2007).

The interviewee does not identify in a way the South African state envisaged for its trans* citizens:

"I've never wanted to kind of go from one box to another box. Hmm, so it was a questionable... uh, how do I then reconcile wanting to be both and altogether or neither male nor female" (35 years old, 07 Feb. 2007).

nor does ze[12] agree with the current practice of the Department of Home Affairs that ensures that the physiognomy of South African trans* citizen matches their gender identity while it ensures at the same time that there are only two sexes and genders.

"I get a sense that if, if there was a different world, if we had a different social structure, that those people would not necessarily be attached to their identity, they would be, they would be more fluid and just identify [...] the kinds of self that they feel they need to be without having to, without feeling the need to transition to become what they want. [...] some people feel as though there is something very, very different from the role they're sort of encouraged to perform and therefore make a transition. Other people do this in a [...] different way and don't feel a need to transform themselves physically to match their emotional state" (35 years old, 07 Feb. 2007).

---

12 | Ze, hir, hirself, etc. pp are gender neutral pronouns. They are used as a step in the direction of gender-neutral language and an attempt to work against a linguistic consolidation of the gender-binary in order to make trans* and intersexed people visible.

The interviewee seems to argue here in accordance with Foucault who maintains with respect to homosexuality and not transgenderism, "I think what the gay movement needs now is much more the art of life than a science or scientific knowledge (or pseudo-scientific knowledge) of what sexuality is" (Foucault 1989: 382). Instead of accommodating the knowledge of official stakeholders to achieve subjectivity, ze envisages a world where people distrust that the question of identity needs to be reflected visually in a prescribed and fixed gender. Similarly, Foucault critiqued the modes through which people are tied to specific identities and advised "[...] not to discover what we are, but to refuse what we are" (Foucault 2000 [1982]: 336). He urged to question identification-labels and to create oneself as an object of art as power lies in creative activities.

Due to the powerful sex-binary structures mediated through biomedicine and implemented through the state, or in short, due to biopolitics, it becomes quite difficult to express ones identity when it is in opposition to state policies. This means the interviewee could not access surgery through a state hospital. Ze accessed surgery via a private surgeon who was only willing to perform the surgery after several years of hesitation.

"It only happened when I was about twenty eight, [...] I mean I've been wanting breasts for a long time, but I never allowed myself to imagine that that would be a possibility [...] and then I realized that it actually is a possibility. [...] I'd stretched my ear lobes and they'd gotten thin on the inside so I needed to go see a plastic surgeon to go, to get them fixed. So I went in and I just suddenly, as I was sitting there, thought I want breasts and I want to see if I can ask this person if he would do them... so and as I was sitting there it suddenly kind of bubbled up from the inside—I know I've always wanted this, hmm, but I can actually possibly have it... and so I'd asked and it was a whole long kind of process from then in terms of actually getting them" [ze received the surgery four years later] (35 years old, 07 Feb. 2007).

Breast enhancement also belongs to the technologies that were originally intended for a different cause. Even though this technology has a long tradition of being used in gender confirmation surgery, it has only been performed in state hospitals on trans* citizens who identify firmly as female. As has become quite apparent in hirs statements, the interviewee does not identify as a woman nor can ze place hirself in a bi-gendered system.

Another example of unforeseen and un-accommodated citizens (though explicitly not gender outlaws) are pregnant trans* men. As there is no homogenous trans* community, pregnancy in trans* men was discussed very controversially. This was especially the case as Thomas Beatie, the American trans* man falsely celebrated by the press as the first[13] pregnant trans* man, made the headlines in the South African Press. Comments within the trans* community ranged from dismissive:

"What do you guys think of Thomas Beatie being pregnant again? The outrage from 'normal' crowd saying he went too far, calling him a mutilated lesbian on the Barbara Walters show. I think he just screwed up the TS cause for us very badly and put us back a few years" (MtF, 20 Nov 2008).
"Maybe FtM should be sterilised. After all MtF are. It would make the playing field even and then Thomas Beatie things won't happen" (MtF, 1 Dec 2008).

to supportive:

"I think it's very brave. Personally I wouldn't do it, because I didn't want any female body parts. [...] I think he is very brave to come out doing it in public and maybe it's high time!" (FtM, 40 years old, 27 Apr. 2008).
"I thought about this issue again in terms of what I can argue and what not. I cannot argue that men don't have babies. Men don't have babies. [...] Being transgender though... FtM's can have babies. [...] So anti-Beatie people would like to argue that FTM's should NOT be PERMITTED to have babies? [...] You get to be of the opinion that FTM's should not have babies. I am also free. I get to think that FTM's SHOULD have the OPTION of having babies" (FtM, 38 years old, 23 Nov 2008).
"I would say that is the ultimate trans experience. (..) I think it is a very, very bold, very enlightened step. Because he is offering his whole self. You know? And yeah, it is not [...] compartmentalizing, he is not saying that 'This is what I was and I don't want anything to do with it!' You know? Now I'm this! He is saying, 'This is who I am'" (MtF, 65 years old, 02 Apr. 2008).

Those who were dismissive feared in most cases that their rights as fully acknowledged citizens would suffer due to gender identities or bodies outside the socially accepted norm. Their arguments are strongly reminiscent of the 1970s discussions in the US on how to have homosexual people be recognized as respectable citizens by mainstream society which resulted in the (attempted) exclusion of gender non-conforming homosexuals (effeminate gays and masculine lesbians) in the gay liberation movement.

13 | Trans* parents or pregnant trans* men are not such an unusual case as is depicted by the press. In 2005—three years before Thomas Beaties pregnancy—filmmaker Jules Rosskam featured the experiences of 19 female-to-male transgender parents in his documentary film "Transparents", broaching the issue of the invisibility of transgender parenting in contemporary discourse. And already in 2000 the Village Voice provided an article about the parenthood of two trans* men in 1999 (Califia-Rice 2000).

"We have to remember that the DSM V [Diagnostic and Statistical Manual of Mental Disorders] is about to be discussed and will be put in place. The doctors who write these guidelines will have a look at what is happening and the criteria can become stricter because of one individual's action. [...] People see this as a joke and view TS issues as weird and unnatural. We want to be accepted as part of society and *therefore need to play by society rules*" (MtF, 27 Nov 2008, emphasis mine).

This comment demonstrates likewise in an exemplary way Foucault's conceptualization of governmentality, where individuals through the internalization of external authority turn themselves into subjects and police their selves in society. Thus governmentality points equally to state actions and the 'conduct of conduct'. The conduct of trans* citizens is not just governed by governmental institutions and biopolitical standardizing bodies such as the American Psychiatric Association, which publishes the Diagnostic and Statistical Manual of Mental Disorders, but also through trans* citizens themselves and their cisgendered surroundings. Many interviewees monitored themselves very closely; not necessarily due to legal regulations but due to fear of discrimination, harassment and assault.

"I'd never go out [dressed] like this [in 'male' clothing] if I was going out with my friends, because that's unacceptable. Like then everyone would be like staring at you if you go to a female toilet, and you would not enjoy yourself at all, and I don't want to make it all awkward for my friends, like if they bring other friends or if they introduce me, so I don't want to make it weird for them" (FtM, 23 years, 10 May 2008).

Even though it was acknowledged that the case of Thomas Beatie might be used to harm the rights of trans* people, it was also pointed out that it might in fact benefit the trans* cause.

"Society wasn't ready for slavery to be abolished, or for women to gain the vote, or for racial equality, or for any other big revolution. Let's face it folks, society has to be dragged into the future kicking and screaming. And it is brave individuals like Mr. Beatie and his wife who do so. The only reason any of us find this abhorrent is because of social conditioning–the very same conditioning we rail against when we try to get people to accept us" (MtF, 24 Nov 2008).

When Mr. Beatie gave birth to his third child in 2010, this was still discussed in the media but with less sensationalism. His three media-covered pregnancies informed the wider public on trans* issues and allowed for questions and discussions in cisgendered circles which would otherwise have never come into contact with this topic. It also allowed for familiarization and illustrates how new technologies alter views on an individual and social level concerning how trans* citizens' bodies are or ought to be. This familiarization process was, however, not facilitated through a queer narrative but instead through an account of normality: the Beaties, like the average heterosexual family, wanted to have children; they were like everyone else in their universal longing for a child with the small exception that Mrs. Beatie had a hysterectomy and therefore was unable to become pregnant. Conveniently, her husband was able to carry a child to term because he had kept his ovaries and uterus during gender confirmation surgery.

Although this illustration deals with narratives of normality, the (dis)use of certain technologies (here, the use of gender confirmation surgery without the removal of ovaries and uterus) it leads to the possibility of new subjectivities (pregnant male). And even though trans* citizens, as users of medical technologies, are configured (and many configure themselves) in a bi-gendered model, these citizens are not always passive subjects of biopolitics and governance. Instead, as seen in the examples above, they are quite active participants. User agency in the re-shaping of their bodies and identities as consumers in markets is often overlooked when analysing them solely in their role as citizens of states. In the following section I will move on to explore their local and global agency within the realms of supranational citizenship, citizen science and medical tourism.

SUPRANATIONAL CITIZENSHIP, CITIZEN SCIENCE AND MEDICAL TOURISM

Citizenship is increasingly perceived as more than the legal rights and duties one gains through the membership in a political community; instead it has become defined in terms of a social process through which rights are expanded and claimed. One of these claims entails the right to be healthy, achieve health or transition in ways that might be in opposition to state policies. In the process of claiming rights in opposition to state policies, international courts gain importance; "where citizenship rights fail to provide protection of individuals from the state, the individuals will appeal to international courts for protection of human rights" (Isin/Turner 2008: 7). Similarly, the significance of supranational citizenship increases. Linklater states in his extensive discussion of cosmopolitan citizenship that "the universal human rights culture is deemed to be evidence of the emerging law of world citizens; cosmopolitan citizenship is thought to be exemplified by the increasing global role of INGOS[14] and by efforts to promote the democratisation of world politics" (Linklater 2008: 330).

Without diverting into the discussions around cosmopolitan citizenship, the importance of international non-governmental organizations (such as the

---

14 | International Non-Governmental Organizations

Trans Secretariat[15] of the International Lesbian and Gay Association (ILGA) and the International Gay and Lesbian Human Rights Commission (IGLHRC)), international conferences (such as the Yogyakarta conference of November 2006 and the Global Arc of Justice Conference of 2009) and the possibility for individuals to invoke international law against their own state has clearly become an important factor for the work of trans* activists and has led, if not to a cosmopolitan trans* citizenship, at least to international trans* activist networks and movements. I have demonstrated elsewhere (Klein 2009) that South African trans* activists are in any case involved in a broader international social movement addressing gender and sexuality.

"As a simple matter of law, nationality is the primary axis by which peoples are classified and distributed in polities across the globe. However the continuing rise of new forms of cultural politics has challenged modern understandings of belonging and has contributed to rethinking the meaning of citizenship" (Isin/Turner 2008: 4).

This internationalization has led to an extension of the idea of citizenship to an international level and is already reflected, for example, in the European Union and within the Commonwealth of Nations. Both, the European Union and the Commonwealth of Nations offer citizenship to South Africans of European descent. This is interesting for trans* citizens who would like to transition, for example, in the Netherlands or in the UK. Thus, the idea of citizenship as connected to a specific political niche such as a country has increasingly expanded through international human rights to encompass larger entities. "In the last two decades of the twentieth century, postmodernization and globalization challenged the nation-state as the sole source of authority of citizenship and democracy" (Isin/Turner 2008: 4). Trans* citizens not only visit other countries in their capacity as supranational citizens, they also have the possibility to receive the surgeries they desire as medical tourists. Many South African trans* women travel to Thailand; Thailand has very experienced surgeons who carry out a great many more surgeries than the experienced surgeons in South Africa. As of January 2006, Dr. Suporn, a Thai surgeon frequented by some of my interviewees, had performed almost 1,100 primary cases of reassignment surgery. In the same time period, the team of surgeons at *Pretoria Academic Hospital* carried out surgeries on about 8 to 12 people.

"Look, at the end of the day it is your personal choice. I am sure the local doctors are competent enough and are capable of doing a good job. My personal choice was to go to Thailand though as I felt that they are by far more experienced than anything local.

---

15 | The purpose of Trans World Secretariat is to connect all the activists groups around the world who are working on trans* issues.

One thing I am sure about ... when it comes to medical care, nothing we have locally comes even close to what I have experienced in Thailand. Their pain management was absolutely brilliant. They treat you with respect and are gentle and kind. For me, this was something very important to me, so I went what [sic] I thought was the best person for the job. I wasn't about to take any chances. I had no complications and everything went very smoothly" (MtF, 28 June 2005).

Gender confirmation surgery is regarded as a common procedure in Thailand. There are over 170 active surgeons. Two local associations provide education or certification for surgeons doing gender confirmation surgery: the Society of Plastic and Reconstructive Surgeons of Thailand and the Thai Academy of Cosmetic Surgery and Medicine. This is in stark contrast to South Africa where there is no such society and very little training available. During the time of my research, South African trans* citizens who were able to be classified as transsexual by a psychologist, in line with the World Professional Association for Transgender Health's Standards of Care for Gender Identity Disorders (or simply WPATH's Standards of Care, SOC) were only seen at two hospitals: *Groote Schuur Hospital* in Cape Town and *Pretoria Academic Hospital*.

Thai surgeons are also renowned for their skill and performance in very difficult cases. In 2005, I was in contact with a trans* woman who had grasped a rather unorthodox method of getting rid of her male genitalia; she shot her genitalia in order to destroy them. This led to a physique with very little material left to do a penile inversion (part of her gender confirmation surgery. This is how she tells the story in a report to a South African trans* group in 2006 when she finally received surgery.

"My beginnings in Sex Change Surgery began many years ago in a very unusual way: In a twenty year old frustrated fit of pique I tried to do for myself what my ignorance prevented me from finding, and being skilled in the use of certain tools, chose as my scalpel a .357 Magnum revolver, loaded with 158 grain semi jacketed hollow point Norma round. Designed specifically to destroy flesh. Let's be honest and say the results to a mere penis and scrotum were not pretty. Even after reconstruction. So when I finally came to choosing my surgeon for SRS[Sex Reassignment Surgery/gender confirmation surgery], my candid opinion is the 'lucky' surgeon was not starting on level ground, as he would be with most 'normal' cases. Yet my 'want list' now at age 49 was as ambitious as any Girls': Aesthetics, depth, being sensate. Well, perfection would be acceptable.
Several of my South African sisters had been elsewhere, and I was not very impressed with the 'local' talent simply because although there is evidently one good doctor, there were seemingly few willing satisfied customers to testify. Cost was also no-where near realistic for me. The name Chettawutt [a Thai surgeon] did begin to occur rather frequently, and in favourable light. More digging, more favourable results. What particularly hooked my attention was that he seemed to do more than his fair share of

'difficult' procedures, and yet still come out with exceptional results" (MtF, 28 March 06).

A further distinction between South Africa and Thailand is that under existing Thai law, it is not necessary to comply with the Standards of Care (SOC) as set by WPATH. I need to add though that this was never mentioned to me as a positive asset. A much more important factor is money.

"On FFS [Facial Feminization Surgery]: I guess the USA has a few good plastic boffins around with Hollywood and the likes of Michael Jackson but obviously at a nice juicy price. Having looked around I found more affordable offerings in Thailand with the likes of Dr. Suporn (most expensive and two stage SRS [Sex Reassignment Surgery / gender confirmation surgery]) and Dr. Chettawut (more reasonable pricing). Their websites give you a good idea of before and after results as well. In SA we apparently have some of the world's best plastic surgeons but at a nice stiff price if you can find one who will do specifically FFS. I have not found one locally to be honest. For folks like us with little money to throw around I think Thailand will be the best option if you consider FFS" (MtF, 17 Aug. 2005).

Surgery in Thailand, including the recovery period, bringing a partner along and doing some sight-seeing is still cheaper than going to a private surgeon in South Africa.

"It cost me R65 000 (@ R7 to the Dollar) things are better now. I also went to Dr. Chettawut and would recommend him. The R65 000 included my partner which I feel is a must. It is not something to [sic] even if you are surrounded by English people. Local would have cost me more, about R90 000 if I went from Cape Town to Dr. [...]. His fee alone = my whole trip to Thailand including some sightseeing and shopping! The best is that you can deduct all the expenses including travel from tax" (MtF, 16 Aug. 2005).

The kinds of surgery available, the procedures used by different surgeons, the outcomes and experienced problems of surgery are discussed on the internet and at private gatherings. The same is true for experimentation with hormones, how to circumvent official procedures and where to get the best medical treatment for little money. Medical science and technologies are discussed without the institutionalized presence of surgeons, endocrinologists and other medical experts. Trans* citizen science has become well established outside South Africa's public health care system, with the internet playing an important role in the collection, dissemination and organization of knowledge. It is peers, and not the established medical community, who have taken over the medical information and education of each other. Citizen science provides the answer to the question of how far the state or society may impose or limit medical intrusion on their bodies. Through it, technologies of the self can be employed in the desired sense of the individual and not necessarily as intended by the respective government.

It is clearly the case that the state's executive organs use medical technologies as objects of identity projects to stabilize hegemonic representations of gender. Nevertheless, trans* citizens as users of these technologies in a world market are also able to destabilize these representations, even if the latter is especially true for the more affluent and wealthy. That trans* citizens from poorer economic backgrounds experiment in similar ways has been shown in the examples of the birth control pill and hormone-replacement therapy.

CONCLUSION

Foucault's power-diagram, his power/knowledge thesis and the concept of "co-production" from Science and Technology Studies prove to be helpful when rethinking governance and biomedicine in South Africa with respect to the configuration of trans* citizens. Scientific knowledge is at all times inseparably linked to power relations and is, in turn, co-produced by them. The net-like organization of power (power-diagram), which allows for actions upon the actions of others, is not fixed. Changes may occur when new identities and social relations (such as the pregnant male) emerge in biomedical classifications due to new somatechnics or when new communication technologies allow for fast, concerted action and a wide distribution of information. Thus it is not so much a question of whether technology will bring about progress (Karl Marx) or a dehumanized bureaucratic society (Max Weber), but of how technologies alter the power-diagram and in turn shape systems of knowledge as well as truth discourses. Rabinow and Rose suggest that biopower operates through three elements:

> "truth discourses about the vital character of living human beings articulated by a number of competent authorities (which do not necessarily have to be from within the discipline of biology); strategies for interventions into the collective existence of whole populations or subgroups in the name of health and life; and, the modes of subjectification by which individuals work upon themselves in relation to the above. The precise nature of these elements may, however, vary over time" (Raman/Tutton 2010: 717 citing Rabinow/Rose 2007).

As I have pointed out (when, for example, discussing pregnant trans* men), South African trans* citizens have access to numerous discourses. This applies not only to global discourses disseminated through the internet, supranational citizenship and medical tourism but also to the inconsistent discourse between the South African legal system and the Department of Home Affairs. Despite a progressive legal background, the silent background norm of a sex/gender binary carries on in administration. Bodies and genders outside the binary of male and female are not accommodated for by the Department of Home Affairs even though they are protected by law. There are different South African truth discourses available such as the following examples: Department of Home Affairs: sex defined as something inherently physical that does require the absence of reproductive organs for trans* citizens; Legislature: a binary sex order that rests on gender identity and acknowledges intersexuality as an exceptional sex; and trans* sub-cultures: sex as something fluent.

However trans* citizens are not solely passive subjects of governmental legislative, executive and judicial organs as well as public health care interventions, but rather active agents in the (re)shaping of their identities through their appropriation of sexing/gendering technologies. One has to keep in mind that they are neither fully subjected nor can they freely choose from expanding opportunities for self-development. According to Burr, identity is "constructed out of discourses culturally available to us and being achieved by a subtle interweaving of many different threads" (Burr 1995: 51). The interaction and intersectionality[16] of various socially and culturally constructed categories leads to very different levels of (in)equality in society and produces huge differences in access to knowledge, medical assistance and legal help.

Furthermore, there exist different modes of subjectification and resistance by which individuals work upon themselves. The existence of different discourses opens up a space that allows some to escape the disciplinary measures of a single cohesive regime of truth or a dominant regime of truth, as maintained by the Department of Home Affairs in the case of South Africa. With regard to this some aspects of (unruly) trans* citizens' local and global agency within the realms of supranational citizenship, citizen science and medical tourism have been explored. I have shown how trans* citizens (try to) protect their right to procreation (threatening the Department of Home Affairs with court cases and getting vague reports from sympathetic surgeons) and their human right to self-identification (accessing technologies through supranational citizenship, medical tourism and citizen science).

On the other hand I have also demonstrated that

> "Contemporary governmentality [...] operates in the 'contact between the technologies of domination of others and those of the self' (Foucault, 1988: 19), where individuals govern themselves as well as being governed by others" (Oster/Cheek 2008: 216).

---

16 | The term intersectionality was introduced by Kimberlé Crenshaw (1989) to point out the ways in which different social partitions are enmeshed.

Therefore these technologies of the self cannot be read exclusively as forms of resistance. This is demonstrated, for example, by some of the unfavourable comments made by trans* people on the pregnancy of Thomas Beatie. The remarks illustrate how the commentators turn themselves into subjects (having internalized external authority) and police their selves in society. Besides the internalization of the values of the more conservative parts of South African society, they also took on the standards of the American Psychiatric Association (APA) as a further external authority. The APA's view of trans* people was considered as especially significant at the time, as it is working on its fifth edition of the Diagnostic and Statistical Manual of Mental Disorders that will include a new definition of "gender incongruence". To be publicly regarded as 'normal' (men/male identified people do not become pregnant according to the hegemonic binary gender script) was for many trans* commentators of great importance as the APA discussed whether the new definition should entail a reference that "gender incongruency" is not a mental disorder. This kind of anticipatory obedience is part of governmentality; it should not be forgotten that governmentality cannot solely be understood as the organized practices through which subjects are governed but also as the ways in which governments try to produce citizens best suited to fulfil their policies. Legal and administrative procedures regulate and simultaneously create identities.

In contrast to Weber, who conceived power as the ability to realize one's will against the resistance of somebody else, Foucault has made every endeavour to clarify that power is held by no one, but is inherent in all relations (Foucault 2003: 168). Thus, the answer to the question of who holds the power over a citizen's body or gender identity is not a question of dominance, but one of relations, as I have shown above.

Politics again

Biomedical Hype and Hopes: AIDS Medicines for Africa

Anita Hardon

Health activism is ascendant around the world and its specific instances have attracted much scholarly attention.[1] This interest comes at a time of transition for health care more generally: from a classical public health model where governments are expected to oversee public well-being, to a neo-liberal model where patients are expected to be informed, self-mobilizing biological citizens (Petersen/Lupton 1996). Health activism feeds into—and is reinforced by—a new mode of governance, what Rose and Novas (2007:442) have termed the "political economy of hope". By this, Rose and Novas are referring to how life itself has become wedded to the generation of wealth, involving alliances between medical practitioners, patients hoping for effective treatments, and pharmaceutical and biotech firms seeking greater profits and shareholder value.

This chapter focuses on transnational activism to make AIDS medicines widely available in Sub-Saharan Africa. It describes the origins of the AIDS treatment movement, the concerns of its activists, the kinds of subjectivities and frictions the movement reflected and created, and its material effects on health systems in Africa. More specifically, I focus on the hype and hopes that accompanied this transnational activism, showing how these contributed to the transformation of AIDS care, first in the US and then in Africa.[2] Only ten

1 | Health activism incorporates proactive and reactive contests over biomedical technologies, recognition of health problems and the restructuring of healthcare. Most case studies on health activism over the past decade have focused on Europe and the US and have not looked beyond national boundaries. See Epstein (2008) for a good overview of health movements.

2 | I have been inspired by Nguyen's 2004 study on AIDS activism in Ouagadougou and Robins' 2004 study on the South African Treatment Action Campaign. See also Beckmann and Bujra (2011) for a critical analysis of the political economy of treatment activism in Tanzania.

years ago, most people diagnosed with HIV in Sub-Saharan Africa faced a death sentence; now they can have access to life-long anti-retroviral treatment.

In the early days of the epidemic when treatment was unavailable, AIDS activists formed support groups for people infected or affected by HIV. They advocated disclosing one's status to promote a positive self-image and to fight stigmatization and discrimination (Epstein 1996). American and European activists in the 1980s and 90s shaped a social movement based on shared interests and identity, experiences and solidarity (Melucci 1989; Taylor/Whittier 1992; Johnston/Larana/Gusfield 1994). The movement also spawned its own social practices. But what happened when these activist care arrangements and ideas—along with antiretroviral drugs—were transplanted from North America and Western Europe to East and South Africa? Were they adopted by those infected and affected by HIV? Did they help to de-stigmatize the illness?

Recent ethnographies in Sub-Saharan Africa have pointed to the power relationships in health facilities where AIDS medicines are made available. Patients face rigid procedures that determine access to the drugs as well as strict treatment adherence regimes. Patients' lifestyles are morally reframed with the aim of producing *docile bodies*, thereby submitting them to biomedical– and ultimately, state–authority (Ssewaya 2010; Mfecane 2010; Mattes 2011). Docile bodies are necessary to ensure treatment adherence; if the medicines are not used properly, the virus becomes resistant, threatening the life-saving efficacy of the drugs. How did the social practices that accompanied AIDS medicines to African settings intersect with the biopower[3] evident in the disciplining of its users?

Through genealogical excavation, I describe how AIDS treatment activism emerged in the USA and spread around the world, involving numerous groups with varying agendas that changed over time.[4]American activists in the early 1990s were able to influence research leading to the development of life-

3 | Foucault (1978) introduces a bipolar diagram of biopower in his analysis of the modern European state's growing preoccupation with control over vital forces of its population. One pole focuses on the management of individual bodies; the second is that of regulatory control, i.e. biopolitics of the population. In AIDS care programs, global health donors and African states introduce new care modalities that aim to both discipline HIV-positive individuals and to regulate the body politic to prevent further transmission. In this article, the emphasis is on the power asserted over individuals within African health care systems (see also Nguyen 2010 for an analysis of the way in which biopower is asserted in AIDS care in Cote D'Ivoire).

4 | Few scholars have studied transnational activism. Keck and Sikkink (1998) and Khagram and colleagues (2002) are exceptions who, as political scientists, have focused on how transnational activist groups develop shared beliefs and seek to transform these into norms accepted by governments and international agencies.

saving anti-retroviral treatment (ART). They subsequently catalysed political commitment among world leaders, enabling the large-scale initiatives to improve access to AIDS medicines in Africa that we know today.

Following the journey of AIDS activism across time and space is easier said than done. I did so by working with a team of PhD students conducting fieldwork in various local settings in East and South Africa (Kyakuwa 2010; Ssewaya 2010; Mfecane 2010) and by collaborating with activists in research aimed at improving access to AIDS medicines. This chapter presents insights from these various endeavours, including a policy analysis conducted for the World Health Organization (Hardon et al. 2007), a rapid assessment I directed for Health Action International (Hardon/Daniels 2006), and a collaborative project with the East African Treatment Access Movement/International Treatment Preparedness Coalition (ITPC). Through the years, I participated in the meetings of the International AIDS Society, and organized in January 2009 an 'expert' meeting to document the history of AIDS activism and to explore the connections and disconnections between activist priorities and repertoires in East Africa, Europe and the USA.[5] I also negotiated funding for one of the leading activists of Médecins Sans Frontières'Access Campaign to document its recent history ('t Hoen 2009).

EARLY TREATMENT ACTIVISM

The AIDS treatment movement began within the American gay community in the mid-1980s. At the time, support groups exchanged scarce information and experimented with different treatments. In the words of David Barr:[6]

"There was nothing that we could use from government at that time. AIDS treatment information flowed from patient to patient. There were rumours about cures in Paris and Israel. There was a drug called AL721, an egg-based lecithin product. You could make it in a bathtub. We produced and distributed it, but then it didn't work. Some of the support-groups bought drugs, and sold them to people who needed them. We made newsletters, which provided treatment information. Patients brought these newsletters to their doctors. One of the groups made a directory of clinical trials and it was updated all the time. Clinical trials were the only way to access potentially life-saving drugs.

---

5 | This meeting was reported in the documentary: *Living Positively: A Conversation with East African HIV/AIDS Activists*. CRAMARK Productions, directed by Mark Crama and Eileen Moyer (2009).

6 | Barr, a pioneer within the AIDS treatment movement, gave a presentation at the expert meeting in January 2009.

As more experimental treatment became available, the community networks became the source of information. The patients became the experts. We had to care and support people who were sick. We started conducting weekly treatment literacy workshops to educate each other on the rapidly changing treatment options. We discussed side-effects of treatment and were concerned with resistance." (Expert Meeting, January 2009, Amsterdam)

Epstein (1995) suggests that treatment activists at the time were caught in a "hype cycle" where the urgency of the AIDS crisis meant that both researchers and people infected with HIV tended to invest preliminary results with more significance than they warranted. Activists not only distributed information on clinical trials, but were involved in their design. AZT was the first drug that was proven effective in a clinical trial and activists immediately recommended it to all HIV-positive people, though longer-term follow-up studies showed its efficacy could not be sustained.

Pharmaceutical companies then suggested the dual therapy of AZT with ddC. Many activists, however, raised concerns about its longer-term efficacy; they also mistrusted the researchers conducting the trials. The debate over whether the AZT/ddC dual therapy actually 'worked' went hand in hand with dispute over how efficacy should be established. Rather than requiring proof of efficacy through what activists termed 'body counts'—higher numbers of deaths in the placebo group—activists pressed for quicker and more humane methods. They argued that short-term increases in CD4[7] counts could serve as surrogate markers for decreased mortality, thus reducing the time needed for clinical trials (Epstein 1996).

Treatment activists won this battle: they were able to exert significant influence on the development trajectories of new pharmaceutical substances. Drug companies and clinical researchers had to compromise on study design and means to evaluate clinical outcomes; they needed AIDS patients to pursue their work.

The annual (and later biannual) meetings of the International AIDS Society became venues for activists to discuss their concerns with scientists. This did not come without a struggle, as the following report on the New York ACT UP website suggests:

"In 1989, ACT UP and its Canadian counterparts, AIDS Action Now! and Réaction-SIDA, stormed the Fifth International AIDS Conference in Montreal. Up until that June day, the conference was a members-only event for the AIDS establishment, a chance

7 | The CD4 count is a lab test for the number of CD4 cells (also called T helper cells) per cubic millimetre of blood. Because HIV infects and destroys T cells, its progression is typically marked by a decline in the CD4 count.

for scientists to hobnob with their fellow wizards while dispensing wisdom and press releases to beleaguered doctors and a fawning press. PWAs were presented mainly as abstractions, their lives reduced to statistics on spread sheets, their needs and desires mere sidelights to the noble pursuit of science. Of course, if they wished to make their presence more concrete, they were welcome to do so, for a $500 registration fee.

And then came Montreal. I'll never forget the sight of our ragtag group of 300protesters brushing past the security guards in the lobby of the Palais de Congress, the fleet of 'Silence=Death' posters gliding up the escalator to the opening ceremony or our chants thundering throughout the cavernous hall. There we were, the uninvited guests, taking our rightful place at the heart of the conference. And when PWA Tim McCaskell grabbed the microphone and 'officially' opened the conference 'on behalf of people with AIDS from Canada and around the world,' even the scientists stood and cheered. We were there to hold science itself accountable to PWAs–to demand, in the words of ACT UP's 'National AIDS Treatment Research Agenda,' that 'people with AIDS and their advocates participate in designing and executing drug trials,' and that research be driven by people's needs and not just by the interests of drug companies. This meant broadening research priorities to include treatments for the opportunistic infections that actually killed PWAs, and ensuring that the full range of people with HIV be enrolled in the studies. The drug trials themselves needed to be designed for the real world–'prophylaxis permitted, placebos avoided, efficacy criteria and end points humane'–and people intolerant of standard therapies and/or ineligible for on-going clinical studies still had to be given access to these experimental treatments." (ACT UP New York website, accessed 2009)

Since the 1989 meeting in Montreal, AIDS treatment activists have attended International AIDS Society conferences in ever larger numbers. They often take the floor during scientific sessions and meet in separate 'global villages' to share their experiences and to plan joint actions. Activists, for instance, have been championing the principle of Greater Involvement of People Living with HIV and AIDS (GIPA) since 1983—for their *right* to participate as equal partners in response to the epidemic. While their calls elicited little response from governments for a decade (GNP+ 2000), 42 countries at the Paris AIDS Summit in 1994 agreed that GIPA was crucial for responses to HIV/AIDS to be effective and ethical (UNAIDS 1999). In a review of GIPA practices, UNAIDS (1999: 4) suggested that "greater involvement" meant many things, from sitting on the boards of international funding agencies to involvement in national-level programs and policy-making, to membership in community-based organizations engaged in prevention and care. Activists stress that GIPA is not only a right, but an *organizing principle* from which "we can shape our involvement as networks and groups connected at the national and international levels". More fundamentally, it is "a necessary reminder of the importance of taking active control of our lives and our health" (Morolake/Stephens/Welbourne 2009: 2).[8]

Post-HAART access activism

Highly active antiretroviral treatment (HAART), involving a combination of three anti-retroviral drugs, finally became available in 1996. In the meantime, the concerns of AIDS activists had changed. In the absence of life-saving drugs, HIV-positive individuals had relied on self-care and mutual care; they now increasingly adopted a clinical gaze, with CD4 counts and viral loads as the key markers of health. AIDS activists jointly constructed the clinical routines to which they voluntarily gave up their bodies. In the field of AIDS activism, the hegemony of biomedicine was achieved through consent.

Once they had gained some stability in their own lives, treatment activists turned their attention to the global inequities in accessing the new life-saving drugs. New York-based activist Evan Ruderman:[9]

"As I began to recover, and I felt I had time and a life, and I am actually not spending every moment of my day in this complete survival kind of thing, like how I am going to wake up, walk across the room...I really began to see, pay attention to the fact that the majority of the people outside in the world didn't have what I had. It is amazing that I survived and yet I have the best health care in the world. I really saw the disparity of, even in this country, the access that I have, and the access that this married woman, in her late fifties, in the middle of Nebraska, who has just been diagnosed has, where she has to drive 60 miles to the nearest clinic to find a doctor that has never treated a patient with HIV. And then I met Shatinka who was HIV-positive and coming out, and told me what was going on in Africa. And I was stunned... It didn't have any meaning for me as an individual to be alive and to continue to have such privileges if there was a whole world out there that didn't have access. That was something so unfair to me that in my heart I couldn't really live with it."

In the late 1990, AIDS medicines were unaffordable for the poor in Africa and Asia. Though development donors were willing to invest in prevention and

8 | This definition of GIPA echoes the 1978 declaration on primary healthcare adopted by the WHO in Alma-Ata, which encouraged community participation at every stage from needs assessment to implementation. Like GIPA, the Alma-Ata Declaration defined community participation not only as a right, but as a process whereby individuals come to view health as a responsibility.

9 | The quote is from the documentary film directed by Anne-Christine d'Adesky, *Pills, Profits, Protest: Chronicle of the AIDS Movement*.

palliative care, they were unwilling to invest in antiretroviral drugs (ARVs). American and European AIDS activists therefore sent limited supplies of ARVs to their counterparts in Africa through solidarity networks. But as described by Nguyen's seminal study on biopolitics and therapeutic citizenship in Ouagadougou (2004), only a tiny fraction of people living with HIV in Africa could gain access to ARVs by positioning themselves as model activists—living positively, attending discussion groups, and caring for others through humanitarian networks and AIDS activist organizations. The majority in Africa did not even know ARVs existed.

By the end of the 1990s, AIDS treatment activists were part of a vocal and global social movement, including militant groups such as ACT UP with branches in Paris, New York and Chicago, the South African Treatment Action Campaign, and similar groups in Thailand, Brazil and elsewhere. They blamed pharmaceutical companies for lack of access to life-saving AIDS medicines, as seen in the cartoon below by the well-known South African graphic artist Zapiro.

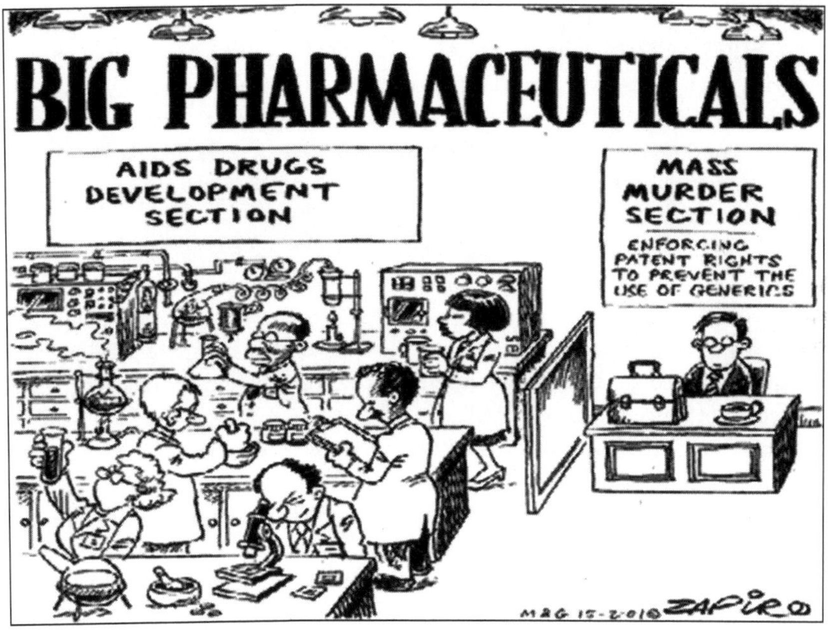
BIG PHARMACEUTICALS
AIDS DRUGS DEVELOPMENT SECTION
MASS MURDER SECTION
ENFORCING PATENT RIGHTS TO PREVENT THE USE OF GENERICS
M&G 15-2-2010 ZAPIRO

The internet facilitated communication between activist groups while the biannual International AIDS Society meetings provided a venue for face-to-face meetings. Militant activists formed alliances with health and development organizations involved in AIDS care, such as the Geneva-based Médecins Sans Frontières (MSF) and Partners In Health at Harvard University ('t Hoen 2009). They framed the issue of access to antiretroviral drugs as follows (Hardon 2006):

- access to ARVs is a human right;
- greater access will increase uptake of HIV testing, thereby helping to prevent transmission;
- greater access to treatment will diminish the stigma and discrimination surrounding HIV/AIDS.

Public health experts, however, were not immediately convinced. In early 2000, their counter-arguments were as follows (Hardon 2006):

- underdeveloped health systems may not be able to provide the quality of care needed for effective ARV use;
- poor adherence to treatment may lead to rapid increases in drug resistance;
- providing ARVS may be less cost-effectiveness than prevention programs (Creese et al. 2002) and will divert resources from other health priorities.

The appeals to human rights prevailed. Transnational activism played a key role in this, contributing to a series of interventions that cumulatively led to a dramatic change in the global AIDS landscape. Before HAART, northern activists had focused on mutual support and experimental treatments; after HAART, the movement switched its focus to universal access. Northern activists now worked together with their counterparts in Thailand, Brazil and South Africa, where national battles for access to AIDS medicines were raging ('t Hoen 2009).

In Brazil, activism led to legislation ensuring universal access to AIDS medicines. The Brazilian ART program saved the government money it would otherwise have spent on care for AIDS patients (Biehl 2007). The Thai government followed the Brazilian example with its national AIDS care program, linked to a universal access insurance scheme. Significantly, both countries produced their own ARVs.

In Africa, national networks of people living with HIV/AIDS confronted governments with demands for universal access to AIDS medicines. The South African TAC was perhaps the most vocal; its charismatic leader Zachie Achmat drew global media coverage by denying himself treatment so long as the medicines were unavailable to his countrymen. The Ugandan AIDS Service Organization (TASO) also played a key role; it was set up by Noerine Kaleeba and modelled on the support structures she witnessed among people living with HIV in the UK, where her husband was diagnosed with AIDS in the early 1980s. TASO provided counselling and social support; once AIDS medicines became available, it also trained 'expert clients' to introduce antiretroviral treatment in Uganda (Grebe 2009). TASO became a model for ART provision in Africa.

Activist doctors in Médecins Sans Frontières' (MSF) Access Campaign worked together with TAC and TASO to begin AIDS treatment trials in

Africa. Contrary to what public health sceptics had feared, their early results indicated that treatment with—and adherence to—ARV regimes was possible in settings with underdeveloped health systems (Kasper et al. 2003). Adherence strategies, developed by MSF to avoid drug resistance, were the key to success. The strategies included pre-treatment triage to define 'good patients', intensive adherence counselling, support groups and treatment buddies whose task is to help patients adhere to the treatment regimes. These adherence instruments were later copied throughout Sub-Saharan Africa as necessary elements of successful AIDS treatment programs. The findings of a trial in a poor township near Cape Town were impressive, and were presented at the 1998 Global AIDS Conference in Barcelona. The MSF doctors reported:

"To date, 180 patients have been placed on this therapy, selected from among the 3,000 patients who have attended the MSF clinics in Khayelitsha. These patients were extremely sick when they began therapy... However, on antiretroviral therapy, their survival was impressive. After nine months of treatment, 88% of the patients were alive. These encouraging results occurred with very few serious adverse events." (Kasper et al. 2003)

MSF identified community involvement as critical for success at three levels:

"(1) At the political level, when politicians have questioned the validity of using antiretroviral therapy in resource poor settings, it was the patients who responded, writing letters to newspapers and speaking out in the media; (2) At the community level, they play an important role in the support groups run for patients on antiretroviral therapy, with those who have been on therapy for longer periods of time helping mentor those beginning; and (3) at the individual level patients have educated themselves on the importance of adherence, allowing them to take responsibility for their own therapy, making it unnecessary to use medical staff to observe them taking their pills." (Ibid.)

MSF also negotiated a reduction in the price of AIDS medicines. Early in 2000, the Indian generic drugs manufacturer CIPLA offered to provide MSF with ARVs for 10% of the cost of the patented medicines, reducing the cost of HAART to US$ 350 per person per year.

In the meantime, major international for a including the UN Security Council were discussing the political risks of the AIDS epidemic in Africa. Leaders compared the effects of AIDS, especially for political stability, to the effects of war. Secretary General Kofi Annan stated at the January 2000 meeting of the Security Council:

"By overwhelming the continent's health and social services, by creating millions of orphans, and by decimating health workers and teachers, AIDS is causing social and economic crises which in turn threaten political stability [...]. In already unstable societies, this cocktail of disasters is a sure recipe for more conflict." (UNAIDS 2000)

UNAIDS Executive Director Peter Piot stated at the same meeting:

"Visibly, the epidemic is eroding the social fabric of communities... in its demographic, social and economic impact, the epidemic has become more devastating than war, in a continent where war and conflict appear to be endemic." (UNAIDS 2000)

Appearing before the UN Security Council, World Bank President James D. Wolfensohn called for a "War on AIDS". Stating that AIDS was contributing to instability in societies and creating fertile ground for both internal and cross-border conflicts, he emphasized the need for greater international support for prevention and also suggested that every war needs a war chest (UNAIDS 2000).

Proof that ART could work in Africa, the reduction in the price of AIDS medicines, high-profile demands for universal access, and the UN's concerns about security in Africa– all paved the way for global action. 2001 witnessed the birth of the Global Fund to Fight AIDS, Tuberculosis and Malaria, following Kofi Annan's proposal for a global 'war chest' to fight these three major diseases of poverty. Annan called on donors to provide an annual minimum of US$ 10 billion; US President George Bush responded with the President's Emergency Fund for AIDS Relief (PEPFAR). In 2003, the World Health Organization launched its "3 by 5" initiative: 3 million people under treatment by 2005. Serving as director of the WHO AIDS program when these targets were set, Jim Kim had worked alongside activist doctors, including Paul Farmer, through Partners In Health.

Multi-layered AIDS treatment activism, the bold experiments of the Brazilian and Thai governments, and UN action made unprecedented resources available for the world's poor. The ARV landscape in Africa changed dramatically. Up until around 2003, only a lucky few could access ARVs; with limited reserves of the costly drugs, health professionals, policy-makers and families had to decide who deserved treatment (for Uganda, see Whyte et al. 2006). One researcher in Zambia estimated that 40 to 50% of adult hospital bed-days were used for HIV/AIDS patients; for every terminally ill patient in hospital, there were probably 10 to 20 people living in the community suffering the symptoms of early HIV-related ailments and turning to help from first-line health services (Foster 1994).

The magnitude of the illness and death caused by HIV/AIDS was overwhelming for both nuclear and extended family systems. Ntozi/Zirimenya (1999) had observed dramatic changes in Uganda's household composition, with mortality rates among 15 to 64 year olds leading to surging, dependent, younger and older populations (WHO/UNAIDS2008). Families and communities alike framed HIV/AIDS in moral terms (Whyte 1997; Dilger 2005; Hardon/Dilger

2011). Individual cases of illness were often ascribed to witchcraft (Yamba 1997; Ashforth 2002) or the violation of taboos (Mogensen 1995; Wolf 2001; Dilger 2008; Prince/Geissler 2010).

Aiming to meet the WHO's goals—and now enjoying greater access to global resources—governments in East Africa were among the continent's first to make ambitious plans to scale up treatment. The WHO's "3 by 5"program aimed to deliver ARV treatment to 110.000 persons (based on 50% of estimated need) in Kenya, 130.000 persons in Tanzania, and 55.000 afflicted individuals in Uganda (WHO 2006). The Ministries of Health in these countries set out to accredit AIDS care centres, enabling them to provide ART to populations in need.

Funds to scale up antiretroviral therapy in Africa came from the Global Fund and PEPFAR. The former provided funds to African state institutions; the latter channelled funds through various non-state 'prime' partners, many of them based in the US. The 2005 PEPFAR plan aimed to treat two million people with ART by 2008 (60.000 people in Uganda; 150.000 in Tanzania; and 250.000 in Kenya). Unlike most previous efforts in Africa, the targets this time were met: 92% for Kenya; 96% for Tanzania; and 241% for Uganda (PEPFAR 2009). In the meantime, the WHO had shifted to reporting estimated coverage (the percentage of people in need with access to ART). As of December 2007, the estimated coverage for Kenya was 38%, for Tanzania 31%, and for Uganda 46% (WHO/UNAIDS 2008).

ART programs had become islands of abundance within public health facilities hit hard by reforms (Sullivan 2011). They offered frontline health workers the magic bullets to do what they were trained to do: treat people in need. AIDS medicines provided the promise of life to East African populations which had come to equate HIV infection with death—both socially and physically.

MAKING IT HAPPEN

Once resources for AIDS treatment had been committed, activists turned to prepare communities for treatment. In 2003, a number of New York pioneers, together with their partners in Europe, South Africa and elsewhere, established the International Treatment Preparedness Coalition (ITPC). Its first meeting was held in 2003 in Cape Town. Founder Greg Gonzales:

"ITPC is a network of hundreds of people. But they are tied together as a sort of global coalition. A lot of early AIDS activism was about identity politics. Now it's broader, not just about being an HIV-positive person. It's about health care and human rights. We conduct treatment literacy, but the big issue is for national groups to get their governments to do the right thing. Treatment literacy is incredibly labour and resource intensive. We're still not reaching the far grassroots. We still only have 30% treatment coverage, but it's much more than just getting pills into bodies." (Expert Meeting, January 2009, Amsterdam)

Linda, one of the activists I met in Cape Town, introduced me to how the Treatment Action Campaign (TAC) combines local awareness-raising with national advocacy for treatment access:

"If you understand how your body works, you will understand that you need to finish the treatment, what you need to do when you have side-effects. We also use our educational sessions to empower women. When women are empowered to understand treatment they are able to say what kind of side-effects they have and negotiate better with doctors. We wear t-shirts [that say] 'I am positive—how are you?' to start discussions, and we use our treatment literacy talks to talk about what our government should do, and what the G8 has promised. We have set new targets for our government: 500,000 should be on treatment in South Africa, there are now 700,000 that are in need. So we are pushing them to keep their promise." (Fieldwork, July 2008, Cape Town)

Annett from Kamuli Young Positive, a member organization of ITPC, spoke at our workshop on treatment literacy:

"It's important for young people to have their own organizations, because young people feel more confident talking to their peers than to old people. We have different problems and we need to bring them up. Young people who are positive like dating, but health workers and people in the community consider this wrong, as it could lead to falling in love and wanting to have babies. We educate health workers about the sexual and reproductive rights of young people and we provide counselling and prevention of mother to child transmission advice for young people. You see, young people who have been tested HIV-positive want to have a life." (Expert Meeting, January 2009, Amsterdam)

ITPC member organizations typically combine peer-support and educational activities with advocacy aimed at governments and other healthcare providers. These groups have ensured that, alongside ARVs, ideas regarding empowered patients and rights to healthcare have entered local healthcare institutions in Sub-Saharan Africa. While these ideas were previously present in the empowerment and HIV prevention activities of community-based organizations, they were new to the domain of biomedical health.

In 2005, the ITPC report *Missing the Target* and an assessment I conducted with Health Action International (Hardon/Daniels 2006) pointed to major problems in the global scale-up of HIV treatment. The WHO goal of providing ART to 3 million people by 2005 had not been achieved. By the end of 2005, an estimated 1.3 million people in low and middle-income countries had access to

ART, or only about one in seven of those thought to be in need in Africa (WHO 2006). There were significant shortfalls in contributions to the Global Fund to Fight AIDS, Tuberculosis and Malaria, reducing its capacity to finance national programs. Locally, numerous obstacles stood in the way of patients seeking access to free ART, including transportation costs and user fees as well as lack of social support and support for treatment adherence.[10]

These surveys revealed how health systems in Africa were experiencing difficulties delivering the goods on the ground, and that costs unrelated to the medicines themselves were acting as barriers to treatment. We were furthermore concerned that these barriers would undermine adherence and that resistance to drugs would therefore likely emerge sooner rather than later (ITPC 2005; Hardon/Daniels 2006).

DOCILE BODIES?

In 2006, four PhD researchers began their fieldwork in health facilities in South Africa and Uganda. Their aim was to follow AIDS medicines to the local settings where access was then being achieved in the context of ambitious ART treatment scale-up programs. Their field notes describe how social practices (i.e treatment buddies, support groups and adherence counselling) developed by activist organizations such as TAC, MSF, and ITPC to help patient adhere to the life-saving drugs, became rigid disciplining tools when introduced on a nation-wide scale in African health systems.

Achilles Ssewaya (2010) studied adherence in two peri-urban health facilities in Uganda: a state-run district hospital and a well-known mission program. Clients in the two facilities were obliged to enrol in ART education classes with their treatment buddies to receive their prescriptions. Once ART was prescribed, clients received follow-up counselling involving a monthly pill-count to check adherence. If clients were found to be failing, they received further counselling, and if they continued to fail they risked being excluded from the treatment program.

Ssewaya's vignettes describe an educational session in the mission health facility (the state facility conducts similar sessions):

"At Mbuya Reach Out Headquarter, the counselling venue was surrounded by a toilet structure in the rear, an open compound to the left, and a main road across the hedge to the right. The counsellor had to shout at the top of his voice to outdo the background

10 | ITPC (2005): Missing the Target: A Report on HIV/AIDS Treatment Access from the Frontlines; ITPC (2006): Off-Target for 2010: How to Avoid Breaking the Promise of Universal Access.

noise from the high-pressured water tap near the toilet, whizzing toilet doors, climbing vehicles and indistinct noise from the crowd in the open compound. Each client had a plastic chair. In principle, one's treatment buddy is supposed to attend at least one of the three repeated ART education sessions in order to acquaint oneself with the adherence standards and responsibility. The client composition is heterogeneous, comprising men and women, but women form the majority. A female co-facilitator starts pinning up the pictorial visual aid at 9:35 am; thereafter, an expert patient walks into the open venue and introduces himself as the co-facilitator. The session follows a question and answer approach; the expert patient, in his role as counsellor, answers the questions himself.

[...] I should begin by emphasizing the importance of coming with a treatment partner. If you have not come with your treatment supporter today, I will allow you to attend this time, but make sure you come with one next time. If you have a question [during the session], please feel free to ask.
Before I talk about ARVs, we should start by talking about HIV/AIDS itself. True, I am here to teach you about the new medicine, but first of all you will need to know the reasons for taking the medication. Why are you here today? We are sick and craving to live longer. What health problem brings you here today? HIV/AIDS. What is the difference between HIV and AIDS? HIV is the weevil (Kawuka); while AIDS is a condition in the form of multiple diseases.
[He continues] With AIDS, the symptoms are obvious, but avoid pointing a finger unless tests have been done.

What is positive living?
[...] Avoid sex, feed well and take your medicines. You should avoid the habit of eating red meat, thinking that you are eating a balanced diet. Eat food that is readily available. Avoid sexual behaviour that can lead to re-infection.
We are here in order to know the amount of blood soldiers we have in our body, and to seek medicine. [He introduces the illustration and starts explaining the biology of the virus.] Mr. White Blood Cell [WBCs] is armed with a gun, the CD4 fights the enemy. When the number of body soldiers goes down, the body becomes exposed to any kind of infection—for instance, flu—that infection becomes persistent. The ARVs restore the number of body soldiers. The WBC—or for our purpose, the CD4, which we shall refer to as 'body soldiers', which defend our bodies- are restored. When the number of 'body soldiers' substantially decreases, the enemy wins the battle. The medicines you will take will restore the CD4 cells.

What are ARVs?
ARVs are powerful medications that fight the virus and can improve your health. ARVs stop the virus from making more copies of itself. They help the body army to fight the invading enemy thus prolonging our lives.

Do the ARVs cure HIV/AIDS?

[The rain disrupts the session.] You should know this, ARVs do not cure HIV, they only put an enemy to sleep. If you take the ARVs you can still infect other people, especially if you have unprotected sex. The new person [re-infection] awakens the virus. [He displays another illustration of the ARVs and the 'sleeping' virus.] The moment you stop taking ARVs, the virus will wake up. If it wakes up, it will be more ferocious than ever before.

How should we take ARVs?

ARVs should be taken as the doctor tells you. If you miss a dose or share your ARVs, the medicine will not work. You cannot economize ARVs by taking half a dose—that is wrong. Always take a full dose.

How long should I take the ARVs?

ARVs do not cure HIV/AIDS. They must be taken for life. ARVs do not work when taken for only 2 weeks or 1 month. Do not start ARVs unless you have enough money [for transport] to continue [with medication].

How do ARVs work?

[The counsellor displays another illustration of the cell structure.] The virus leaves its coat at the entrance and escapes through the first gate (cell membrane) up to the second gate. It further slips into the second gate, reaching the inner training ground (nucleus). It takes control of the 'soldiers'. The virus disorients the command chain and it asks the soldiers to produce many copies of the virus. It eventually ruptures the shell, releasing numerous enemies. It is at this stage that your body becomes weaker and weaker. Because your body soldiers have been either killed or disoriented, the body becomes exposed to all sorts of attacks. It takes three stones to cook a pot. It takes three medicines to fight the HIV. When you try to boil a pot on two stones, it will certainly topple its contents and you will end up starving that day. One of the drug components intercepts the enemy at the quarter guard. The second medication neutralizes the virus that must have slipped through the quarter guard. The third drug neutralizes the enemy who is already deep inside, thus stopping the enemy's reproductive activities. If you take your medications properly and consistently, it will certainly restore the ability of your body to fight the invading enemy, and eventually become productive. If you stopped taking ARVs for a while, it is as though you are locking up a dog and starving it for three days. If it broke free, it would bite any object standing in its way. It is the same with starving the virus of medications.

Are ARVs really strong?

They [ARVs] cause side-effects and, at the same time, are difficult to take. Fortunately, when your body is extremely down, ARVs will help you gain more years. If you happen to develop side-effects, do not lay back or stop taking ARVs. You should tell the CATTS [Community AIDS and TB Treatment Supporter] as well as report to the clinic immediately.

Is it OK if I have one Nile Special [brand of strong beer]?
ARVs and alcohol do not go together. If alcohol is a problem, I implore you to discuss such a problem with us so that we can help you. It hurts if you take alcohol. Lastly, drink a lot of water so that ARVs circulate well in your body. Drink, but not alcohol. Feed well on the available food. Mukene [small high-protein fish] is good for your body. Do not fry food. You do not need a sack of money to eat well. Avoid [sexually] reckless behaviour. But also kneel down and thank God that he has given you this opportunity of accessing the drugs for life.

Note how, in the course of the sessions, those planning to start treatment are given an immunological lecture on how treatment works and are told they need to adjust their lifestyles, including eating and sexual patterns. Note that an 'expert patient' is relaying these messages—one who has adopted the hegemonic biomedical discourse and is educating his fellow patients on how to live. Whereas AIDS activists like David Barr in New York and Linda in Cape Town had voluntarily submitted their bodies to a medical gaze to self-monitor their health, medical professionals and expert patients in the Ugandan health centres observed by Ssewaya gave their clients scant opportunity to share their own views and experiences, or to exercise control over their own lives. Medical prescriptions on when and how to take the drugs were merged with social prescriptions on how to live one's life.

Mattes (2011) observed similar disciplining practices in a care and treatment centre in Tanga, a large city on the Swahili coast of Tanzania. The centre, which provides antiretroviral therapy with support from PEPFAR, the Global Fund and other donors, requires patients to follow adherence classes with a treatment buddy to gain access to treatment. The classes resemble those described by Ssewaya, though in Tanga they are given by nurses and are followed by an exam. Mattes (2011) shows how the hospital monitors its patients and punishes non-adherence. But as Foucault argued, power is never absolute; where there is power, there is resistance. Mattes describes how one of his informants resisted the message from nurses that ARVs are the only way to prolong life. Haruna instead wanted to try an herbal concoction. Mattes (2011: 159) reports:

"'Willing to start ARV's: Do I tick it or not? The nurse is almost shouting. 'I ask you not to tick, so I can investigate the other medicine', Haruna replies in a low voice. The atmosphere in the small room is tense […]. After a short discussion, she finally concedes that the treatment is voluntary. She welcomes him back any time to verify the effect of the herbal medicines by means of a CD4 test, and notes 'patient not willing to start ART' on the checklist."

Sakhumzi Mfecane's (2010) ethnographic study in South Africa's Limpopo province reveals the gendered effects of the new social practices: men experience participation in HIV-positive support groups as challenging to their masculinity. Celebrated 'masculine' practices–drinking, smoking, having multiple sexual partners—are criticized by counsellors, expert patients and participants as being irresponsible. Drinking is associated with lax adherence; having multiple partners is seen to increase chances of re-infection. Mfecane (2010: 224-225) reports:

"In one of the support groups that I attended I witnessed an occasion where a man, who said he was still drinking, was treated harshly by other clients. Senzo, whom I was recruiting into the study at the time, said he does not drink regularly or heavily '[...] but there will be this day; this day when I feel like 'No, today I really need it, I can't live without it... Just one'; if I take just one beer, you will see me walking by myself to the pot [...].' His confession was met with a barrage of disapproval from other men who warned him against the dangers of drinking. One of those criticisms came directly from a male facilitator who used a Xhosa phrase 'Isiqhelo siyayoyi's ingqondo (if you do something once, you will do it again, and again)'. Another man added 'The doctor advised me to think of stopping alcohol, and smoking. So he told me if I don't stop I might have problems with my medications [...]. So from that time onwards I decided the best way for myself would be to just stop completely [...]. I advise you to do the same my friend!' Senzo was quiet when such censure was aimed at him, and then he responded by saying, 'No, I will try; I will try.'"

Mfecane shows how such criticism can pressure men to stop drinking, provided they are invested in being seen as 'good patients' by fellow support group members. Those who continue drinking do so in secrecy. The same was true for other 'masculine' practices such as smoking and having multiple sexual partners.

The disciplining actors in Ssewaya and Mfecane's ethnographic vignettes are 'expert patients'—people living with HIV/AIDS who have been empowered through the new social forms that have travelled with AIDS medicines to East and Southern Africa. In training programs, they have been taught how to conduct adherence counselling and provide support to others living with the virus.

Beckman and Bujra (2011) argue that the rapid influx of funding has led to factionalism and infighting within the HIV-positive community in Tanzania: those able to access resources have become facilitators, marshalling the infected for treatment. But in her study in Masaka where expert clients have been trained by the pioneering AIDS care program TASO, Kyakuwa (2009, 2010) presents a very different picture. She shows that frictions occur between nurses who tend to discipline patients and expert clients who side with them. One of the expert patients in her study reports:

> "We tell our personal tales of suffering with the disease and with the drugs to fellow patients to encourage them and to give them hope... We tell of our beginning with ART, of the side-effects we suffered. You know we are not angels. We consider ourselves patients first and experts second." (Kyakuwa 2010)

Kyakuwa (2010) shows how expert patients in this setting collaborated with nurses to develop a herbal cream that patients can use to treat the rashes that they suffer when taking AIDS medicines. In doing so, they go against the medical norm that herbal medicines should not be used alongside ART.

Conclusion

This chapter has traced the role of health activism in bringing antiretroviral treatment to Sub-Saharan Africa. American and European activists in the epidemic's early days forged a collective identity for the movement—by living positively, disclosing their status, caring for each other and informing themselves about experimental treatments. AIDS activists aligned themselves with pharmaceutical companies, and co-produced the biomedical markers that were used to test efficacy of drugs. We have seen how when effective drugs had been developed, activists adopted a medical gaze, in their attempts to live healthy lives with AIDS medicines, using biomedical markers to monitor their health. Nowadays, in North America, Europe and elsewhere, those who can afford treatment and/or are well insured, have access to a wide range of AIDS medicines. Side-effects can be avoided and adherence failures can be overcome.

When in the North, people infected with HIV stayed alive, AIDS activists shifted their attention from identity politics to human rights and the global inequities of access to AIDS medicines. They were remarkably successful in reducing the prices of drugs and in mobilizing resources for AIDS programs in Africa. Activist doctors within Médecins Sans Frontières played a key role in furnishing evidence that ART could work in places with underdeveloped health systems. The stakes at the time were high. Public health critics argued against the widespread distribution of ARVs in Africa, fearing that health systems would be unable to administer the drugs, leading to poor adherence and the emergence of resistances. Following the GIPA principle, MSF recommended a specific form of bio-sociality to reduce these risks: that ART programs be accompanied by peer support and community involvement. In developing this model, MSF not only proved that AIDS drugs could work in under-resources health systems, they also presented a new ethics of care: people living with HIV were expected to engage not only in their own healthcare but that of others.

Whereas the social practices of peer support and community involvement empowered AIDS patients in the US, and were instrumental in the MSF trials that provided 'proof of concept' for ART programs in Africa, they also discipline people's everyday lives. As we saw in the fieldwork conducted in diverse health care settings in Uganda, Tanzania and South Africa, ART comes with what amounts to a new moral code: take your medicines twice a day, eat well, abstain from alcohol, and do not use traditional treatments. This mode of governmentality excludes patients who do not adhere to the medical, social and lifestyle recommendations. To gain and sustain access to treatment, patients in clinics need to present themselves as disciplined therapeutic clients[11], regardless of whether this is really the case in their daily lives. In this they have little choice: they risk losing access to the life-saving medicines.

Where in affluent settings patients can voluntarily consent to the medical regime of ART, in these African settings, ART doctors and nurses define *who* gets access to life-saving drugs and who is excluded. Biopower is not only asserted in the triage conducted in clinical settings, but also in the educational programs where patients are invited to adopt a medical gaze, in the adherence programs that count patient's pills every month and demand that patients adopt treatment buddies to help them adhere to drugs, and in support groups where patients are socialized into being responsible citizens.

Though the ethnographic vignettes suggest that 'expert patients' often work with nurses and doctors to discipline their fellow patients, Kyakuwa (2010) shows that the social forms accompanying the routine provision of antiretroviral therapy in Africa also create potential for change.[12] As ART becomes more accessible, and more and more people find out that they have a life with AIDS, 'expert patients', treatment buddies and others involved in the ART programs may increasingly side not with health professionals but with their fellow patients, demanding for example access for example to second line drugs when resistance to the first line regimens occurs, introducing complementary medicines to treat side-effects, and calling for access to AIDS medicines for those who are excluded. Through the internet and at regional and international AIDS conferences they link up with activists elsewhere confronted with similar issues, thereby increasing their expertise and countervailing power.

In analysing governmentality and biopower in AIDS care the power of pharmaceutical agents should not be overlooked. If AIDS medicines did not cause dramatic improvement in health, people living with HIV and AIDS would not so easily consent to the medical regimes that they entail. However, the power of AIDS medicines is not a given. A recent report in the Lancet reveals that in Uganda, where ART roll-out started early, one out of ten new AIDS patients are now resistant to first line drugs (Hamers et al. 2011). Patients in Sub-Saharan

11 | See Whyte forthcoming.

12 | See also Illife (2006) who argues, the mobilization of people with HIV/AIDS has introduced patient power into medical systems in Africa.

Africa do not have to pay for first line drugs as they are provided through large grants, but the grants do provide for free second line regimes, which are still very expensive. If resistance to the current first-line regimes increases—a likely scenario—the African AIDS treatment hype may soon be over. Interestingly, the agencies and donors involved in the African treatment programs have done little to monitor resistance levels in the ART programs that they fund (they focus on success), perhaps because bad news could dry up the commitments of the private and public sector donors, as well as that of the tax payers in the North.

The Politics and Anti-politics of HIV interventions in Kenya

Ruth J. Prince

Introduction

Following the disputed elections of December 2007, the price of food in Kenya rose steeply, as the ensuing political violence disrupted food production and distribution networks. During 2008, the price of a kilogram of maize flour doubled.[1] At the same time, the Kenyan media reported on several large-scale corruption scandals, involving government officials and politicians with financial links to maize brokers. It was alleged that maize had been sold at discounted prices to brokers, who hoarded it until prices rose. These practices continued in spite of a growing food emergency in the arid north and east of the country.[2] By the beginning of 2009, famine was gripping these regions, with reports of people being forced to eat the roots of plants.

Allegations of government corruption in the face of huge price hikes in the cost of basic foodstuffs produced a lot of anger in a country already battered and disappointed by the post-election violence. Editorials in Kenya's mainstream newspapers as well as the letters and comments sent in by citizens heavily criticized the coalition government, pointed out the gross disjuncture between

1 | This price rise was the subject of numerous newspaper articles. See for example, "Children with AIDS helpless victims of Food Crisis", by Professor Wilfred Mlay, *Daily Nation*, 29 November 2008.

2 | See, for example, articles in the *Daily Nation:* "Maize Scandal: Briefcase Agents Profit" by Bernard Namunane, June 27th 2008, http://www.nation.co.ke/News/-/1056/525430/-/u1vwhs/-/index.html; "MPs Face Arrest Over Maize Scandal", by Fred Mukinda and Bernard Namunane, January 1st 2009, http://www.nation.co.ke/News/-/1056/517864/-/u1bugf/-/index.html; "Government Dissolves Cereals Board" by Oliver Mathenge, 26th January 2009, http://www.nation.co.ke/News/-/1056/519988/-/u1d9x4/-/index.html; and in Afro News: "First Lady Implicated in Maize Scandal", by staff writer February 5th 2009, http://www.afrol.com/articles/32359.

the lives of politicians and those of Kenya's citizens, many of them unemployed, struggling to survive from day to day. In the streets of Kisumu, Kenya's third largest city[3], in local government and NGO offices, among shop-assistants, street sellers, market women, men providing bodaboda (bicycle taxi) services and mothers taking their children to the clinic, the price of food and the maize scandals were constant topics of conversation. Food was a political issue.

During this time, I was conducting ethnographic research on the expansion of large-scale HIV treatment and care programmes in Kisumu.[4] Since 2004, with vast amounts of money provided by PEPFAR and the Global fund, these programmes have offered free antiretroviral treatment (ART) and other medicines to HIV positive people, organized through complex 'partnerships' between the Ministry of Health and various NGOs and international organizations.[5] The aim

---

3 | Kisumu's population is estimated to be half a million; it is the capital of Nyanza Province. (http://www.unhabitat.org/content.asp?cid=2275&catid=206&typeid=6&subMenuId=0).

4 | Research was conducted between October 2008 and May 2009 with additional visits in April 2008, December 2009 and September 2010. Research focused on the interface between HIV/AIDS interventions and people's lives, relations and identities, and with local economies. In a city with over 24 clinics providing HIV tests and antiretrovirals, I focused on two NGO-run and two government PSCs. I conducted over sixty open-ended interviews and numerous conversations with staff members and volunteers associated with the HIV clinics; observed clinic practice; regularly accompanied one of the staff in his 'follow-up' work with patients, and occasionally followed other community health workers and volunteers. I visited eight patient support groups in the city (there were many more), and regularly attended the meetings of two of these groups. I also built up a network of twenty families with HIV-positive members whom I (and later mostly a research assistant, Biddy Odindo) visited at home, and followed in and out of clinics and hospitals. No members of this latter group had formal employment. My competence in Dholuo aided work with these families; I mostly conducted conversations and interviews with more middle-class patients and staff members in English. I am grateful to Dr Eric Nyambedha and the Department of Sociology and Anthropology, University of Maseno for hosting me as a visiting researcher, and to the Provincial and District Medical Officers, the District Commissioner, the staff of the NGOs and government clinics in Kisumu, and the group members, families and individuals who supported my research. Special thanks to Biddy Odindo for her follow-up work with the families.

5 | In 2009, HIV prevalence in Nyanza Province was 13.9 of the population aged 15-45 years (the national average was 6.3%), according to the 2008-9 Kenyan Demographic and Health Survey (UNICEF: http://www.unicef.org/infobycountry/kenya_statistics.html). Since early 2005, the free delivery of ART has been expanded, first in the city and later into rural areas, through government health facilities, private and mission hospitals, NGOs and selected faith-based groups. See http://www.unaids.org/en/CountryResponses/Countries/kenya.asp. By September 2009, almost 300,000 people

of such programmes is to enable positive people to live a 'normal' life through suppressing virus levels and promoting immune defences with daily doses of antiretrovirals, multivitamins and antibiotics.

According to the message of the clinic, surviving HIV requires strict 'adherence' to the medication, orienting one's life around the requirements of the pharmaceutical regime and taking on the messages of 'positive living': responsibility for one's health, awareness of risk, and self-care. Antiretroviral treatment is indeed often experienced as a miracle, enabling and extending life for those who were facing severe illness and death. Yet, as I followed people into the clinics and into their homes, and attended the meetings of the various groups to which they belonged, it became obvious that matters of survival involve much more than sticking to medical regimens, attending one's clinic dates and thinking of one's body as carrying the HIV virus. I found that for many positive people in Kisumu, ART programmes may extend life but they do not necessarily support living. Doing well on antiretrovirals depended as much on finding an income, feeding a family, and paying school fees as on the treatment itself (see Morris 2008; Meinert/Mogensen/Twebaze 2009; Meinert *forthcoming*).

This paper considers the consequences of the increasingly medicalized economy of health care and welfare in Kisumu, where access to medical treatment and to material benefits and means of making a living are organized to a large extent around HIV. It examines the intersections between humanitarian interventions, organized by non-governmental groups and directed at poverty alleviation for those "affected and infected by HIV", with medicalized regimes of care offered by ART programmes, and with the moral economies of family life and urban survival. HIV-positive people and their families are the target of not only medical treatment but also of funding flows and projects offering various forms of material and 'livelihood' support.[6] For many families and individuals struggling to make a living in the city, being HIV positive has, ironically, opened up pathways to scarce material resources. However, accessing such resources is often dependent upon one's visibility and legibility to the official world of NGOs and government programmes.

This situation raises questions about the economic as well as moral *value* of being HIV-positive and about the *worth* of HIV positive and negative lives. It also raises questions about the 'politics of life' (Fassin 2009) in contemporary Kenya. The politically tense issue of food prices was played out daily in concerns about

---

in Kenya were receiving ART (up from 10,000 in 2003); about a third of them lived in Nyanza Province. See http://www.aidskenya.org/Programmes/Treatment--Care-&-Support/ART, and the PEPFAR website http://www.pepfar.gov/countries/kenya/index.htm.

6 | These include training programmes run by NGOs that give people skills in HIV-related knowledge and thus possibilities of finding 'grassroots' work in HIV-interventions.

hunger, expressed by many of the patients I met in the HIV clinics and followed in their homes. They pointed out that their ability to survive was as much about food and income as about medicine. Yet the politics that reared above the anger at food prices and maize scandals, deeply felt and hotly discussed on the streets, in people's homes and in offices, reached neither into the clinic nor into the NGO world. In the latter spaces, hunger was constructed as a problem of poverty, to be addressed through specific projects targeting poor people. It was not considered as an outcome of the wider structures of inequality in Kenyan society, whether those highlighted by the corruption scandals or the huge gaps in income between NGO staff (especially expatriates) and the people targeted by their projects. The struggle for survival was thus not so much ignored in the massive drive to extend ART in western Kenya as deflected into humanitarian interventions organized by a plethora of different non-governmental organizations and directed at those 'affected and infected by HIV'.

Antiretroviral therapy programmes and HIV/AIDS interventions are examples of what Li describes as "vast schemes to improve the human condition", which seek their goals through working on the practices and desires of their target populations (2005: 383). Through ART programmes, individuals in Kenya are being encouraged to think of themselves in terms of the virus they carry, and HIV positive populations are being managed through bureaucratic and scientific procedures. As such, they can be described in terms of Foucault's ideas about 'governmentality' and 'biopower' (Foucault 2004 [1976]), and as an example of our modern 'politics of life' (see Rose 2007). Here, a biological definition of life is becoming central to our notions of self and to politics as the site of governing bodies and groups, but also—as biology becomes a means of assessing and claiming rights to healthcare or welfare benefits—of negotiation and debate (Rabinow/Rose 2006; Biehl 2007; Fassin 2009). The scale of ART programmes, together with the fact that funding medical care for HIV positive people in Kenya now far exceeds that provided for the health needs of the rest of the population, gives credence to the argument that citizenship—in the sense of rights and responsibilities characterising membership of a sovereign, political entity—is being reduced and circumscribed by biological conditions that open up claims to specific medical therapies (e.g. Petryna 2002; Arendt 1958). Such trends, described in terms of 'therapeutic citizenship' (Nguyen 2010) or the 'pharmaticalization of public health' (Biehl 2007), are defining a new era of global health and development interventions, especially in Africa. Here, project-specific 'archipelagos' of humanitarian interventions, organized by non-state and non-national groups, have become the order of the day (Hearn 1998; Redfield 2005; Rottenburg 2009; see also Mkandawire 2001).

The framework of Foucauldian biopolitics as developed by scholars such as Nikolas Rose provides a productive framework through which to understand the relations between health, biomedicine and governmentality in Africa today. Yet, recent characterisations of the response to HIV-AIDS in terms of 'experimental politics' (Rottenburg 2009) or 'government-by-exception' (Nguyen 2009) tend to situate their analyses within these frames, rather than explore their edges.[7] This paper addresses the question of how such a 'politics of life' unfolds under specific social, economic and political conditions. Drawing upon ethnographic research in clinics, community based groups and patient's lives it offers insights into emerging practices of 'biosociality' (Rabinow 2005[1996]) in Kisumu, and their intersections with moral economies of NGO interventions as well as with pharmaceutical regimes of care.

'Lets Pull Together'

On a hot Saturday afternoon, in a community hall on the outskirts of one of Kisumu's informal settlements, members of the 'Lets Pull Together', an HIV-positive 'patient support group', arrive for their fortnightly meeting. The hall belongs to a Catholic organization, which has been active in the city for the past thirty years. During the week it functions as an HIV clinic and is packed with patients, but on the weekends it is used for meetings of various groups attached to the Catholic centre: church groups, youth and women's groups as well as two patient support groups. The members of 'Lets Pull Together', many of them women, greet each other and settle into the chairs arranged in a circle near the open door. I recognize MinAchieng', MinAnna and MinJacinta—they are members of another patient support group I had myself attended the previous day, on the other side of this provincial city. Their long skirts and blouses are newly pressed, but their feet are dusty—they have walked a long way to attend this meeting. Some of them are 'clients' of this Catholic-run clinic, but many get their HIV treatment and checkups from other HIV clinics.[8]

7 | As Li reminds us "(g)rand schemes [...] are contingent on a tangled set of practices, processes and relations" (2005: 383), not the outcome of a single vision, but of a complex assemblage of ideas, institutions, knowledge, science, technology, practices. Analyses of global health interventions echo earlier critiques of development as a tool of western domination (Escobar 1995), which frames problems in terms of technical expertise rather than political-economic relations (Ferguson 1994). Such critiques uncover a truth, yet leave the interesting area between policy and practice (see Mosse 2005) unexamined.

8 | During the past 30 years, this Catholic organization has provided health and other services to the low-income population surrounding the centre. In 2006, with funds from PEPFAR, the US Presidential Emergency Fund for AIDS Relief, it began to offer HIV testing and counseling, and in 2008, it entered a partnership with the American NGO

Ochieng', the chairman of 'Lets Pull Together', is a father of four, whose wife and youngest child are also HIV positive.[9] He is one of the founders of the group, having discovered his own HIV status in 2006. He begins the meeting by asking MinJacinta to pray. He then suggests that members introduce themselves and give a short history of their HIV status and ARV medication. This procedure is part of the routine of support group meetings, but its elaboration on this day seems to be more for my benefit (it is my first visit to this group, although I've attended the meetings of other support groups attached to this clinic); most of the members already know each other and each others' situations well. Talking mostly in Kiswahili, Ochieng' then announces the agenda: the secretary—a large middle aged woman who used to be a teacher—will read the minutes of the previous meeting; Ochieng' will then introduce the visiting anthropologist to the group and afterwards give a short talk about how to "live with HIV". Finally John, the treasurer (a tall man, who, like Ochieng' and the secretary, speaks both Kiswahili and English with ease) will announce some news. It is this last piece on the agenda that many of the members are eagerly anticipating. The treasurer has attended a meeting organized by the government's National AIDS Control Council, in which 'community-based' and 'self-help' groups were invited to submit written proposals to a donor for what has become known as 'income generating activities' (IGAs) targeting those 'infected or affected by HIV'. If the application is successful, the group will receive some money to start small businesses (such as selling vegetables or trading fish). In his recounting of this meeting, the treasurer stresses that the group has to show it is serious and "accountable", well organized and committed. The group is already registered with the government's social services department; it has a bank account and a bureaucratic structure. "We can show our accounts, and we have minutes and lists of our members", he said, and suggested these bureaucratic details should be included in the proposal, as should the (un)employment and family situations of members. The group had discussed their needs for "IGAs" (everyone uses the acronym) in previous meetings: today, members talk about their lack of income, their material needs, and the challenges of feeding a family and sending children to school. Some members direct this talk directly

---

that receives PEPFAR funds to organize and support HIV treatment centers in Nyanza Province.

9 | Pseudonyms are used for names of people and groups. The names chosen by patient support groups -in English, Kiswahili or Dholuo—often emphasize virtues of working together for one goal, mutual support, and combating stigma. Western Kenya has a long history of what is today termed 'community-based' groups, which in colonial and postcolonial times acted as mediators between state or church authority and 'community' (see Haugerud 1993; Lewis 2000; Shipton 2007). People today often speak of how working in a group produces better results than "standing alone".

to me, assuming I am associated with an NGO, but Ochieng' skilfully turns the direction of the meeting back to proposal-writing. He talks about the many "OVCs" (Orphans and Vulnerable Children—another widely used acronym) in the community, and suggests that the group could also apply for funds to help these children's caregivers with school fees, uniforms and even food. As someone who has worked in HIV clinics, both as a volunteer and lately as a 'community health worker', and as a family father whose neighbours include many families looking after orphans, Ochieng' knows what he is talking about. He points out that many of the members are themselves already taking care of orphaned nephews, nieces and grandchildren. The treasurer suggests that the group use some of the money it has saved up to hire a proposal writer (someone who knows how to use official language, who can couch the group's intentions in a way that funders can recognize). He already has a particular person in mind who can do the job for 3,000 shillings, and he suggests that the group uses its collective funds for this purpose.[10]

The NGO city and the HIV economy

Residents of Kisumu jokingly refer to their city as a "NGO city". "This city survives on NGOs", Alan, an unemployed teacher told me. This is of course an exaggeration. Most of the city's residents survive in the 'informal' economy of market stalls, vegetable selling, domestic work, tailoring, fish-smoking and charcoal-making, water-selling, bar work and transportation—and informal market stalls line the streets outside the city's central business district. The city also has some small industrial manufacturing and many small businesses, and, as Kenya's third largest town, it is an important administrative centre, housing many government bureaucrats, as well as teachers, nurses and medical staff, clerks and cleaners. Yet the number of NGOs has risen exponentially since the mid 1995s and particularly over the past decade. The last survey by the 'NGO coordination board', in 2008, lists 907 NGOs with operations in Kisumu; these range from global organizations such as World Vision to nationally-established

10 | 3,000 Ksh was about £30 at the time. Like many of the support groups I visited in Kisumu, 'Lets Pull Together' also functioned as a rotating credit group. Members contributed a small amount of money at each meeting (usually 20 shillings or 20p), which was put into a collective kitty, and either kept for collective activities or drawn upon by each member in turn or in times of special need. Rotating credit is a long-established practice of groups in western Kenya (and has been widely documented in both colonial and postcolonial Africa). Women in particular are avid members of groups, which are usually formed among people of similar income. The practice of rotating credit underlines the multiple activities and functions of groups.

NGOs to local 'self-help' or 'community-based' groups, which register themselves as NGOs with the government and hope to receive funding from the bigger NGOs.[11] Many of the international and national NGOs are involved in HIV-related interventions such as the introduction and expansion of anti-retroviral treatment to HIV-positive people; projects providing school fees, food and care to orphans; income-generating activities and micro-finance projects; hospice care; youth interventions, and 'HIV prevention'.[12]

The funds that NGOs receive mostly come from outside Kenya; and these funds flow into the buildings and vehicles, salaries, and workshops associated with international and national NGOs. In Kisumu they produce signs of wealth that are strikingly absent from other spaces in the city, and they circulate resources, albeit in circumscribed ways. Thus, most of the larger four-wheel drive cars one sees on the city streets display logos of non-governmental organizations or external aid agencies. Many of the well-heeled middle class of Kisumu, those who draw a salary at the end of the month and who enjoy lunches of chicken and fish in the cafes that have sprung up in the centre of town, are employed by NGOs. Accessing this NGO world through formal employment is difficult (if not impossible) for most of Kisumu's residents. However, as part of current donor interest in 'community-based development', NGOS channel a portion of their funds to 'community-based groups' and they target those with specific needs, if they can present themselves as organized and accountable. This has resulted in an explosion of community-based groups of all kinds—youth groups, women's groups, widow's groups, even men's groups—all jostling to gain visibility and thus access funds.

In this city of groups, HIV positive Patient Support Groups are particularly prominent. These groups are attached to 'patient support centers' (henceforth PSCs), clinics providing free HIV tests and counselling, where HIV positive people receive free antiretroviral medicines, multivitamins and antibiotics as well as regular, if basic, medical check-ups. Since PEPFAR and the Global Fund made commitments to funding ART, the number and reach of PSCs has expanded in Kisumu.[13]

---

11 | See the 2007-8 report by the NGOs Coordination Board (set up by the government in 1990): http://www.ngobureau.or.ke/Publications/National%20Survey%20of%20NGOs%20Report.pdf. It shows that there are 117 NGOs with their headquarters in Kisumu, and 790 operating in Kisumu but with their headquarters elsewhere. The survey staff could not physically locate or interview many of the smaller NGOs, raising questions about how they operate and indeed whether they still exist.

12 | See also http://www.kanco.org/KANCOmembers.php, which lists NGOs working in western Kenya.

13 | By 2010, there were 25 PSCs within the city (64 in Kisumu district), ranging from the large PSC attached to the provincial hospital, to small clinics run by local

By 2008, every PSC in Kisumu had at least one 'Patient Support Group' attached to it. These groups varied in size and membership, as people joined and left, but usually contained a core group of committed HIV-positive members. Most patient support groups have a similar bureaucratic structure and similar procedures as the one described above: chairperson, secretary, treasurer; minute-taking, membership lists and registration cards. This bureaucracy is important: it lends the group status, gives it weight, and demonstrates its accountability. It reproduces known forms, making the group legible to others organizations—governmental and non-governmental—that control funds or access to them. Most groups try to register with the government as a 'community-based organization' or a 'self-help group', which makes them visible (group members may be invited to official meetings as representatives of 'the community') and gives them access to funding opportunities. To do this, they should have a bank account and a written constitution, and they have to pay a sum of money.[14]

Thus, while support groups like 'Lets Pull Together' provide a social location for the encouragement and management of 'positive living', where people can 'share' their experiences and challenges, they also have to a large extent become locations where people can access funding, material goods, as well as training and even employment opportunities. Through joining a support group, people learn that articulating their positive identity can open up economic opportunities.

How has this situation developed? Starting in 2000, positive lifestyles were actively cultivated in HIV positive people by NGOs and donors, backed up by the government, as part of a strategy to address discrimination and encourage people to go for HIV tests.[15] HIV positive people were given something people refer to as "appreciation" money to stand up and 'witness' about their HIV positive status. They were also encouraged to start up patient support groups. Living and spreading the "HIV gospel", as Ochieng' described it to me, became a career path for the early members of support groups in Kisumu, many of

---

NGOs. PEPFAR provides funds to a host of 'prime partners' (http://www.pepfar.gov/partners/103021.htm), which organize and monitor PSCs (e.g. Global AIDS Programme (GAP): http://www.cdc.gov/globalaids/Global-HIV-AIDS-at-CDC/countries/Kenya/; Family Aids Care and Education Service (FACES): www.faces-kenya.org); the Catholic Relief Services (CRS): http://crs.org/hiv-aids); Academic Model for the Prevention and Treatment of HIV/AIDS (AMPATH): http://www.iukenya.org/pdfs/ampath.pdf); and Liverpool VCT (LVCT): www.liverpoolvct.org). See also Madiega 2011.

14 | National NGOs have to pay the Board 11,000Ksh; International NGOs pay 22,000. They are issued with a certificate, but have to pay extra for it; they also have to pay 500 shillings for the approval of their name. see http://www.ngobureau.or.ke/servicefees.aspx.

15 | See "Reversing the Trends: the Second National Health Sector Strategic Plan of Kenya". Ministry of Health, June 2006.

whom went on to receive 'training' in HIV counselling or community work, and even employment in HIV-related work. During the same period, there was a proliferation of NGOs providing funds for those 'infected or affected by HIV'.[16] Support groups became the natural target for NGOs searching for HIV positive people in need of material support. Sacks of food and loans of money encouraged more people to join support groups and their membership numbers increased substantially. As HIV gained economic value, at least for the unemployed, there were even reports of people claiming to be HIV positive in order to join a support group. One group I knew began demanding that members bring their PSC cards with them in order to ensure there were no fake identities.[17]

When I first attended support group meetings, the leader or 'chairperson' would usually set off a round of introductions with each person giving a short history of their encounter with HIV and ARVS (for example: "I learned my status in 2006. I have been on ARVS since 2007."). Often the chairperson of the group would ask one or two members, usually women, to tell their stories. Often involving sickness, the death of husbands and rejection by agnatic family, these stories were very emotional, with the teller sometimes breaking down in tears.[18] After attending several meetings and several support groups, however, I realized that these narratives, while genuinely felt and articulated, were called up more for my benefit as a visitor. They could be called upon—members had learned how to tell the story of life before they came to 'know' HIV—but they were not part of the routine of group meetings. Instead the meeting would be devoted to more urgent matters—to discussing worries about school fees or ill family members, conflicts with in-laws, and lack of food. Other matters

16 | For example, 'Orphans and Vulnerable Children' (OVCs) and 'Widows', as well as HIV positive people, emerge in this global AIDS discourse as categories of persons in particular need of, for example, food, school fees, income generating activities, or 'home-based care' (see Epstein 2007).

17 | Support group membership was clearly class- (or income-) based. Those who enjoyed salaried employment did not need the material benefits associated with group membership. At the same time, due to perceived discrimination of HIV people in many workplaces, they had more reason to hide their HIV status. I met some HIV positive people who were teachers, nurses or civil servants at the PSCs, but none were members of a support group.

18 | Many of these women discovered they were HIV positive during a period of sickness, or after the death of a spouse and subsequent conflict with in-laws (Prince 2011). In these narratives it was through being tested, accepting their status, becoming clients of a PSC and members of a support group that these women managed to gain a sense of worth and rebuild their lives. In this patrilineal society, married women belong to their husband's land and family. A rejection by the husband's family thus amounts to a refusal of a woman's social identity and her future (Geissler/Prince 2010b).

included information about members who were too ill to attend or who were caring for sick family members; requests for contributions to the funeral expenses of a former member of the group; discussions about whether group members should form a credit-rotation group or "merry-go-round"; exchange of information about microcredit organizations operating in Kisumu; and the exchange of news about which NGO or church group was this week or month supplying bags of flour, mobile phone credit or start-up cash for IGAs.

Not all groups are successful. 'Let's Pull Together' is a particularly well-organized group, whose leaders are educated and articulate and passionate about "helping our community" and "fighting HIV/AIDS in our country", as Ochieng' put it. They also have good connections with both the Catholic NGO, and with other NGOs in Kisumu. For example, Ochieng' had worked for several years as a 'volunteer' HIV counsellor in both the provincial hospital and the Catholic clinic, and in 2008, he had managed to get formally employed by the clinic on a one-year contract when it expanded its HIV treatment activities using PEPFAR money. Other groups lacked such well-connected leaders, although many had leaders and members who were enthusiastic practitioners of what they referred to as the "HIV gospel".

Several months after the meeting described above, Ochieng' wrote an email telling me that the group had been successful in its bid for funding from PEPFAR, and that it had received some money[19], some of which was earmarked for IGAs for each member, and some of which was to support orphans and vulnerable families identified by the group. He was brimming with enthusiasm and elation at their success. When I returned to Kisumu for a visit in 2010, I found that several other patient support groups had become attached to the Catholic NGO, hoping, I suspect, to emulate the success of 'Lets Pull Together'. These groups had not been successful in applying for PEPFAR funds. But they had received a one-off gift of a few thousand shillings for IGAs from an NGO supporting people living with HIV.

Thus, the better-organized group—with well-connected leaders who knew how to write or solicit proposals—received funding, while those who lacked such skills did not. Like the village groups in the World Bank scheme described by Li, what was being offered was "equality of opportunity to compete for funds, not equality of outcome" (Li 2007: 248). In a situation in which every group is able to demonstrate a need, accessing funds depends, crucially, on a particular expertise: the ability to write a proposal or to keep records, to demonstrate accountability and efficiency. This expertise is both generated and sought

19 | Some 50,000 Ksh or £500.

after by NGOs[20], and pursued by individuals who need to learn the particular language and material culture of development.

Some of the NGO projects focusing on HIV affected people in Kisumu have enjoyed a degree of success. For example, some of the early members of 'Patient Support Groups', those who agreed to stand up to 'witness' about their status, invested the money they received into 'training' or small businesses.[21] Like Ochieng' and his wife, some of them found work, first as volunteers for NGOs and later as employed 'counsellors' or 'community health workers'. However, many of these NGO-led interventions are rather transient and short-term, as they are subject to the changing concerns of donors. NGOs must continually make funding applications, and their operations are limited to circumscribed spaces. Recipients of such interventions thus experience them as extremely patchy and unstable. For example, the self-help group that MinAchieng', MinAnna and MinJacinta were members of, located on the other side of town, had for a time received funds from a UK-based charity for a project supplying food and school fees to widows and orphans. After two years the charity had suddenly withdrew its support, leaving the children they were supporting half way through secondary school with no means to pay the fees. According to leaders of the group, this abrupt change was due to the shifting priorities of the charity's donors, and thus it was not even within the control of the charity itself.

Such stories underline the fact that while NGOs may provide some basic services, these are oriented more to the requirement of donors and their funds than to the people they target. Like the healthcare interventions I will turn to below, such welfare interventions are organized through an archipelago of short-term projects and interventions, producing a patchwork of services that are limited both temporarily and spatially (see Hearn 1998). Moreover, success itself is often ephemeral. The funding of groups like 'Lets Pull Together' is supposed to make them into 'income generating' and 'self-help' groups, which can then stand on their own (see Boesten 2011). However, this rarely happens, as their 'income-generating' activities are economically insecure. And while groups like 'Lets Pull Together' may get funding for one year, they may fail to get further funding (and consequently often lose members, as people migrate to more successful groups).

---

20 | People learn such skills through training workshops and seminars, organized mostly by NGOs.

21 | Sometimes undergoing a training programme was a condition of the exchange they entered into.

HEALTHCARE AND 'WELFARE'

Support groups are places where the pharmaceutical regime of the clinic meets the humanitarian economy of welfare organized through NGOs and directed towards those living with or affected by HIV. They are imagined as places where people learn to live positively with HIV and to organize their bodies and lives in terms of the requirements of antiretroviral therapy. Support Groups indeed encourage a solidification of identity around being HIV positive. People learn to tell the story of their lives within a certain genre—that of HIV—and to articulate their needs in terms of being HIV positive. Through joining a support group, people living with HIV also become visible to others. Encouraging this visibility as a way of combating stigmas and 'normalizing' HIV has been important to HIV positive people, and to those working to improve their lives (Ogot 2004). Yet visibility has another, economic, value for those surviving in this NGO city. It makes you visible to organizations that control the flow of funds and the projects. As the leader of another support group in Kisumu joked, "We hope that scientists do not find a vaccine for AIDS. We need HIV!"

This material suggests that the 'new' subjectivities inscribed by 'positive living' and new technologies of care, often remarked upon in the literature as life-transforming (e.g. Robins 2004; Comaroff 2007; see also Whyte 2009), are grounded in an economy in which being positive has a material value. As AIDS projects and NGOs converge on the city, having HIV is proving to be a resource. While the conditions of life in the city that I described above face all those who lack a regular income, being 'infected or affected by HIV' is a recognised form of suffering that NGOs respond to. Projects supporting income generating activities, micro-credit, orphans and vulnerable children, and the distribution of food all respond to the recognition that the poverty experienced by many families has been exacerbated and to some extent created by HIV/AIDS. HIV makes one eligible for interventions. Just being poor does not.[22]

Joining a group and making oneself visible as a HIV positive person with certain 'needs' requires a certain ability to recognise opportunities. However this does not mean that group members are simply opportunistic. Life in the city is tough if you have no formal employment. There is no public housing scheme for people outside government employment; landlords erect barely finished rooms with mud walls and leaking roofs, and charge high rents for them; schooling is expensive, and many families take care of orphaned grandchildren, nephews and nieces (Nyambedha/Wandibba/Aagaard 2003; Nyambedha 2008). For many, giving the family a solid meal is a daily struggle. Many of the women who come to the 'Lets Pull Together' group are members of other support groups

22 | Although a pilot study by UNICEF in Kiusmu introducing cash transfers to 'vulnerable families' has recently been introduced.

because these provide some of their few opportunities to access food or money. Many of them live alone, are widowed or separated from their husbands. They cultivate their membership alongside other 'income-generating' activities, such as selling vegetables, doing laundry for wealthier patrons, or making and selling chapatti; while the male members provide *bodaboda* (bicycle taxi), cart water for sale, sell sodas or tailor. All these ways of earning a living are unstable and transient—vulnerable to price changes, weather conditions, the ability to buy on credit, and the uncertainties of donor funds—and one has to be constantly alert to changes and new opportunities and able to switch between different activities.[23]

In the next section I explore how the ability to survive with HIV is imagined by the clinic with its focus on pharmaceutical regimes of self-care, and juxtapose this with the realities of daily life in the city, where many people struggle to find enough food to feed their families.

REGIMES OF SELF-CARE

As a 'community health worker' (CHW), Ochieng' spends his weekday mornings in the community hall, which acts as the PSC of the Catholic NGO. Together with three other CHWs, he registers new 'clients', updates their medical forms and takes their vitals—weight, height (for children), and pulse rate—before sending them past the curtained-off partition to see the nurse and clinical officer who ask about the patient's health, prescribe drugs and sometimes send the patient on to the laboratory for further tests. On Wednesday mornings Ochieng' also conducts 'adherence classes'. According to Ministry of Health guidelines, before people can be initiated on antiretroviral therapy, they must attend three adherence classes, where counsellors teach them about HIV and 'positive living', the importance of taking care of your health and living 'responsibly' (through eating a 'balanced diet', not passing on the virus nor exposing oneself to re-infection), as well as how to consume the daily doses of multivitamins and antibiotics, and the various combinations of antiretroviral drugs.

Ensuring the success of the ART programmes—initiating and keeping large numbers of people on antiretroviral medication—relies to a large extent on instilling particular habits and attitudes towards medicine, one's body, and ideas of risk. Antiretroviral medication must be taken twice at day at exactly 12-hour intervals. The strict adherence to the medication suppresses the replication of the virus and its mutations that can become resistant to the drugs (WHO 2003, 2009; Castleman/Seumo-Fossil/Cogill 2004; Laing/Hodgkin

23 | See Guyer 2004 for an ethnographic analysis of trading and other economic activities in the informal economy.

2006). Hence there is much focus on giving the patient what is referred to in the clinic as 'correct information'. Health should be achieved through the patient knowing about the virus; such knowledge allows her to 'take control' of her viral condition, through close monitoring of her own health and care of herself. The use of the term 'client' underlines the attempt to move HIV from its associations with illness and patienthood, towards 'autonomy' and 'choice': you are not a patient, passively accepting your condition, but a person who can act upon it. Counselling and education about HIV and ARVs, about diet, medication, sexuality, the importance of keeping time, and keeping one's clinic dates—reiterated in counselling sessions such as those led by Ochieng'—aim to produce this ideal client, at once obedient (to medical and clinic regimens) and 'empowered' (able to take responsibility for her own health). That this stance or orientation is normative, entwined with moral judgments, is underlined by the term used by the clinic to describe a client who does not conform to these medical regiments: 'defaulter'.[24]

EMPOWERMENT AND DISEMPOWERMENT

Ochieng' is an example of how successful a decision to embrace 'positive living' and the regimes of the clinic can be. Both he and his wife quickly embraced their positive status, joined support groups, and through being 'active' members, gained access to the training in HIV counselling and community health work that was being offered by various NGOs in Kisumu. After several years of precarious survival, during which they worked as 'volunteers' for the clinics, they both managed to gain paid employment as 'community health workers', albeit on one-year contracts. On their combined monthly salaries, they are able to rent a solid three-roomed house and to put their oldest child as well as Ochieng's younger brother through secondary school.[25]

24 | This (English) term is used for those who do not turn up to appointments, who do not take their medicines, or do not take them properly. The etymology of 'defaulter'—'nonpayer', 'debtor' 'cheat', 'absentee from court'—illustrates the connection made in these new medical regimes between health, economy and legal regimes. While the PSC often make quite an effort to follow them up and staff is often sympathetic, there are clear guidelines concerning their inclusion. As one of the Ochieng's co-workers explained to me: "The defaulters are given another chance. They have to enrol again in the Adherence classes and attend all three of them again. If they don't come, and if they drop out again, they are out."

25 | However, they are also vulnerable to increased demands from extended families members, for help with school fees, medical expenses, and looking after children.

However, when I accompanied Ochieng' on some of his 'home' visits, I was stuck by the contrast between his experiences of 'empowerment' and those of many of the people he visited. For example, Rose, a young mother of two, was struggling with her HIV status and with her treatment regimen. Her husband, a fisherman, had left her after she had disclosed her status. Having no place to go to, she had stayed on in their rented room on the lakeside of town, earning some little income by buying fish at the lakeshore and selling it in town—but she was continually on the verge of being thrown out by her landlord. According to Ochieng', Rose's health deteriorated after her husband's departure. When she missed several clinic appointments in a row, Ochieng' went to visit her and found her in a weak state. She admitted to him that she had not been taking her medicines because there was little food in the house, and taking them on a empty stomach made her feel sick. Ochieng' encouraged her to come to the clinic and continue with the medicines, but he later admitted that he felt uncomfortable offering only advice "when the problem is food". Knowing her HIV status and being initiated on ARVs had not 'empowered' Rose in the way it had Ochieng'. Moreover, the strength and life promised by ART had, in the absence of an adequate diet, failed to materialise.

TALKING ABOUT HUNGER

Food is a constant worry for many Kisumu residents. In our ongoing study of 20 families with members on ART, most of them living in Kisumu's 'informal settlements', people reported that they were often hungry and ate only one meal a day. Sometimes there would be porridge in the morning (made with flour and water, and rarely milk); sometimes only black tea with sugar. Living conditions were precarious as many had no steady income to rely on.[26]

Many of the HIV positive people we followed reported an initial weight gain and rise in energy during the first weeks of taking ART. During this period of ART initiation, the PSC usually gives underweight 'clients' a flour supplement, particularly if they had suffered from tuberculosis or other opportunistic infections. The flour and the medicine gives them an initial weight boost, which they experience as a shift from being ill and weak to a feeling of increased strength and the ability to be mobile, work and function normally. However, the flour supplement is usually discontinued once the person reaches a 'viable' weight[27], and many experience a sharp rise in hunger and an intolerance of

26 | For example, selling vegetables may give one an income of 100 shillings on some days, and twenty shillings on others. Compare this to the cost of a basic family meal: 10-20 shillings for vegetables and 50-100 shillings for maize flour.

27 | For women, the cut-off point is fifty kilogrammes.

certain kinds of food. "Since I started taking these medicines I just want to eat a lot. But the challenge that faces me is, how do I get food? The ARV medicines need a lot of food", Elizabeth told us. She was the mother of two girls, the youngest of whom she had just discovered was also HIV positive.[28] Irene, whose husband and child were also positive, told us: "Food is not easy to get. At times my husband goes to the market (to trade) and comes with nothing, and this makes us sleep hungry."'[29] We often heard people commenting: "Taking ARVs without proper food is like committing suicide"[30]

Eating a good meal each day is a challenge facing many families, HIV positive or not. However HIV positive people reported that ARVs introduced an intolerance of hunger and a dependence on their body's need for food to a degree they had not experienced before. At the same time, they found it difficult to ask for special treatment from family and neighbours: "People will say, 'Why you? We are also hungry!'", as Elizabeth once explained. In western Kenya, bodily needs should not be expressed—children are taught not to complain about hunger even if they spend a day without food—and in a situation where everyone gets one meal a day, it is hard to claim that having HIV gives you the right to more or better food. Self-care is here not a virtue but a form of selfishness.[31]

---

28 | (E. Atieno, Sat 12th December 2009). Elizabeth told Biddy that her husband had refused to take an HIV test, and that she had taken her daughter to get tested without his knowledge.

29 | (Irene Akinyi 14th December 2009).I am grateful to Biddy Odindo for recording these conversations.

30 | This expression seems exaggerated yet it was commonly used. To some degree people's talk of hunger was oriented to us, as outsiders, particularly as we were initially associated with the world of NGOs and groups. However, this does not make it less real. Tragically, Elizabeth died in June 2010, and although her husband then got an HIV test and took great care of his positive daughter, at the time of writing, I have just heard from Biddy that the little girl has died. This underlines the continued problem of medication in a situation of economic precariousness. It also underlines that in the context of limited government welfare, NGO projects provide inadequate protection to such vulnerable families.

31 | Hunger is not a novel experience in rural Nyanza. During the 20th century, labour migration combined with the introduction of maize as the staple crop, led to this area experiencing a huge decline in food production (Hay 1976; Cohen/Odhiambo 1989). During the 1980s and 90s, infant malnutrition was a prominent concern of donor agencies and medical research. From the 1990s, rural hunger has been exacerbated by the deaths of economically productive household members due to AIDS, and the decline of labour migrants' cash remittances (Francis 1995; Nyambedha/Wandibba/Aagaard-Hansen 2003; Geissler/Prince 2010a).

Paradoxically, it is in this situation that the clinic becomes a space where people can talk about food and thus about hunger and material needs. This is because here it was recognized that HIV positive people needed to eat well in order to do well on the medicine. Ochieng' spends one morning a week counselling people who are about to start on ARVs. He shows them the medicines and their strengths, but also mentions side-effects. "You have to eat well if you want to do well on these medicines", he says, "they are very strong". He points to the poster on the wall which displays the ingredients of a "balanced diet": proteins, carbohydrates and vitamins. The interaction between food and diet is also underlined in the provision of fortified flour to HIV-positive children and to severely underweight adults. This flour is given for a limited period (usually three months), often when the person is initiated on ARVs.

Flour supplements are not a response to hunger, but a medical intervention to prevent unacceptable weight loss and deterioration. However they make a huge difference to many families, who fiercely cling on to them. A nutritionist employed at a PSC told me about arguments he had had with grandmothers and mothers who refused to give up their flour supplement. One HIV-positive child in his care had been (against regulations) receiving the flour for over a year:

"This child has been receiving supplements for too long—the limit is three months. So this came to the attention of our funders and they insisted that the supplement should be stopped. I had the grandmother here, she could not understand. 'How am I to feed my grandchild?', she asked me. I told her, 'Would you die if the funders left? What were you eating before? You cannot rely on this. It is not food aid. Donors come and go.' It is difficult..."[32]

There is a large gap between the forms of self-care expected by the clinic and people's everyday struggles to get enough food. Flour supplements are no solution to the problem of making an income. And like other HIV counsellors, Ochieng' is well aware that few of those attending his ART adherence classes have the means to eat 'balanced' diets. Yet, the focus in the clinic on the relations between ARVs, diet and nutrition opens up a space for talking about hunger and thus about living conditions. While this talk does not enter official space—questions concerning daily diet are not included on patient's medical forms—patients do tell the clinic staff "I cannot take this medicine when I have not eaten!" This is often done in a humorous rather than a confrontational way, but the message is clear: "We cannot survive on medicine alone."

In voicing their hunger, people pull the conditions of their survival into the clinic. However, the political challenge that lack of food and income poses seems to stop short there. During interviews with staff at patient support centres

32 | Interview with R.O., 27th September 2010.

in Kisumu, I asked what solution there could be to the problem of food faced by people on ARVs. In most cases, I was referred back to NGOs and proposal writing. "Patient support groups could write a proposal to ask for funds from a donor or well-wisher for Income Generating Activities", staff suggested. The inequalities that the geography of hunger makes visible are channelled into requests for aid from foreign funders and NGOs. And, as the example of 'Lets Pull Together' demonstrates, this aid is directed to groups and individuals who can demonstrate a particular expertise.

THE POLITICS AND ANTI-POLITICS OF HIV INTERVENTIONS

ART programmes tend to construct survival as a matter of adherence to medicalized regimes of care, thus overlooking conditions of life in the city that may be more important to whether medication is successful or not. By framing matters of adherence as matters of knowledge and access to information, they exclude political questions about why some people can't do well on medicines, not because of knowledge but because of poverty and inequality. As James Ferguson observed of development projects in Lesotho, ART programmes may "effectively quash political challenges to the system [...] by insistently reposing political questions of land, resources, jobs, or wages as 'technical' problems responsive to the technical 'development' intervention" (1990: 270). Issues of hunger and access to food are not within the province of treatment programmes: "This is not food aid."[33] Yet to stop here would be to present too simple an analysis of what is going so. For at the same time, ART programmes bring matters of hunger and access to food into view, into the space of the clinic, where they can be articulated, albeit obliquely.

There is potential, then, for programmes that provide treatment to HIV positive people to point to the inequalities in survival chances that exist despite access to medication. When patients link their survival to food and hunger as well as to medicines, there is an "opening", for the ignition of political practice, as "expert discourse is punctured by a challenge it cannot contain, moments when the targets of programmes reveal, in word or deed, their own critical analysis of the problems that confront them" (Li 2007: 11).

However, in Kisumu, the recognition of hunger and inequalities did not translate into a political issue in a public arena, beyond private observations and complaints. This is despite the tense political atmosphere in which food prices and economic inequality were debated in Kenya during 2008 and 2009.

33 | As I was recently told by Kenyan and American doctors and directors of the Global AIDS Programme in Kisumu during a presentation of a version of this paper to KEMRI-CDC seminar, October 1st 2010, Kisumu.

Why not? Asked what could be done about hunger and lack of food, staff at the patient support centres suggested that patients should join a group and make proposals to 'well-wishers' and 'donors'. The problem of hunger is channelled into the humanitarian economy of NGO interventions, which encourage HIV positive people to form groups and write funding proposals. As for the groups themselves, any independent thinking and grassroots activism is quickly submerged by the need to account upwards. Despite the 'grassroots' rhetoric of interventions, groups such as 'Lets Pull Together' do not decide which projects and activities should be funded and where welfare should be directed. Instead they have to orient their activities to the requirements of the donors. This humanitarian economy of short term, project-specific and patchy welfare interventions thus does not encourage people to think of their health care and welfare in terms of their rights as citizens and the responsibilities of the state, but rather to think of themselves as recipients of charitable donations from 'well-wishers' and as sufferers having 'needs'.[34]

34 | The tension between responding to immediate suffering and pushing for social transformations that would target the source of suffering is much discussed in relation to humanitarianism (Calhoun 2009).

Inherent Failure and Contradiction

Experimental hubris and medical powerlessness: Notes from a colonial utopia, Cameroon, 1939-1949[1]

Guillaume Lachenal

Turning the political command over to doctors—the utopia of 'medical governance'—has been a recurrent dream in the history of public health. This chapter examines an extraordinary attempt to materialize this dream. Between 1939 and 1948, the French administration of Cameroon handed over the direction of an entire province to doctors. For nearly a decade, the Haut-Nyong territory was placed under the responsibility of a handful of young colonial doctors, to the exclusion of any other administrative or military authority. The stated objective was to conduct experimentation in colonial administration, namely to set up a medical utopia where public health would blend into policy-making. Rediscovered thanks to the work of Peter Geschière (1982: 39; 1983) and the Cameroonian historian Wang Sonné (1998), this experimentation is worth studying for at least two reasons. First of all, this extreme case lets us glimpse colonial medicine's political horizon in a pure state, we might say: a medical government turned toward population growth and the fight against epidemics, and guided solely by medical techniques, scientific knowledge and humanism. This case illustrates how colonial doctors envisioned in material terms the inaccessible ideal of European hygienists since the 19th century (Murard/Zylberman 1996)—the ideal of a 'social medicine' directly ruling and reforming society, as it applied verbatim Rudolf Virchow's saying: "Politics is nothing other

1 | Article translated from French by Noal Mellott (CNRS, Paris, France). The original French version of this chapter was published in Annales Histoire Sciences Sociales, January-February 2010, 65, 1, pp. 121-156: "Le médecin qui voulut être roi. Médecine coloniale et utopie au Cameroun". The author thanks the Annales for graciously authorizing this translation. The author also wishes to thank Richard Rottenburg, Julia Zenker, John Manton and an anonymous reviewer for their comments on the English manuscript.

than medicine on a grand scale" (Virchow 1848; McNeely 2002).[2] Secondly, the Haut-Nyong utopia was designed as a literal experiment to be discussed and reproduced, but it was also a quite real place and a decisive episode in the history of colonial medicine. Despite the evidence, accepted by the doctors themselves, that this experiment was a nearly complete failure, it would inspire how health actions were imagined, planned and institutionalized after the end of the war in French Africa.

This empirical case will, herein, serve to reconsider how historians and anthropologists have approached the medical government of Africa and, in particular, how this issue has been frequently described with metaphors such as 'experimentation' and 'living laboratory'. The purpose is not simply to object to these metaphors as being exaggerations or simplifications or to recall that a gap always exists between the intentions (experimental, humanitarian, disciplinary) voiced by doctors and actual realizations. That approach has become relatively classical nowadays and has even defined a research agenda in colonial studies (Stoler/Cooper 1997). Instead, this paper elaborates methodological propositions for moving beyond the alternative between a naive, literal description of biopolitical projects and a critical stance that amounts to showing that reality is more complicated or that big projects never work.

This paper proposes to reconsider the historiographical status of failure. It argues that hygienist or experimental utopias were productive in their failures, because they opened up a space of critique, reform or reaction. The paper begins with a review of the question of failure in the history of medical government, and suggests to avoid two historiographical pitfalls: forgetting the existence of failure (when we literally interpret doctors' claims about making Africa healthier, or about rationalizing the continent); and presenting the failure as the outcome of research by historians (when we concentrate exclusively on the contradictions and stalemates of colonial, experimental or medical 'governmentality'). After presenting a few theoretical points and the case of Haut-Nyong, I shall draw up a hypothesis about the *positivity* of this failure. How was the (systematic) failure of biopolitical utopias—instead of being a 'discovery' made by historians—a crucial factor in: their design, the rhetoric surrounding them, their implementation and their aftermath? By placing failure at the centre of analysis, this approach enables us to directly address the questions of medial powerlessness and hubris, not as retrospective assessments and ex post facto critiques of doctors' governmental ambitions but as positive and central aspects of the relationship between biomedicine and governance.

2 | Virchow (1848): "Die Politik ist weiter nichts als Medicin im Grossen."

REVISITING THE 'COLONIAL LABORATORY'? A REVIEW OF THE LITERATURE

Experimentation has been a favourite theme in the history of colonial medicine. Even though experimental medicine in the colonies has not been the subject of many studies as such (exceptions being Pelis 1995 and Bonah 2007), the term 'experimentation' has met with success in historiography, where it serves as a loose metaphor for government interventions in the colonies. Bruno Latour's (1984) thoughts on the Pasteurian revolution have been influential in interpreting colonial medicine as a 'living experiment'. According to him, the Pasteurians saw the colonies as a field where they could give free reign to their reformist ambitions (Dozon 1985). The "Solons of the tropics" were able, in these new lands, to come near to a "pasteurization of society" (which they had vainly sought to achieve in their homeland) by turning a whole society into a laboratory in the sense of a controlled, controllable place organized by scientific rationality and devoted to producing evidence and order.

Other authors, inspired by Michel Foucault's (1997: 89) well-known proposal about the "reverse effects" on the European world of colonialism's political techniques, have also described colonies as laboratories. For example, Paul Rabinow (2005: 289-317) has portrayed colonial Morocco (in particular, the Rif War) as a "laboratory of modernity" for French military officers, technocrats and planners. This phrase has even become a commonplace in the history of colonial sciences and techniques. Countless dissertations, articles, chapters and books have borrowed this figure of speech (e.g. Tilley 2001; Eckart 2002; de l'Estoile 2004; Braun/Hammonds 2008). Most of this research, though well documented, uses the word "laboratory" in a lax way (an exception being Anderson 2006). As a convenient metaphor, the word has had echoes in recent condemnations of using Africa or the "South" as fields for "delocalized" experiments (Shah 2006). Recent studies have precisely, yet problematically, described the colonial world (Africa, in particular) as the place of an "experimental governmentality" where political rationalities, though initially restricted to the domain of scientific research, were expanded to the scale of a whole society and population (Bonneuil 1999 and 2001), or even as the ultimate phase in a process of "experimentalization of the world" that had started in 18th-century Europe (Chamayou 2008).

There are several problems with adopting these ideas and metaphors. A general critique points to the confusion of intentions with realizations (Stoler/Cooper 1997: 6). Some studies, though excellent in other respects, treat the colonial doctors' writings as self-fulfilling discourses (Dorlin 2006; Chamayou 2008). They fail to take into account the internal incoherence of such declarations, the criticisms levelled against them or the material factors restricting their application. This version of an experimental governmentality that was "ordering and disciplining the tropics" (Bonneuil 1997) should be qualified by taking seriously the study, as initiated by Mbembe (1996), of indiscipline and disorder in the colonial context.[3] In like manner, Foucauldian interpretations of colonial health actions as a laboratory or "matrix of subjectivation" should be reassessed given that colonial medicine was, in most areas on the continent, satisfied with interventions quite limited in time and space, as Megan Vaughan (1991) has pointed out.

A second problem is more important. Simply put, the metaphor of experimentation was a favourite figure of speech used by colonial authorities themselves. For instance, the Pasteurian Charles Nicolle (1934: 142) referred to his medical surveys in Tunisia as "experimentation in action"; and Louis Tanon, the director of the Institute of Colonial Medicine at the Faculty of Medicine in Paris, wrote: "The hygiene of our lands [...] has every reason to draw inspiration from the experiments carried out in vast territories, where relatively primitive races dwell whom European civilization has not yet transformed." (1930: ii) Commenting on colonialism's life-size experimentation thus amounts to paraphrasing the writings of colonial science.[4] This is not a problem in and of itself, but this calls for a careful discussion of the role of this metaphor in the colonial context. The question of experimental metaphors, in other words, must be tackled pragmatically (Sibeud 2002: 12-13), by analyzing their force in the negotiations conducted within the colonial administration; their appropriation by professional groups such as doctors; their function as a source of legitimacy in the eyes of French public opinion; and the critical, ironic or indifferent reactions to them.

Several strategies can help to renew the study of the colonial laboratory and of medical and experimental utopias in Africa without merely dismissing the metaphor as an abusive simplification of a much more 'complicated' reality.

To formulate the question differently, a first possibility is to discuss the actual function of colonial utopias in imperial societies, in particular: how were the colonies presented to public opinion back home as an ideal place for public health interventions? For instance, campaigns against sleeping sickness or the experiments in social engineering conducted in leper-houses often had

3 | Mbembe: "In colonial disciplinary plans, as in what has been called native 'responses', there was always a proportion of 'misses', of the 'unexpected' and of 'disorder', which research has, till now, described with an incredible lack of precision. This proportion of 'misses', of the 'unexpected', of 'disorder', of the 'unforeseen' and of 'aborted efforts' or, in more positive terms, of the use of reason, is what we call 'indiscipline', especially in cases where it is consciously constructed, and without taking into account the results and effectiveness of the actions undertaken." (1996: 33)

4 | For examples of colonial doctors using this metaphor, see Anderson (2006: 113-114); and on Cameroon as a "field of experiments", Martin (1921: v-vi).

an inordinate impact on opinion in the colonizing country (Dozon 1985 and 1991; Lyons 1992; Edmond 2006; Lachenal/Taithe 2009). However these experiments, which usually went under that very name, had a 'materiality' as important for us as their 'posterity' back in Europe, where they were seen as ideals for public health interventions. Rather than being living laboratories or life-size experiments, the colonies were different and differentiated spaces that provided doctors with rhetorical resources. To pursue a classical analysis in line with Foucault (1994), the colonies would have to be seen as "heterotopias" or "counterspaces" rather than as a laboratory—as a constellation of projects both material and rhetorical, real and theatrical, that public health activists could use back in the homeland as a mirror, as a desired and idealized reflection.

What I would like to propose is a complementary but pragmatic approach to the idea of a laboratory. This approach should be limited neither to observing a gap between grandiloquent intentions and reality (Fassin 2001) nor to contriving variants on the theme of a "thwarted utopia" (Murard/Zylberman 1996). We might simply set the idea of a living experiment opposite the list of the thousand budgetary, theoretical and practical difficulties encountered by colonial health services and doctors. But this "analytics of failure", to borrow from Gary Wilder's (2005: 78) critique of colonial studies, is not satisfactory. It takes no notice of the fact that the gap between discourse and reality was, in part, positive. It is possible to move beyond the alternative between paraphrasing experimental metaphors and rejecting them as mere normative prescriptions that complicate understanding a much 'truer' everyday reality. How did the claim of conducting a living experiment weigh on daily actions? What effect did the publicity given to colonial experiments have on practices? How did the experimenters refer to, and interpret, the gap between plans and practices, especially when they depicted the failure in political, scientific or aesthetic terms? What we need to understand is this experimental governmentality's materiality and performativity: what did it mean to govern and be governed in a place said to be a laboratory?

A last proposal: taking seriously colonial medicine's experimental claims (in both their materiality and rhetorical effects) also implies accounting for the hubris rife in them. Since the 19th century, at least, the growth of experimental medicine had been associated with a critique of mad scientists and the insanity of science (Bonah 2007). Likewise, a reflexive approach to the colonial laboratory entails acknowledging an immanent critique, omnipresent in colonial literature, of the megalomania underlying the very idea of a living experiment.[5] Understanding medicine or, more broadly, the colonial government as a thwarted or frustrated utopia spares the rationality of such plans even though they were—at the time—

5 | Colonial megalomania evidently makes us think of Rudyard Kipling's short story, *The man who would be king* (1888), and Joseph Conrad's *Heart of darkness* (1902). Louis-Ferdinand Céline's *L'Église* (1932) includes a satire on colonial medicine.

the target of criticisms ranging from ironical remarks on the ineptitude of "pilot projects" (Mazenot 1996: 21) to public scandals (Taithe 2009).

In a pioneering study, Warwick Anderson (2006: 9, 74-103) has shown that the first impediment to realizing the colonial doctors' hygienist dreams was "colonial nerves", i.e., cases of "neurasthenia", "Congolitis" or "delusions of grandeur" among staff members, including doctors. Such cases were so frequent that, in the colonies and homeland, medical-psychiatric institutions—and many a publication—were devoted to them (Abatucci 1910; Martonne 1930: 109; Martin 1932; Jennings 2006; Dozon 2008: 50). Johannes Fabian (2000) has proposed an incisive reinterpretation of the history of the late 19th-century ethnology of Africa. According to him, the vast operation whereby anthropology was to put the continent "in order" was a task undertaken by explorers who were exhausted, alcoholic, addicted to morphine, madly in love or sick with malaria, and whose means of knowledge had more to do with ecstasy (to use a positive word) than cold rationality. This has opened the way for shifting the critique of colonialism "from the question of guilt to that of error" (Fabian 2000: 281). In the case treated in this chapter, it opens onto a hypothesis about the function—not just anecdotally in terms of blunders—of delusions, irrationality and nihilism in the biopolitical government of colonial Africa.

AN INITIATION IN HUBRIS: THE HAUT-NYONG EXPERIMENT, 1939-1948

"We are neglecting no measure capable of interesting natives and rousing them to pursue, despite themselves, their own well-being." (David 1942:70)

The metaphor of the colonies as laboratories of modernity fits well to the history of medicine during World War II (Gaudillière 2002; Harrison 2004). Techniques used decisively in Europe, such as DDT or mass blood transfusions, were experimented through colonial Africa (Rabinow 1999: 84; Fintz 2004; Schneider/Drucker 2006). Furthermore, Allied campaigns in the tropics tapped new technologies—jeeps, jerry cans and bulldozers—that would come to symbolize international public health after the war (Amrith 2006). New forms of organization and governance also emerged during the war. Mark Harrison (1996) has cited as an example how a generation of British military doctors represented a new "culture of command" defined by its "managerial ethos" and a style of leadership freed from the code of military bravery.

Experimentation represented a key value in this new governance. In the army, a specifically colonial ethos set store on inventiveness and individual initiative. Colonial doctors—the majority of doctors in the Free French Forces—enjoyed talking about "their war" in Africa without gasoline, alcohol or drugs, and about the thousands of ways of making up for shortages (Lapeyssonnie 1982). Doctors thus had the opportunity to learn their trade. This was especially so for young specialists like Henri Laborit, who referred to colonial hospitals as "an absolutely astonishing field of experiments" for surgery (Laborit/Grenié 1997: 19; Keller 2007: 229-230). The situation led to seeing the empire as a world without limitations, where genuine experiments in policy-making could be carried out. Indeed, extreme tests in governing territories and peoples were conducted, as in Anchau, Nigeria, where British colonial doctors displaced populations, founded a town and tried to invent a new native society (Nash 1948; McKelvey 1975). Far from hamstringing the ambitions of colonial public health, WW II reinvigorated them. As Dominique Pestre (2004: 14) has argued, the war was often an initiation in hubris for scientists and statesmen. This is the angle from which I would like to tackle the case of Haut-Nyong.

Time for utopia

In early 1940, Richard Brunot, governor general of Cameroon, explained his approach to the governing council:

"I placed the Haut-Nyong region fully in the hands of medical authorities. By giving these doctors the leadership of this region, I wanted to signal my determination to grant in all matters an absolute priority to all that is human. Before developing the land, it is necessary to produce people; and to this end, what better method than to confer the task on health technicians? Their policy will mainly center on developing bodies and families. They will, in a word, make a medical administration. Planning, breeding, feeding, healing, thus is defined their role." (Journal Officiel du Cameroun 1940:118)

This project borrowed slogans from the improvement (mise en valeur) policies that, imagined since the 1920s, had sprung from the same mixture of colonial humanism, demographic obsessions, techno-scientific optimism and references to France's generosity (Coquery-Vidrovitch 1979; Conklin 1997; Wilder 2005: 43-117). This was not the first attempt in French colonial medicine to create a sanctuary where public health would reign. In fact, the Haut-Nyong medical region had the same bounds as the "sector of prophylaxis of Haut-Nyong", the principal area of activity during the 1920s of the Mission against Sleeping Sickness. The head of this Mission, Eugène Jamot (1935, quoted in Froment 1988), had demanded to be granted "in the infested zones [...] the authority of a surgeon in his operating room". The "camp" at Ayos had become a "medical campus", base of logistics and centre of research for the Mission. It even enjoyed an extraterritorial status, since it was placed directly under the authority of the governor of Cameroon with no interference from the local administration (Tantchou 2007). Owing to the emergency legislation in French Cameroon, everyday medical, administrative and police powers could be merged. Doctors in the countryside were granted "disciplinary powers" (CAOM 1924). Furthermore, the Indigenous Code on the legal status of colonized peoples contained a few ad hoc offences, such as the misdemeanour of "not executing prophylactic measures".[6] Whether the fight against sleeping sickness was an administrative or a medical question was a topic of discussion between the two World wars, both in French imperial circles (Martin 1931) and on the League of Nations's Hygiene Committee, which officially recommended granting police powers to doctors (LNHO 1925).

Turning the whole area into a medical region in December 1939 signalled a change of scale. Dr. Jean-Joseph David, a colonial army doctor (alumnus of the Naval Health School of Bordeaux and of the School of Application at the Pharo in Marseille), was appointed to head the region, assisted by six other doctors in charge of the region's subdivisions. Marcel Vaucel, head of Cameroon's Health Service, summed up the situation: "The Haut-Nyong, worked for years now by doctor-prospectors familiar with all its nooks and crannies, was already a region of medicine. Thanks to Governor General Brunot, it is now a medical region where everything will be done for the sake of the native's health." (1940: 162)

The project was launched in a propitious political environment. In French Cameroon, doctors had, since the 1920s, managed to obtain a political and financial backing without parallel in Africa, usually by brandishing the threat of Germans coveting their former colony, which had been made a French and British mandate after WW I. The French administration's health policy in the former Kamerun was a favourite target of procolonial lobbies on the other bank of the Rhine. It was an international issue and a subject of long debates at the League of Nations (Eckart 1997; Callahan 1999 and 2004; Essomba 2004). Cleverly blown out of proportions by French colonial doctors, the German menace was used to justify health programs that had no equivalent in the French Empire (Headrick 1994: 405-406). The argument was never as plausible as in 1939, with the looming spectre of Germany coming back to Cameroon.

Besides, the ambitious, pragmatic formula of a medical region served to govern at a lower cost, since savings were made on assigning administrators to an enclave that was the historical centre of sleeping sickness in the colony and, too, an underpopulated area. Throughout the period between the two World wars, underpopulation was seen as an insurmountable obstacle to development (Geschière 1983). The idea of a medical region was not new: the German campaign against sleeping sickness, suspended by the Allied takeover in 1914, foresaw handing over to doctors administrative responsibilities for the most

6 | "Infractions spéciales à l'indigénat", order of 4 October 1924. Special offences were published in Gazette du Cameroun, 14, 15 November 1924.

infested zones, the aim being to avoid frictions between administrators and the service in charge of the campaign (Kuhn 1914).

The war breaking out in 1939 did not change the situation, quite to the contrary. When Cameroon and French Equatorial Africa tipped to the side of Free France in 1940, colonial doctors stood in the front ranks (Sicé 1946). The director of the Institute of Hygiene in Douala, the Pasteurian Jean Mauzé, and the head of Cameroon's Health Service, Marcel Vaucel, won renown by rallying Cameroon to the Free French cause in late August 1940; they then joined the French Resistance in the Sahara. In French Equatorial Africa, Colonel Adolphe Sicé, an army doctor and director of the Pasteur Institute in Brazzaville, was among General de Gaulle's first supporters. In 1941, de Gaulle appointed him *haut-commissaire* of Free French Africa, the name given to the new imperial territory encompassing Cameroon and French Equatorial Africa. For the colonial medical corps, the time had come for military heroism, administrative responsibilities and policy innovations. The Haut-Nyong experiment was a project where men could prove their mettle.

Dr. David drew up an action plan defined as a "social undertaking with demographic aims" (1942: 57). Haut-Nyong's medical administration was not intended to merely facilitate the work of doctors by leaving them to freely organize public health campaigns. The intent was—and this moored the experiment in a hygienist utopia—to give doctors as much freedom as possible including in matters of political and social organization. The project adhered to the "social medicine" ideals that the Rockefeller Foundation and League of Nations (Weindling 1995) had advocated during the interwar period, but without referring to them outright. When David warned in the first report, "No demographic recovery can be imagined without introducing thoroughgoing reforms in native society" (1942: 58), he was not trying to list the levers of actions beyond his control but, instead, to enumerate the priorities for his "direct medical administration". The head of the region was trying to administer a political medicine, not simply a public health program. He insisted:

"It would be vain to think that an isolated medical action suffices for re-establishing the demographic equilibrium if it is not completed with major works in hygiene, education and economic infrastructure. Cleaning up the country, building model villages, developing individual resources, in a word, improving the native's social situation are ultimately the most effective weapons. That is, on the administrative level, the task that falls on the medical region." (David 1942: 40)

This program stands out owing to its experimental ambitions. A twofold objective, political and cognitive, ran through it: lift the population but also meticulously describe this lifting and thus test the worth of administration as a method for improving public health. The medical region was a test in scientific government: not only were enlightened technicians in charge but, even more, the government itself was an experiment (Murard/Zylberman 1984, Bonneuil 2001). This justified support for the project, in particular the large number of qualified persons assigned to it. According to Dr. David, this price had to be paid if the "Haut-Nyong region is to favourably pursue its destiny. This is the price for collecting what might be unique documents." (1942: 109) But he worried lest, lacking the means for endowing the project with a scientific dimension, "this experiment loses most of its interest and its genuine significance".

A telltale fact: the reports on Haut-Nyong not only circulated inside the local administrative pyramid but were also sent to specialized circles back in France. The Sleeping Sickness Committee in Paris, on which colonial doctors and the mandarins of Parisian parasitology sat, greeted the project in 1941 as "evidence showing the administration's full interest in the native's well-being" (Commission de la Maladie du Sommeil 1941: 14). For these experts, it was a trial run since "the creation of medical regions should multiply on a large scale" (ibid.).

Actions were planned and assessed scientifically. An "action plan" was submitted to the governor and the Ministry of Colonies in February 1940 (David 1940) and again in 1942 as a four-year plan. The results were published. A new journal in Brazzaville, stamped with the Gaullist Lorraine Cross, Revue des Sciences Médicales, Pharmaceutiques et Vétérinaires de l'Afrique Française Libre, served as a forum for the Haut-Nyong doctors. An administrative routine changed: the yearly report was replaced with a "study on the direct medical administration of a distressed demographic [sic] region" (Médecin-Chef de Région 1944[7]). Besides the usual policy reports, doctors published their medical/sociological diagnoses and their reflections on the program and its results, which were quantified and discussed.

The medical administration was, indeed, an enterprise for producing documents and records. Individual health records were systematized; "rounds of screening and inspection" (a medicoadministrative technology par excellence) were expanded beyond vaccination campaigns and the fight against sleeping sickness so as to count and follow up on pregnant women, syphilitics and infants or even inspect cacao plantations. By 1940, the Haut-Nyong medical region was routinely said to be an experiment or experimentation. This was much more than a metaphor. It shaped actions and made the utopia into something material, starting with all the paper used for documents and records.

---

7 | The other existing report, which I have not consulted, bears the same title: Médecin-Capitaine Souhde, chef de la subdivision de Messamena, extrait d'étude médico-administrative de la subdivision de Messamena, 1940-1946, Archives de l'Institut de Recherches Scientifiques du Cameroun, Yaoundé, dossier H, Haut-Nyong. Geschière (1982: 161) has mentioned it.

The medical administration as social therapeutics

The documents produced by Haut-Nyong's medical administration provide a clear-cut (indeed, astonishing) example of how a policy was implemented that not only focused on the population but also proposed subjecting all administrative actions to demographic requirements. Control and transform the bodies of persons, manage and reform the body of society, rationalize government actions: Dr. David and his colleagues were striving to design and apply what, in Foucauldian terms, can be called biopower: a combination of disciplinary institutions at the scale of the individual with biopolitical regulations at the scale of a territory (Foucault 1976: 177-191; Foucault 1997: 213-234). Let us review this total approach—as the doctors imagined and described it—to demographic recovery and, coincidentally, to the invention of a new society.

Child care with the goal of "fighting against denatality and forming a physically and morally healthy generation" (David 1940: 2) was proclaimed the priority. Maternity was to be medicalized. Pregnant women were systematically tested during doctors' rounds in villages: each one examined, registered and summoned to go a month before the due date to a maternity centre. In the towns serving as subdivision seats, 36 new buildings were erected for creating maternity hospitals. Women were to be hospitalized for 45 days in order to spare them "the customary chores and [to receive] advice about elementary hygiene for the new-born" (David 1942: 7). A regional circular fixed their diet down to a gram of salt during this period "when they only eat and rest" (David 1942: 39). More than a thousand women in Haut-Nyong were following this regimen in 1940; and more than 2000, in 1943 as compared with fewer than 700 in 1939.

This medicalization of maternity was a classic objective in public health programs in colonial Africa (Hunt 1999, Hugon 2005); still, its experimental ambitions were especially striking in the Haut-Nyong. The program's success was to be judged by the fact that the "influx of women and children made it possible to gather information" (David 1942: 10). Besides records on pregnancies, an individual record was made for each infant and filled in during the "visits of control at home", which were part of the precisely planned monthly rounds. These rounds served to follow up on the survival and growth of infants and on their gradual infestation with helminthes and malaria. Infant mortalities were recorded with an accuracy seldom reached in Africa at the time (Bonnecase 2008). Graphs of weights were drawn for each administrative subdivision, and compared with European data. Even better, the program's effects were quantified: doctors assessed how the length of mothers' hospital stays affected the weight of infants at birth, and concluded the program had a "healthy influence" (Médecin-Chef de Région 1944: 3-4).

A second part of this program was education. Dr. David planned to fully reorganize schooling so as to serve the "genuine goals of educating adolescents and teaching them how to live" (1942: 43). To reach this "humanitarian goal", the program provided for weekly conferences on hygiene by doctors or their assistants, monthly visits for tests, the individual health files to be kept, work in fields and workshops, and meals in cafeterias where pupils "will learn to eat properly and healthily". The ultimate goal was to take "the native at the age when he is the most receptive" and, David imagined, prepare "a class of small farmers and ordinary village craftsmen, open to our ideas and trustful of our methods" (1940: 44). The region's nine schools were rebuilt; three more were opened in rural areas; and a new regional school was set up in a "nice building" in Abong-Mbang, the seat of the administration (David 1942: 48). More than a thousand pupils between seven and fifteen years old, wearing khaki shorts and shirts, were enrolled. David remarked that "nudity, rags and dirtiness are disappearing" (1942: 45).

Sports, which David defined as a "sanitary discipline", completed this program. Although this was not exceptional at the time (Bancel et al. 2003; Cantier 2004), the Haut-Nyong experiment even stood out in this respect owing to its clearly stated ambition to group "the totality of native youth under medical control" (David 1942: 2). The 1940 action plan announced: "The number of pupils being limited, many young people run the risk of not escaping from their isolation. Sporting associations seem to us the organization best suited for subjecting youth to our medical and administrative surveillance." (David 1940: 44) Every morning between 7:00 and 8:00, a lesson in physical fitness was given in all the medical region's centres. A thousand young people were thus assembled every day. The practice of sports was compulsory in schools (Chef de Région 1942: 52). 26 soccer teams, wearing football shirts and shorts, played against each other for the title of regional champion. According to a circular, the year was to be punctuated by events leading up to the championship. At the end of a semester, qualifying matches involving all pupils were held in each subdividision's village seat in the presence of David himself, who supervised a long series of events ranging from 100-meter races to javelin-throwing. The finals, organized every year at the time of delivery of the certificates marking the end of primary school, brought the best pupils to Abong-Mbang, where a big stadium had been built. This was a success, as David wrote: "The young natives keenly appreciate matches; they thus acquire health and the spirit of discipline wherein they are lacking." (1942: 53)

To "some day give to the fertile land of Haut-Nyong the sturdy arms that it requires", an equal effort—just as ambitious and planned—had to be devoted to adult health care. Proposed in 1940, this program included a "range of administrative and health measures inseparably dependent on each other" (David 1942: 58), most of which were applied by the end of 1942. It was based on a socioeconomic study that doctors had made of farmers in the region. Taking the Bulu area in southern Cameroon as an example to follow, this study saw the source of prosperity in the development of intensive cacao farming. More than five million cacao-trees were planted by late 1943. To improve the local food supply, soya seed was bought and distributed. In 1941, subdivision heads were asked for a report on livestock: doctors counted all livestock and bought hundreds of sheep for persons who did not own any. The head doctor drew up a plan for improving breeds by selecting rams. The 1940 action plan dwelled at length on "community hygiene". The ideal village was described along with its model homes, field for sports, place for laundry and latrines (David 1942: 71). Major roadwork projects were launched; approximately thirty kilometres were opened in 1942 at Messamena, following an "impeccable layout evincing the qualities of endurance and initiative of Dr. Koch, the young subdivision head" (David 1942: 76).

The next point was demographic: "repatriating emigrants and driving out vagabonds". Once again based on a statistical study, the policy advocated by these administrator-doctors sought to put an end to emigration, which had been at the origin of the "continual losses affecting a population that has already borne the brunt of a reduction owing to major endemics" (David 1942: 92). Dr. David demanded the repatriation of at least two thousand persons from Haut-Nyong who were living in other areas in French Cameroon, and even of prisoners serving sentences elsewhere.

Medical actions as such were more or less secondary in this total conception of a population policy. The fight against sleeping sickness was, of course, to continue as it had "for long years now" (David 1942: 105). Thousands of syphilitics were recorded, treated, followed up on and studied. There were enough cases of leprosy to justify plans for an immense leprosarium near Abong-Mbang, which was to include a maternity, court, prison, centre of commerce and buildings for education (David 1942: 97). This literal utopia in a utopia, to be located at fifteen kilometres from the nearest dwellings, was to lodge two thousand patients.

The "emergency measure that is the medical region" (David 1942: 109) did not pursue the single objective of fighting against epidemics, nor even of sparing these efforts the usual frictions with other fields of government action. As Michel Foucault saw in the "plagued city [...] the utopia of the perfectly governed city" (1975: 232) in 17th-century Europe, we are tempted to see in the Haut-Nyong experiment an ideal form of biopolitical government. During a trip to London in September 1942 for a conference on the "postwar problems in Africa", General Sicé appraised the medical region:

"We have tried [...] an experimentation. It has been done in a region particularly afflicted by sleeping sickness and malaria, the Haut-Nyong. The demographic situation there was so serious that this zone's economic output had lost all value. The decision was made to confer the direction and administration to doctors from the colonial Health Corps. The results seem to overshoot all expectations. Death has stopped decimating villages; the treatment of sleeping sickness and malaria has put an end to sterility in households; maternal and child care have caused a sharp increase in the population in several villages. People, released from their obsession with death, have redeveloped confidence in themselves, and are lively and cheerful once again. In this region, life has won; prosperity has come back; people have overcome the forces of destruction.' (1943: 32)

A Foucauldian interpretation of this medical administration falls short, as does an a posteriori discussion of the project's progressivist aspects, as proposed by Wang Sonné, who sees in all this the starting point of the region's development owing to the introduction of village cacao plantations. Let us make no mistake about the biopolitics of the Haut-Nyong experiment. It comes as no surprise that the implementation of the reforms imagined by David would meet with infinitely more impediments than suggested in Sicé's daydreams. By insisting hereafter on the practical and political limits of this experimentation, the intention is not to discover a failed utopia (a point of little interest) but to show how both observers and the parties involved in the Haut-Nyong experiment diagnosed this failure and reacted to it, often by making the situation worse. The doctors themselves as well as missionaries present in the area spun other versions of the history of this medical region. These versions, in the documents and reports, suggest an other, disquieting image of the Haut-Nyong utopia.

Rubber for the Emperor: A counterhistory of Haut-Nyong

"Commandant David [...] has gone completely crazy", according to the Archives of the Congrégation des Pères du Saint-Esprit (Mission de Lomié 1941b). In late 1941, the fathers of Catholic missions in Haut-Nyong could not stand it any longer: "The head of the region, David, [...] is certainly the biggest fake and nonbeliever we have ever had in Abong-Mbang. [...] What a sad situation, and dangerous too." (Mission de Lomié 1942c)

For the missionaries, the hygienist utopia was turning into a bad dream, because Dr. David had a "horrible character" (Mission de Lomié 1942b: 104) and, above all, because his policy of experimentation was competing with the Catholic missions' core activities: guiding bodies and souls through everyday life. The fathers in Lomié complained that when David did not convene the population on Ascension Day, he "chose on purpose Sunday to come see 600 people [a medical visit]: pregnant women, syphilitics and others. Obviously, anything that keeps them, Christians or catechists, from coming to mass." (Mission de Lomié 1941a). When he came back in September 1942 for a control (Mission de Lomié 1942a), "It's always Sunday!" in Messamena, the subdivision head, Dr. Henri Koch, was not appreciated either. He grabbed pupils from the mission to fill the benches in his own schools and made them work in the fields (Yaoundé/Divers

1942). He even arrested two local missionary instructors during their round of visits, whom he accused of "abandoning their village" (Mission de Messamena 1943)—the fight against vagabondage was taken rather seriously in the Medical Region.

The surveillance and confinement of pregnant women or syphilitics were competing with the missions' *sixas*, disciplinary institutions for girls only, which were a mixture of a boarding school and a work camp where Christian girls spent long months before marriage (Laburthe-Tolra 1999). Doctors accused the *sixas* of sheltering persons carrying trypanosomes who were to be confined to their homes in villages (Yaoundé/Divers 1942). It was of no help that some missionaries felt sympathy with the cause of Pétain and the Vichy government. One of them, driven to despair, complained, "When will the reign of the Freemasons be swept away?" (Mission de Lomié 1941b) Called to the rescue, Graffin, the bishop of Yaoundé, recommended moderation: "We should not enter into the administrators' private lives, as long as there is neither rape nor other acts of violence against our Christians." (Mission de Doumé 1941) To put an end to these conflicts (among other reasons), he decided in 1942 to confer the eastern province, much of it part of the medical region, to Spiritan missionaries from Holland.

Skirmishes between the missions and colonial doctors were nothing exceptional (Daughton 2006), at least not in Cameroon. Mongo Beti's novel Le pauvre Christ de Bomba (1956) contains a burlesque account of a "raid" that the service for fighting against venereal diseases made in a Catholic mission. Through such anecdotes, we see another account of the utopia emerging.

The picture in the reports filed by doctors was also painted in shades of gray. The tone of the very first report was disquieting: "The dwindling number of the European staff has reached a limit" and risked "irrevocably causing the Haut-Nyong experiment to collapse" (David 1942: 120). In fact, the whole medical staff counted initially but six permanent doctors (Vaucel 1940), helped by a few assistants: "poor whites" who learned medicine on the job and an unknown number of Cameroonian auxiliaries. In 1943, only three doctors, including the head of the region, still remained; and no relief was in sight (Médecin-Chef de Région 1944: 5). Drugs were in short supply, in particular the arsenicals needed to treat syphilis. Guidelines were rewritten with the old prescriptions of mercury and bismuth.

Medical humanism had to make tough decisions during this time of shortages. The program planned, for instance, the compulsory confinement for a month of treatment of any syphilitic dwelling more than a day's walk away from a dispensary. How to apply this measure? It was not only severe (carrying sanctions for those who refused) but, even more, expensive (the cost of lodging and feeding hundreds of sick people). Dr. David proposed a radical solution to his assistants—turn the dispensary into a work camp:

"To be able to carry on with your tasks despite present difficulties, you will exceptionally be able to hire the male syphilitics in cure as administrative laborers [sic]. The regulatory withholding on their wages will enable you to feed them. As for the question of accommodations, it can be easily solved by quickly building a few additional huts with mats and bamboo." (1942: 102)

Putting patients to work became widespread: persons afflicted with sleeping sickness or leprosy served as labourers for clearing water holes (an 'agronomic prophylaxis' for eliminating tsetse flies) and the site for the regional leprosarium. Another option was to put children to work on coffee plantations in order to free time for the mothers to devote to household chores.

The labour problem, particularly acute since 1930 following the expansion of big European plantations of cacao and coffee,[8] complicated the doctors' plans for social programs. The first action plan (David 1940) started by aggressively accusing European planters in the region of exploiting the population, fostering a native proletariat and flouting medical authorities. During a dinner, Dr. Koch sparked controversy by calling the mine owners "gangsters" (Yaoundé/Divers 1942). The labour shortage was widespread, and the doctors had trouble finding for their "administrative work" able-bodied men, since the latter preferred wages from the planters. The cause, according to the doctors, could be traced back to a decree issued in 1937 after the French Popular Front ratified the International Labor Office's convention on forced labour. According to it, "Labour is free in Cameroon." For David, this "declaration complies with our principles [...] but is the worst of mistakes since—in the Haut-Nyong where hands are scarce—it has sown, owing to the interpretation made of it, confusion and disorder." (1942: 84)

It was necessary to put an end to this "faltering principle of freedom of labour" (David 1942: 84) and to give the administration full control over the recruitment and movement of manpower. Forced labour, in other words, appeared as colonial humanism's last resort. Although the phrase was not used, the context provided doctors with the opportunity in 1943 to tighten controls over the labour force, controls for which local administrators had been hoping for more than ten years (Geschière 1983: 96; Joseph 1986: 62-70).

---

8 | Geschière (1983) has shown that the development of big European plantations in Haut-Nyong was the official strategy for the "*mise en valeur*" (development policy) in the 1920s. Given the labor shortage during the 1930s, the growth of the plantations came to be seen as a threat to the region's political and economic stability and to the operation of the administration itself, which had trouble recruiting personnel (including for medical campaigns). The colonial administration changed strategies in the 1930s, and tried to control work migration and foster small village plantations. This option was supported by doctors in the medical region and pursued, after 1945, by the population.

Population statistics proved embarrassing, and even vanished from reports after 1942. The infant mortality rate definitely fell the first year, but was not calculated thereafter. The improvement in demographics was not discussed. To observe a real "rise in the social level of the natives", the first report claimed it would be necessary to wait "a certain time". Nothing was known about population trends; but fear was expressed in 1942 about a "poor demographic balance" (David 1942: 119). Pneumococcus—a disease never targeted by colonial medicine—was devastating whole villages (David 1942: 119). One out of two deaths of children from two weeks to two years old had been caused by "lung diseases", a vast category beyond the doctors' knowledge and power (Médecin-Chef de Région 1944: 4). At the end of 1942, "model villages" existed "nowhere" (David 1942: 71). A start, just barely, was made at building the leprosarium in 1944. By 1942, the situation was distressing. The establishment of the medical region coincided with the switch to a war economy.

Latex was being harvested again, after having been nearly abandoned since 1915. World prices, at their lowest during the interwar period because of the expansion of hevea plantations in south-eastern Asia, exploded once Malaya, the Dutch Indies and French Indochina were lost. To deal with the expected shortage, the Allies were building up strategic stockpiles, intensifying research on synthetic rubber and lowering speed limits to keep tires from wearing out so fast (Wendt 1947; Oyebade 1998). Despite its poor quality, African rubber, drawn by itinerant tappers from various species of vines and shrubs in the forest, was indispensable (Giles-Vernick 2002: 159-166). The forests in eastern Cameroon and the Belgian Congo were being tapped.

The doctor-administrators held an ambivalent opinion about this new economic situation. Given the price hike (from one franc per kilo before the war to twelve in 1944[9]), rubber truly occasioned a windfall, which locals (as well as European merchants) knew how to catch. Let us recall that, since the end of the 19th century, the history of rubber in eastern Cameroon, as elsewhere in Africa, was marked as much by acts of plundering and coercion as by a pragmatic adaptation of African peasants and traders to world price trends. This was evidence of an integration in the international economy that colonial authorities often simply followed in order to "tame" or "parasite" it with taxes (Dumett 1971; Harms 1975; Geschière forthcoming). The Haut-Nyong had been one of the first areas where a rubber rush had occurred at the turn of the century before coming to a halt when prices collapsed in 1913. German authorities had had difficulty controlling the trade and preventing violent incidents between tappers and traders, incidents that worsened as the locals who harvested latex acquired more wealth and weapons (Geschière forthcoming).

9 | These were the local prices practiced by European merchants (Mission de Doumé 1944: 129 and David 1942: 63).

Thirty years later, the doctors in Haut-Nyong, whose economic policy sought to accelerate the acceptance and circulation of currency, understood that the harvesting of rubber and palm oil (with a comparable boom in prices) was the only way for natives to pay taxes while waiting for their own crops to ripen for the market. In pursuit of its regulatory ambitions, the medical administration devoted the whole subdivision of Lomié, the remotest area in the region, to rubber and conferred the harvesting on certain ethnic groups (David 1942: 63). The official objective was to limit the impact of the windfall, which would "not outlast the end of hostilities" (David 1942: 63), on the regional economy. Demand for rubber was "dangerously reviving the native's taste for long treks in the woods" (David 1942: 63). To harvest wild latex, long trips were necessary, as well as a botanical knowledge and technical know-how beyond the control of colonial experts. This was the exact opposite of the sensible peasantry that the doctors dreamed of seeing in model villages. David feared a "general return to nature" (1942: 119). As for the missionaries, they worried lest the free-flowing money "lead our people to their ruin"; a priest in Lomié wrote about the "fortune that rubber is leaving in the region and to say that it will be so poorly used" (Mission de Lomié 1943: 124).

Even though it represented an attempt to channel native agencies, the compromise chosen by the administration was rather brutal. To limit the impact of the boom on the regional economy, only a few tribes were mobilized for the harvest. Ever larger quantities of latex were required as of 1942, and force came to be systematically used. The missionaries in Lomié railed against this in their diaries: "A very low attendance at mass because the subdivision head made everyone leave for rubber." In 1943, "all the men are in the forest [...] 62 tons [of rubber] on the market on 30 January. No one at mass." In 1944, the subdivision head was even more severe following a poor harvest: "Everyone is out for rubber, because [he] has used a strong hand: all the chiefs [of cantons and villages are] in prison, the others are afraid." (Mission de Lomié 1943 and 1944)

Doctors and missionaries were well-placed to observe the fallout from the region's economic development. A missionary in Lomié noted in 1943, "the other event is the ravage wrought by sleeping sickness. Several cases have been detected by health officials. There were more than a dozen in Pohendoum alone." (Mission de Lomié 1943: 124) The doctors confirmed in their annual health report the outbreak in Pohendoum, a village "providing shelter to forest rubber-tappers" (Farinaud 1944: 31). Harvesting latex and contracting sleeping sickness were known to be linked since the start of the century. This linkage figured in African accounts of the illness and had been an insolvable dilemma for colonial administrations (Lyons 1992). The latex-producing vines mostly grew along waterways and in swamps where tsetse flies proliferated. The ongoing search for new sources of latex meant long trips across infested areas;

and the meeting of people, when taxes were collected or the latex was brought to market, facilitated transmission of the disease.

Colonial doctors in Haut-Nyong faced the most painful of paradoxes, which was never clearly formulated: the sleeping sickness epidemic—the very reason for the medical region and its founding myth—was proof that their project had failed. Worse yet, the epidemic partly resulted from their own actions. Statistics on sleeping sickness showed a sharp drop in the region since 1935 at least. Between 1937 and 1939 (before the "medical command" was set up), the number of new cases in relation to the total population dropped nearly 50% a year. This trend continued more slowly between 1940 and 1942. But then the incidence of the disease shot back up, from 0,17% to 0,29% in 1943, 0,34% in 1944, 1,29% in 1945 and 4% in 1946—a figure that had seldom been recorded, not even at the peak of the 1920 epidemics (Farinaud 1945, 1946 and 1947). Between 1940 and 1943, the rubber harvest in Haut-Nyong soared tenfold, overshooting 400 tons and probably even more in 1944 and 1945 (David 1942: 73; Médecin-Chef de Région 1944: 11), while American imports of African rubber reached 35.700 tons as compared with 7.300 in 1940 (Wendt 1947: 208).

The problems caused by the rubber boom were aggravated by an upsurge in world prices for minerals, a stimulus in Cameroon and all of central Africa to the mining economy and for mineral prospection (Dumett 1985). The Haut-Nyong was not spared. The alluvium of the Nyong River contained rutile, an oxide of titanium used in the paint for airplanes and automobiles. The rutile rush was a cause of despair for Dr. David, who saw his few remaining workers leave for open pit mines along the river—a location known to harbor tsetse flies. Production reached 2.000 tons in 1944.[10] An irony of history: the discovery of the rutile deposit is still hailed as a contribution that the colonial Health Corps made to Cameroon's development. In effect, two colonial pharmacists, Le Floch and Dufour, discovered the deposit during the war (Oudart 2005).

The recrudescence of sleeping sickness but two years after the enforcement of the emergency regime was made worse by the doctors' own projects. In 1942, Dr. David decided to place the region's future leprosarium in one of the last known strongholds of sleeping sickness, Madouma near Abong-Mbang. The laborers sent to work there in 1943 came down with the disease. Given the labor shortage, they were patients who had been sent there from leper-houses in the region. When they returned back to their leper-houses in 1945, they "caused a new, serious outbreak [of sleeping sickness] at the leper-house in Messamena" that spread to the neighbouring village and Catholic mission. The worst was yet to come however. When the leprosarium in Madouma finally opened its doors in 1946, the decision was made to (this time definitively) transfer there all leprosy

10 | Statistic from the website on present-day plans for mining rutile in Haut-Nyong. http://www.akonolinga.net (accessed 14 July 2008).

patients in the region. According to the health service report, "several lepers who realized that contaminations had occurred the previous year in Madouma ran away: the outbreak in Messamena spread even farther, as new, small outbreaks occurred nearly everywhere at random depending on where the runaway lepers carrying the trypanosomes stopped for the night." (Farinaud 1947: 167-168) Was there any surer proof of how lucid the leprosy patients were about the doctors' generous intentions? The story would be a mere anecdote had the outbreak in Messamena not caused one of the severest epidemics in Cameroonian history.

The final results of this medical administration? Without any doubt: a failure, all the more painful insofar as it left the doctors speechless. As Vaucel wrote, the medical region was supposed to put an end to the "muted conflict that for a few years has set the administration and medicine at odds in the Haut-Nyong region: administrative officials half-heartedly applying regulations they claimed were incompatible with country life, and doctors persuaded of the futility of their purely technical efforts and demanding observance of the texts." (1940: 162)

By conferring the command on doctors, the medical administration deprived them of their favourite enemy: the "narrow-minded bureaucrats" in the colonial administration. The doctors thus came face to face with their own powerlessness.

Conclusion

Following a gradual return to normalcy as the number of doctors assigned there decreased, the Haut-Nyong medical region was finally dissolved in 1948. Besides reminding us that Free France, like Vichy, had its share of biopolitical hubris,[11] the short experiment in Haut-Nyong significantly influenced colonial policy. It was replicated in 1944 in Ubangi-Shari (Giles-Vernick 2002: 101-107), and would be cited as an example to follow in manuals of tropical medicine till the late 1950s. To quote from the chapter on sleeping sickness in the foremost textbook of the times: "In the areas afflicted by the epidemic, the 'medical region' formula, which conferred administrative powers on the health service, is especially to be recommended as achieving a maximal unity of medico-administrative goals." (Vaucel 1952)

The Haut-Nyong experiment served as a reference point for the Brazzaville conference in early 1944, which organized health actions for French Africa (IMTSSA 1944). The convergence between the "reactionary utopianism" of the

11 | The importance given to a disciplinary control of women and youth in the Haut-Nyong experiment was very similar to the Vichy government's colonial policies (Jennings 2001).

Brazzaville plan and the Haut-Nyong experiment cannot be ascribed to chance. There were only two doctors on the conference's health committee: Marcel Vaucel, who headed the Cameroon Health Service when the medical region was created and then later became director of the Health Service in the Commissariat for the Colonies in Algiers; and Lt.Col. David, who had just been promoted to the top of the Health Service in Yaoundé. It comes, therefore, as no surprise that this health committee cited the medical region formula as an example and recommended it "for areas exceptionally afflicted by social plagues" (IMTSSA 1944). Without exaggerating, we can refer to Haut-Nyong as a laboratory and school of hubris, since this experiment foreshadowed the extraordinarily ambitious turn taken by colonial health policies after the war, policies lacking in neither daydreams nor disasters (Lachenal 2006).

Official accounts of the Haut-Nyong experiment should not be seen as mere propaganda that tried to cover up a posteriori the real situation, which has been described herein. On the contrary, this chapter should help us see the gap between reality and utopia not as a historian's finding but as the grounds for critiques, actions and subjectivities. What is noteworthy is not so much the systematic failure of social medicine's vast ambitions—in Haut-Nyong and in experiments conducted elsewhere at the same time (Marks 1997; Cueto 2004)—as the historical possibilities ensuing from this failure when it was recognized by the doctors themselves: an increasing reliance on coercion, the quest for technical solutions and, too, a sense of renunciation, which was the nihilistic counterpart to the utopias of social medicine (Roussin 2005).

Public health has constantly pondered this failure. As Didier Fassin has pointed out, the history of public health can be "described as [...] an endless denunciation of its shortcomings and failures" (2001: 54). What transformed certain major colonial doctors into heroes and models for the profession was, precisely, their failures, and the associated drama. The biographies of Eugène Jamot and Gaston Muraz, who had eliminated a disease during the 1920s and 1930s that would loom again as a menace in 1948, read as a series of victory announcements followed by clashes and dismissals (Bado 1996). Inspired by these unfortunate but adored heroes, and rife with an ambivalent "desire for failure", the ethics and aesthetics of colonial doctors harboured a nihilistic potential, which works of literature, ranging from Céline (Roussin 2005) to Sartre (2007), clearly portrayed. By placing immense hope in the ambiguous Africa (Balandier 1957) taking shape before their eyes, the doctors knew they ran the risk of being disappointed and losing their illusions. Historians reveal nothing by exposing these disappointments and lost illusions. On the contrary, the doctors found in them the very meaning and grandeur of their mission. In conclusion, we wonder whether this nihilistic and sometimes delirious—or rapturous—aesthetics was not the very grounds for breeding the political pretensions of these doctors and humanitarians, both of the colonial doctors of yore and of today's heroes of "global health".

A final question: did Commandant Dr. David actually "go crazy", as the missionaries thought? It is hard to answer. He was promoted to head the Cameroonian Health Service in 1944 but passed away shortly after the war. He was buried near Abong-Mbang, where his grave apparently became a shrine.[12] One piece of evidence, reported in the oral accounts collected by Wang Sonné: Dr. David, a referee in pole-vaulting and foreman at construction sites, an obstetrician and demographer, a cacao-farmer and builder of schools, left behind the memory of a "very dreaded" man. He was known as "the Emperor of the East" (Sonné 1998).

Dr. Koch, his deputy and head of the Messamena subdivision, pursued his career after the war, drawing on the expertise he had acquired. Stationed in the early 1950s at the Federal Hygiene Service's headquarters in Bobo-Dioulasso, he conducted demographic and statistical studies (Koch 1949, Le Rouzic/Koch 1949) before turning to the ethnology of "his" tribe, the Bidjoués of Messamena (whose language he spoke) and publishing a book on them in 1968. Faithful to the ambitions of the Haut-Nyong utopia, he penned, in 1967, an esoteric, meditative reflection on the "medicine of hope". A quotation chosen by chance gives the tone of this book and lets us free to imagine what the medical rationality in power in Haut-Nyong amounted to during the long years of war and the rubber trade: "No sick person and no doctor, no individual and no society, will ever be able to deny that the druid's dolmen is alone in its place in reason on this earth." (Koch 1967: 120)

12 | Fieldwork is needed to corroborate this point and confirm the grave's location. In a private communication, Peter Geschière stated that, in the 1970s, locals said that pupils laid their workbooks on Col. David's grave for luck in passing examinations.

Intellectual Property Designs: Drugs, Governance, and Nigerian (Non-)Compliance with the World Trade Organization

Kristin Peterson

Introduction: the WTO and global governance

The launch of the 1995 Trade Related Intellectual Property (TRIPs) Agreement, a global trade treaty housed in the World Trade Organization (WTO), coincided with a number of key events that tied intellectual property (IP) to global trading governance for the first time. Beginning in the late 1970s, global pharmaceutical industry profits were on the decline. In order to counter decline, the drug industry turned to more speculative practices,[1] which promised high economic growth. Through industry lobbying efforts, TRIPs was implemented to protect both speculative pharmaceutical capital and future drug product sales around the world. It mandated that IP linked commodity distribution be governed by an enforcement mechanism carried out by the WTO. It also mandated that new pharmaceuticals be patented for twenty years.[2] In effect, these rules gave drug companies the right to set the price of products and sell them in competitive-free markets of their choosing. At the same moment that TRIPs was implemented, a massive HIV/AIDS crisis was in full force across the African continent. Moreover, anti-retrovirals for HIV/AIDS were being newly marketed and no generic equivalents were available. As TRIPS, antiretroviral production,

1 | These practices included acquisitions, mergers, initial public offerings on the stock market, and connecting upstream and downstream activity between long established drug companies and start-ups (Sunder Rajan 2006; Cooper 2008).

2 | TRIPs also created provisions that allowed living material such as microbes, DNA sequences, genomic plant varieties, molecules, etc., to be patented, leading to similar global debates (Juma 1989; Peterson 2001; Coombe 2003; Dorsey 2003; Nnadozie et al. 2003; Anderson 2009; Mushita and Thompson 2007).

and HIV/AIDS converged, treatment was widely unavailable or unaffordable in Africa in the 1990s and early 2000s.

All nation-state TRIPs signatories, that is, all WTO nation-state members, are required to recognize this IP linked trade regime.[3] Specifically, signatories are required to rewrite their intellectual property laws at the national level to match globally governed WTO rules. Five to ten years after TRIPs was launched, agencies and organizations including the US Department of Commerce, the World Intellectual Property Organization, the United Nations Development Program (UNDP), and many international NGOs provided competing services to African states to help them ratify TRIPs. Each was invested in drastically different, yet legally allowable, ideas of compliance. What was perceived to be at stake? The US, for example, viewed infringement of U.S. products in different parts of the world to be a threat to U.S. IP driven industries such as pharmaceuticals, music, and film. Other organizations such as UNDP believed that TRIPs would limit the prospect of widespread generic antiretroviral drug circulation to low-income countries.[4] TRIPs allows complying countries to incorporate flexible rules into their national laws, which in turn impacts the potential sales and availability of generic and proprietary drug products. At stake for both health advocates and drug companies was *how* countries would comply.

This chapter foregrounds ethnographic research conducted on Nigeria's efforts to comply with the TRIPs Agreement, where the U.S. 'assisted' the country in these efforts. The U.S. was concerned about pirated products that widely circulate in Nigeria. Pirated products began to emerge on Nigerian markets just after the oil shocks of the 1970s. As oil was, and still is, Nigeria's primary form of revenue, the country garnered a severe economic and debt crisis.[5] The country's creditors insisted upon austerity measures in exchange for new loans, otherwise known as Structural Adjustment programs (SAPs), which

3 | TRIPs, however, allows for a *sui generis*, or alternative notions of ownership, albeit one that is difficult to conceptualize. However, one such attempt, the Africa Model Law, articulates community based ownership, long in existence, as legitimate IP rights (which in orthodox terms, favors individual ownership, including corporations) that is legally binding with TRIPs (Ekpere 2001, 2003; Zerbe 2007); it took nearly ten years to conceptualize reconciling community and individual knowledge within the scope of TRIPs among many Organization of African States (OAU, now the African Union) scientists and lawyers who were charged with this task by the OAU Scientific and Technical Commission (Ekpere, personal communication).

4 | Health advocates, scientists, physicians, legal scholars, and policy makers have made a direct link between TRIPs and the number of people who have died around the world without access to affordable pharmaceutical treatment (Pecoul et. al. 1999; Correa 2000; Trouiller et. al. 2001; MSF 2001; Ford 2003; Cullet 2005; 't Hoen 2005).

5 | For work on oil in Nigeria see Okonta and Douglass 2003; Apter 2005; Watts 2008.

were overseen by the International Monetary Fund. SAP ended state subsidies and devalued the currency leading to a crash in manufacturing and high levels of household poverty.

Indeed one outcome of SAP was the immense growth of an informal economic realm where buying, selling, and trading thrive in the interstices of legality and illegality (Bayart/Ellis/Hibou 1999; Roitman 2005; Larkin 2008). Nigeria became home to one of the largest national drug markets in Africa where millions of drugs—generic, adulterated (referred to as 'fake' in Nigeria), substandard, 'dumped', and to a much lesser extent, proprietary[6]—are imported from countries all over the world (Peterson 2012). Moreover, software, music, and film, many of which are proprietary US products, circulate in this unregulated space. They represent the massive global circulation of goods linking Africa not to North American and European markets, but rather to Asian and Middle Eastern ones.

Critically, state privatization was the cornerstone of SAP. Because the state was massively downsized, existing and future regulatory bodies were incapacitated to do the work of the law. Specifically they did not possess the ability to curtail perceived infringement of proprietary products. And yet, just ten years later, the WTO mandated that Nigeria and other African states perform the robust task of protecting transnational capital by regulating counterfeit capital within the scope of the TRIPs Agreement. As an IP linked trade law is imagined to police and curtail pirated products, what do globally governed patents produce in a legally indeterminate environment?

This chapter considers this question by first discussing understandings of intellectual ownership that vary or inhabit differing legal subjectivities across Anglo-American and Nigerian contexts. Such differences emerge out of histories of market competition and business practices rooted in late colonial and early post-colonial periods. Here I show the legal and historical disconnects between Nigerian and WTO understandings of intellectual protection.

Second, is the role of the U.S. Department of Commerce (DoC) program that 'assists' Nigerian in complying with the WTO. The program constituted

---

6 | My definitions of generic, fake, and substandard follow both biological and legal understandings of these categories in Nigeria. I do not critically review these terms here. Generic is a manufactured non-patented copy of a proprietary pharmaceutical product. The manufacturing process usually attempts to exactly match the chemical make up of the product, referred to as bioequivalence. Fake is a drug, which is deliberately adulterated and is not intended to not meet the bioequivalence standard of a proprietary product; it is widely viewed as hazardous to human health. A substandard product may contain more or less bioequivalent standards in either proprietary or generic form. It is not always considered hazardous to human health. But often concerns arise around questions of especially drug resistance due to the wide variance in bioequivalency.

a series of meetings from 1999-2005 that I attended, which were hosted by several Nigerian actors and institutions. I discuss how over the course of this period, Nigeria's intellectual property law was essentially drafted by the U.S. DoC in a manner that complied with TRIPS, but also favoured U.S. business interests. AIDS activists contesting proposed U.S. patent legislation and musicians supporting the Americans in copyright legislation were the main contenders at these meetings. All of these actors—US representatives, Nigerian lawyers, and Nigerian non-governmental organizations—represent a divergent swirl of interests in considering the contours of a new Nigerian IP law. While TRIPs compliance is often portrayed as a struggle between large corporations and poor people, there are numerous local actors, some who interface with international actors, contesting their own stakes in the making of new rules and trading hegemonies.

LEGAL SUBJECTIVITIES AND DISCONNECTS: UNDERSTANDING PATENTS AND PROPERTY IN AFRICA

When the TRIPs Agreement was launched in 1995, signatory states agreed to adopt legislation within a given deadline, one that had to be harmonized across nation-states. Nigeria's deadline was 2000, the same year I arrived to conduct fieldwork. At that time, Nigeria established conferences and workshops that private lawyers and government workers attended. I was curious why Nigeria had waited until its deadline to initiate compliance. One reason had to do with how the signing of TRIPs was carried out. In my interviews with participants at these meetings, many claimed that the Nigeria's Geneva representatives do not communicate with either the government or the private sector. Some of the most prominent IP lawyers in Nigeria even claimed that no one really knew the names of the representatives who signed TRIPs on behalf of Nigeria.

This disconnect between different levels of government might be indicative of common civil service communication. But it also represents a particular moment in Africa's engagement with international trading disputes. TRIPs was first negotiated at the 1986 Uruguay Round of the General Agreement on Tariffs and Trade (GATT), a former Bretton Woods Institution that was implemented just after World War II. The GATT's objective was to facilitate consensus agreements among empires on global trade. Decolonization rapidly changed the terms of trade as many African countries entered global debates that were once the privy of an old boys' European diplomatic network.

Newly independent African states arrived at the Uruguay Round relatively unprepared to negotiate a new IP-trade framework (UNECA, 1996). The lack of preparedness had to do with practices of production as well as epistemological differences pertaining to the law (Ekpere no date; Sodipo 1997). On the one hand, the U.S. turn to IP driven innovation governed by global trade rules was motivated by a new phase of innovation that matched a neoliberal turn to speculative capital and practices in the drug industry. On the other hand, a small manufacturing industry in Nigeria was in the midst of complete collapse at the time of the negotiations. These industries relied upon relatively unsuccessful import substitution policies and not intellectual property as their driving force.

The Nigerian lawyers with whom I spent time over the years engaged these politics in various ways. Most lawyers do not have the luxury to specialize in intellectual property or other legal arenas, as they may elsewhere. Like African physicians, most are generalists, practicing law for the few who can afford it. Moreover, the public does not widely consider IP necessary to the work of commerce. That is, the primary form of business is trading—buying and selling imported products—and not necessarily IP linked innovated work.

As there are very few Nigerian patents filed in the Nigerian patent office, private lawyers mostly represent foreign IP interests. At the same time, they must juggle their analysis of what a 'negative' TRIPs patent compliance potentially looks like for Nigeria versus their client's interests. Despite being told by a few lawyers that, "I speak for whomever I'm representing," the contradictions of the legal circumstance that they must navigate are always present with them. One lawyer told me:

> "The patent system or the contemporary orthodox intellectual property regime emphasizes individual rights. On the other hand, the knowledge systems that exist traditionally in Africa involve a communal ownership of knowledge as well as some kind of obligation to share the knowledge inasmuch as there are some restrictions or conditions on them. In this case, knowledge and ownership can be shared freely in society. Even where the knowledge is located with one individual, say for a traditional healer, he holds it in custody for the entire community and that knowledge is constituted by virtue of his membership of that community. So it does not give him any personal or private rights to own that knowledge."

While this lawyer identifies one aspect of intellectual ownership in Nigeria, there are other forms. Intellectual property in pre-English civil code Nigeria included the equivalent of copyright, trademark, and patent protection. In the case of patents and marks, works in brass, bronze, gold, and wood had characteristics such that their origins could be identified. Some art often maintained insignias from different regions of the country (Asein 1994; cf. Sodipo 1997). Asein (1994) argues that there was not so much a recognition of individual authors, but rather the actual patterns of textiles, blacksmith work, or designs on pots, for example, could be decoded (via colour, design or quality) and their origins and communal reputations identified. Particular individuals or sectors of society produced certain works and exclusive rights to produce (from industrial inventive works to praise songs) were granted by local governance or leadership (Sodipo 1997).[7] An intellectual property lawyer describes how these systems to protect knowledge have long been in place in Nigeria, but conflict with the WTO system of protection:

"The guys who are in guilds[8] and cults who had inventive and arguably patentable processes, methods, and products had their own way of protecting. They could not read or write. The patent system demands people who can read and write. The patent system encourages you immediately to document it and put it in the patent office. [But] [t]heir own way of protecting is to initiate you into an oath of secrecy, into a system of taboos. And mythology and myths and so on are shrouded in secrecy. Now, since education came, and the patent system came, we want to encourage them to share their knowledge and we'll protect them with patents. The question is whose knowledge is it? Is it the individual's knowledge or the group's knowledge? The patent system doesn't recognize group's knowledge as community knowledge."

Patent law requires that one disclose the secret of one's invention. But in these artistic guilds, the moment one discloses a secret it can no longer be protected. In contrast, patent law protection is only rendered as such the moment a secret is disclosed. The same lawyer continues:

"If you want me to divulge it [referring to the reasoning of those poised to patent their innovations], you are now telling me it does not need standard of lenience because we have been using it. Then that means [the patent] system is not for me. So, that's the disconnect. You've introduced a system and you've not met the fears and the apprehensions of the people who are supposed to use the system."

Indeed, is the patent system meant for Nigerian use? The WTO's epistemological construct of property is adopted from Lockean terms of ownership—the mixing of labour and nature—which holds hegemonic interpretive sway in trade-related IP law (Locke 1698). But in Nigeria, many forms of intellectual labour

7 | Boatema Boateng (2011) argues that in contemporary Ghana, kente and adinkra cloth weavers identify multiple forms of authorship, including individual and communal. The communal aspect acknowledges that patterns and weaving emerge out of previous works of art. This is not uncommon to any works of art but because the author is privileged in IP law, these histories of intertextuality get erased.

8 | Similarly, Stephen Brush (1993: 654-655) describes that IPR grew out of Medieval European guilds. Like their African counterparts, they relied upon secrecy and treated the fruit of their labor as common property of the guild. He describes how the English Parliament in 1623 sought to restrict the power of the Crown's monopolies in order to encourage industry growth by creating a single monopoly, the patent.

are temporally dispersed in a way that cannot explicitly show who precisely did the labouring—a phenomenon that is hitched to practices of custodianship. Moreover some forms are not contributable to the single author, but rather, to multiple forms of authorship. Even though there are many kinds of ownership, trusteeship, and custodianship practiced in Nigeria, the country's IP law—inherited from English civil code—cannot account for these, much less international legal rules.[9] They must inhabit "unfamiliar forms of legal subjectivity" (Boateng 2011: 12).[10]

Built into negotiating frameworks that hitch the term 'global' next to 'harmonization' of IP across nation-states, Marilyn Strathern (1999: 186) argues that there are divisions between multinationals and indigenous people/Third World enterprise based upon ideas of a socialized technological competence. That is, "one side is embued with 'knowledge' made possible through 'technology' and the other side of this division has 'society' made effective through 'community'" (Strathern 1999: 187). Other Melanianist scholars have shown how there is little distinction between ritual and economic spheres of practice, meaning that it is difficult to actually distinguish knowledge through its potential in economic terms, as they are in IP trade frameworks (Harrison 1992; Leach 2000; see also Odell 2006).

Compliance with TRIPs means that there must be a move from domination to hegemony; and at stake are two legal sensibilities and subjectivities. One is mandated to become the main paradigm across nation-states while the other is meant to transform so that the legitimacy of this global model is acknowledged. Complying with TRIPs means installing an infrastructure that is more amenable to protecting foreign capital. It was not designed to protect local innovation. Indeed, in order to police Third World production and trade, TRIPs was designed to outsource protecting intellectual property and combating counterfeiting to the Third World itself.

By the late 1990s—four to five years after most countries signed the TRIPs Agreement—the U.S. became concerned that African signatories were not complying (or going to comply) as expected. What happens when knowledge regimes, linked to technology and geopolitics, are brought together in the realm of compliance?

9 | Nigeria Patent and Designs Act, Cap. 344.

10 | African policy makers analyzing the stakes of TRIPs, and of free-trade agreements in general, saw these differences as a way of establishing new trading hegemonies in Africa (Ekpere 2003; Nnadoze et al 2003).

A NEW NIGERIAN IP LAW: DIVERGING CONCEPTS, INTERESTS, AND INFRASTRUCTURES

In December 2000, representatives from the U.S. Department of Commerce as well as the U.S. Patent Office arrived in Nigeria ready to meet with their Nigerian counterparts. All were attending a conference called "Administration of Intellectual Property in Nigeria: A Stakeholders Conference", which was held in Abuja, the capital of Nigeria. This meeting was one of the first in a series, most of which I attended. On the agenda were two major tasks: the first was to elucidate the current status of IP in the country and the second was to brainstorm and make suggestions on overhauling Nigeria's IP law in order to come into compliance with TRIPs.

Two institutions organized these conferences—the Intellectual Property Law Association of Nigeria (IPLAN) and the Commercial Law Development Program (CLDP), a U.S. Department of Commerce (USDOC) initiative funded by the United States Agency for International Development. IPLAN is a Nigerian association of over fifty law firms and companies, which are either representatives or owners of intellectual property and/or are interested in the development of a regulatory framework. IPLAN's work is based on the conviction that IP rights can encourage local technical growth and foreign investment, and it lobbies the government for future changes. Many Nigerian lawyers attending these meetings have foreign clients invested in overseas IP protection. At the same time, many of the same lawyers have local clients wishing to protect their own IP in-country.

The U.S. Department of Commerce's CLDP mission is to support economic, legal, and political reforms around the globe. CDLP was founded in the late 1980s when the former Soviet block fell. It was tasked with assisting newly transforming states with "commercial law changes necessary for a successful transition to market economies" (CDLP no date). The ultimate goal was to establish the legal requirements necessary to accede to the WTO. These international technical assistance programs also aimed to improve oversight of publicly financed projects, rework regulatory functions, rewrite patent law, and enforce intellectual property rights IPR protection. The team from the CLDP was comprised of employees of the USDOC and the U.S. Patent and Trademark Office. The CLDP emerged out of the 1980s bilateral strategies to get TRIPs in place.[11] Coinciding with the declared 'war on terror' and various Bush II

11 | Peter Drahos describes how the "bilateral strategy had 'nice guy, tough guy' parts to it. The 'nice' guy part consisted of suggesting that proselytizing work be done by intellectual property experts in developing countries preferably under the aegis of some economic assistance program like U.S. Agency for International Development [USAID] (1995: 9)." The tough guy part involved creating strategies that would link foreign administration policy initiatives such as the U.S. Department of State's Middle East Partnership Initiative, CLDP expanded its operations into the Middle East and North Africa.[12] Around the same time, CLDP also expanded into Sub-Saharan Africa—mostly West Africa, where oil and U.S. security interests became increasingly important.[13]

The U.S. presence in Nigeria and other parts of the world was strongly motivated by a number of factors. First, U.S. software and pharmaceutical industries faced increasing global competition during the late 1970s and early 1980s. Instead of working toward improving its manufacturing competitiveness, these IP driven companies lobbied the U.S. government for an enforceable IP regime across nation-states via the TRIPs Agreement. Indeed, patent protection for many drug company products were nearing an end while at the same time global generic companies were outcompeting proprietary products. Second, by the late 1990s—five years after most countries signed the TRIPs Agreement—the US was motivated to protect copyright, specifically for software, and American films and music. It was also motivated to protect pharmaceuticals especially since demands for generic versions of antiretroviral drugs were on the rise. In Nigeria, there are (illicit) markets that are entirely dedicated to pirating and selling pharmaceuticals and software–the biggest in Lagos are *Idumota* (drugs) and 'Computer Village' (software). Indeed, one lawyer's interpretation of the US presence was that:

"[t]he US is pushing very hard to create an environment for companies that want the strongest intellectual property protection possible–interests that are solely driving the current developments. Those in power do not understand the implications. They only see these new developments in terms of getting foreign investment and don't see the impact on social welfare. They are willing to bend over backwards to foreign investors."

---

trade privileges to the quality of a country's work in curbing counterfeits and enforcing intellectual property protections. The U.S. Generalized System of Preferences and African Growth and Opportunity Act (which allows duty free and tariff free privileges in the U.S. market) are examples. Other examples included advocating linking debt reduction programs as well as IMF and World Bank loan programs to the legal infrastructure and implementation of IP law (Drahos 1995: 9; see also Drahos and Braitewaith 2007).

12 | Countries involved all include current US client states for which either oil and the war on terror are key issues of interest: Egypt, Bahrain, Oman, Qatar, UAE, Algeria, Morocco, and Tunisia (CDLP no date).

13 | It has also conducted work in the Southern Africa region, where South Africa has one of the most important markets for foreign goods on the continent. Angola is singled out on CLDP's website with its own description–one of the few sites of Cold War military conflicts that still rages (CDLP no date).

At the Abuja meetings, there were two different dominant discourses articulated by the U.S. team at this conference: first was the role of the law; and second, a correlation was made between strong intellectual property frameworks and economic growth. In my conversations with the U.S. representatives as well as observing and re-reading their presentations, it is clear from their view that the law is an "artifact of state power" or that it is made up of "norms" or a "coherent system" (Riles 2008: 606) that imagines the law to do certain things and not others. U.S. lawyers' understanding of how IP works in actual practice comes from their experience in the US court system—the enforcement mechanism for IPRs, which constitutes legitimate contours of property. While Nigerian lawyers (and perhaps more importantly the Nigerian public) may agree in theory that the adjudication of property is finalized in the courts, this is largely not their experience. For example, in any given legal scenario exercised in the court, settlements may be reached but not always acted upon (such as payments to an offended party, reinstatement of employment when unfairly terminated, etc.). And for the public, the judiciary is widely viewed as corrupt. The "rule of law" is differently encountered and understood.

The U.S. at these meetings explicitly articulated the second issue of economic growth, as a direct outcome of strong intellectual property laws. A representative from the CLDP presented statistical data that correlated this positive relationship:

> "One of the key ways in which IP protection is critical to economic growth is as a *precondition for financial and technological investment* [his emphasis]... In short, moving up the economic ladder is clearly correlated with exercising intellectual property rights. There is good reason to think that the causal relationship goes in both directions: that increasing wealth makes a country increasingly concerned about its intellectual property and increasing attention to its intellectual potential makes a country more wealthy."

Indeed, the data he presented articulated the boom story of the life sciences, whose growth was tied to speculative capital and IP-linked trade regimes (Cooper 2008). Taken as a given, the nuts and bolts of how 'good and harmonized' laws actually increase economic growth was never explained in his or other presentations. But the lack of explanation is built into the logic of the meetings themselves. The entire paradigm for economic growth, one that is connected to trade and investment, is driven by the belief that more economic stability comes when the state is privatized and barriers to foreign direct investment are removed. This discourse is extremely powerful, and indeed the entire structural premise of the WTO. Yet for Nigerian and other African economies it has been detrimental as they have suffered negative growth and difficult debt management under such logics.

At the Abuja meetings, there was no real discussion regarding the capacity of the Nigerian state agencies to operate in a way that would be expected in regards to TRIPs compliance. A lawyer who works closely with the Nigeria Patent Office told me:

"We don't have substantive examination in the Nigerian Patent Office. All they do is make sure that the forms are correctly filled and they grant a patent. So you can get a patent for almost anything in Nigeria today, even if it is expired. I mean it could fall into public domain in some other place and they may not scrutinize it. The reason for this is that there is no infrastructure in place: we need pharmacists, researchers, and so forth to do the examination."

The primary techniques needed for making IP do the work it is intended to do are 'search' and 'surveillance'; and Nigerian law requires that a patent application must be filed where the holder is a resident and expects that holder to seek out infringers. This requires the national patent office to have the capacity to discern questions or notions of infringement. However, Nigerian workers in the patent office have indicated to me that they are more often pre-occupied with a lack of steady electricity or interrupted salary payment. In my time spent there, I found little activity in an empty room of computers. Indeed, the US and European patent offices not only possess the capacity to build and search global data bases of IP awards, but also employ some of the top IP lawyers in the world to carry out search and surveillance.

The capacity to discern notions of infringement is not limited to the patent office. Also required are several state agencies to do the actual surveillance, policing, and punishing, meaning that the patent office, the drug regulatory agencies, drug enforcement agencies, and the courts all must work in concert to make this happen. Bringing Nigeria and others into the realm of enforcement indexes new economic and political obligations of the state, where a politics of enclosing the public realm is integral to regulatory politics.[14] In the new IP-global trade framework, regulation is not so much about how the state will police certain forms of capital over others. Rather, it is about how legal transformations recreate the state and its capacity to function in ways that match the demands of foreign market makers rather than the demands of its own public or private sector. Public expectations and demands on the state versus the state's non delivery of public goods, provides an air of systemic ambivalence that facilitates

14 | By enclosure I refer to how various publics such as the state must be erased or curtailed in the making of new property forms. There are a number of important works that draw on enclosure in numerous ways, most particularly privatization of the state, the public realm, public office, and regulatory politics. See Ake 1996; Mamdani 1996; Bayart/Ellis/Hibou 1999; Mbembe 2000; Chalfin 2010; Roitman 2005; Ferguson 2006.

an ideal US lobbying environment, where social and economic devastation meets promises of future prosperity of stringent IP law.

FAKES AND COPIES: MUSICIANS AND AIDS ACTIVISTS DEBATE COPYRIGHT AND PATENT LAW

At successive US-Nigerian forums on IP law, several organizations lobbied to make their concerns about the content of the IP law known. Especially prominent were AIDS activists organized around patent concerns and musicians organized around copyright concerns. Over time the U.S. developed a friendly relationship with the musicians who had long organized campaigns to raise awareness about copyright violation. Indeed their work is rampantly copied and used without permission, although they themselves buy pirated products because it is often the only way that one can access international film and music. Nigerian musicians, who had long orchestrated protests against the pirated use of their copyrighted music at both home and abroad, generated a particular understanding of IP protection that at the surface appeared to resonate with US concerns over counterfeiting. But the Americans were not so much interested in the protection of locally generated products like music. Rather they were invested in regulating counterfeited US products. Nevertheless, musicians' desires for a strong copyright law converged with U.S. desires for the same and an important alliance was built between the two parties.

In contrast, AIDS activists opposed the drafts on patent legislation. Activist interests lay in accessing much cheaper generic versions of HIV/AIDS medication. In the private markets, both generic and proprietary HIV drugs are not widely available. The main reason has to do with the fact that free drug programs outcompete the private market. But both AIDS activists and drug companies are equally wary of the availability of anti-HIV drugs on the private market. The former due to fears of self-medication, which is widely practiced in Nigeria and the latter because of profit margins as drug companies are subsidized in free programs. However, AIDS activists understood that access to generic antiretrovirals could be secured in future free drug programs including the potential for Nigerian companies to manufacture generics, rather than be limited to proprietary drugs.

Activist demands conflicted with U.S. desires to develop strong intellectual property protection for the U.S. based pharmaceutical industry. The U.S. DoC hired Nigerian and other attorneys living in the U.S. to write new drafts of Nigeria's patent law that restricted the circulation of generic copies of proprietary drugs in ways that exceeded the requirements outlined in TRIPs. At that time, the Nigerian government had initiated one of the first free HIV anti-retroviral programs in Africa, initially meant for 20.000 patients. All the drugs came from the Indian company *Cipla*. If the government had implemented the first draft, it would have made its own national HIV treatment program illegal.

An important issue at stake at these meetings was parallel importation laws. Once a more or less obscure concept in patent law, it had been harnessed in social movement slogans ("Demand Parallel Import Laws Now!" was adopted by the Treatment Action Campaign in South Africa). Parallel importation is significant because global pharmaceutical companies set different prices for the same products being marketed in different countries. The prices match what country elites can afford especially in the absence of widespread health care coverage. This means that the same anti-retroviral drug that sells in Nigeria can be cheaper than what it sells for in Spain or India. Parallel importation as outlined in TRIPs legally allows for a country to 'shop around' for the lowest price on the same product wherever it may be distributed in the world, so long as the parameters of such circulation are revised and stated in a country's IP law.[15]

For AIDS activists, the U.S. proposals were not the only obstacle to accessing generic HIV treatment. Nigerian patent law does not allow for any kind of parallel importation. The main reason is that among pharmacists and regulators, the term 'parallel importation' is used interchangeably with smuggling of usually adulterated (referred to as 'fake' in Nigeria) drugs. While this may sound like a minor problem, I witnessed several disputes including a great impasse on this definition at a 2005 conference on access to HIV drugs in Lagos where drug regulators and pharmacists could only make connotations to fake drugs and smuggling, and AIDS activists to generic drugs and patent law.

The resistance by pharmacists and regulatory officials is understandable. Products that sell well and fast are identified by international 'faking' companies and their Nigerian counterparts[16] for manufacturing and are priced lower for distribution. There are several countries that the public and regulatory agencies associate with fake products (India and China mostly) and those with what Nigerians refer to as 'original' or proprietary (Britain and the US, for example).

15 | These parameters of circulation in TRIPs are referred to as "national," "regional," and "global." If a country chooses "national" it means that parallel importation is essentially not allowed as proprietary products are limited to consume only what is marketed in-country. "Global" allows for the greatest circulation where products from around the world can be imported to compete with in-country marketed products. Activists argued for global circulation offering the widest possible search for cheaper version of the same product or its generic equivalent.

16 | For drugs, most of these companies are located in China and India, according to regulatory agencies and drug enforcement officials who have created "partnerships" in these countries in an attempt to stop piracy. Nigerian counterparts are those who work with such companies to import fake products.

If generics hit the market at already lowered prices, the potential for faking poses extraordinary regulatory challenges. Therefore, reconciling legal room for parallel imports with fake drug flows remains difficult with a state infrastructure that cannot entirely secure drug safety.

Fake drugs are born out of an infrastructure that developed at the height of structural adjustment. In this environment commodities linking West Africa with Middle Eastern and Asian markets, circulate on Nigerian markets that straddle licit/illicit and formal/informal realms. For instance, pharmaceuticals are considered legal products if they are copied or substandard, but not faked. They travel through legally defined 'illicit' markets, which are protected by organized unions and officially registered professional organizations. The substance of drugs and their routes of travel bestride realms that are never easy to discern by either pharmacists or regulatory agencies.[17] Yet, the global drug companies derive the bulk of their income from such markets and heavily rely upon them. Even though they are sites for which many fake drugs pass, global companies do not want these markets to disappear.

During one of the conference breaks, a doctor friend, who attended because of his interest in access to generic drugs, was agitated about the discourse of the discussion. He rhetorically asked me, "how many of the people on the panels, who claimed that piracy was evil, could actually avoid purchasing music and video in Nigeria that are not pirated?"

FINAL LEGISLATION IS DRAFTED BUT NOT IMPLEMENTED

With different interest groups contending the anatomy of a new law, the U.S. kept returning to Nigeria. It continued to set up different forums and conferences, all of which were financially supported by USAID (about $1.2 million total).[18]

---

17 | Others have reported the same kind of effects in different market sectors: Guyer 2004; Meagher 2007; Larkin 2008. The proliferation of second hand products that have "migrated into the mainstream" (Larkin 2008)—like spare parts, pirated video, etc—gives the WTO free trade anxiety yet is part of an infrastructure that got built out of SAP policy when many people were ejected from the formal economy. AbdulMaliq Simone (2006) demonstrates how notions of piracy help to understand the everyday practices of African urban residents attempting to create resourcefulness in cities that lack resources.

18 | At that time, AIDS activists had organized themselves in NGOs almost for the sole purpose of gaining access to HIV treatment, which was not widely available in Nigeria at the time. Yet, the donors to which they were linked, provided funds to organize workshops on human rights for people living with HIV and not on the possibilities of IP and access to drugs in Nigeria. Indeed, for US based donor agencies, the idea of commencing such

Lawyers and policy makers throughout West Africa were invited to a significant 2001 meeting. This meeting was advertised in the national newspaper, *The Guardian*. Among many items on the advertised agenda was a panel called, "Problems with Parallel Importation." When I arrived at the meeting, I was surprised to see that the panel was taken off the agenda. Presentations made by the US contingent directed attention away from parallel importation and instead focused almost exclusively on patents connected to internet and genetics technologies.

On the one hand, giving presentations on patents and genetics makes sense to the U.S. contingency. The reason is that patents under TRIPs were designed to protect new molecular technologies in order to promote financial growth for the pharmaceutical and biotechnology industries. Yet, on the other hand, West African lawyers and policy-makers at the meeting did not have clients or contingencies that were concerned about cybersquatting and single nucleotide polymorphisms.[19] The question and answer period during such presentations continued to bring up the issue of parallel importation, and more generally, generic drug circulation, which received virtually no attention. This was a crucial turn in these meetings—it was the point at which the U.S. limited its invitations to Nigerian musicians. When it came to patents, no invitations were extended to the Ministry of Health, state health agencies, drug authorities, or to local health and HIV NGOs.

After 2001, the meetings focused on finalizing IP legislation. The U.S. introduced stringent measures to draft legislation other than parallel importation. One of these measures was compulsory licensing—a government directive that can issue a license to a drug company to manufacture a patented drug without permission. Under current Nigerian law, a compulsory license can be issued by a government official to a drug manufacturer of its choosing for almost any reason. But this draft, written by the U.S., made it illegal. The TRIPs Agreement stipulates that compulsory licenses can only be issued in the case of health emergencies. There is still a dispute over what constitutes health emergencies at the WTO: the U.S. and European countries argue that a health emergency should be limited to malaria, tuberculosis, and HIV. African and other countries argue that a health care emergency should not be limited to three specific diseases. Despite disputes over these definitions, the TRIPs Agreement outlines a series of long and drawn-out steps that must be taken before a compulsory license is issued. Moreover, compulsory license rules apply to manufacturers, exporters, and importers; crucially, the change to one

activities were in contrast to US foreign trade interests. That is, access to generic drugs was viewed as impinging on the proprietary rights of the drug industry.

19 | SNPs are DNA sequence variations that occur when a single nucleotide in the genome sequence is altered.

country's IP law could impact not only domestic markets, but global circulation patterns—this especially true of Indian generic drug companies which are the largest exporters to Africa.

With health and patents off the public meeting agenda, Nigerian AIDS activists found out by accident about the meetings and muscled their way in. While activists could not successfully demand parallel importation, they did manage to keep compulsory licensing in the draft law, which was viewed as a great victory. But less than a year later the US returned apparently dissatisfied with this outcome and produced a new draft, this time under less public circumstances. That is, no announcement of the meeting took place and AIDS activists and even government health officials informed me that they did not know about it until its "successful conclusion" was announced on the evening news.

I acquired this new draft and it should be noted that one never knew where the real draft was actually located—even those people who appeared to be responsible for its existence. At several points I was literally chasing 'latest drafts' or pieces of them across ministries, hotel lobbies, and the National Assembly, more often in vain. This new draft turned up at the poolside of a posh hotel on Victoria Island in Lagos. It kept the compulsory licensing intact but now included "data exclusivity" otherwise known as an anti-Bolar provision. When a patent is awarded, an inventor must disclose how an invention is made in order to get a patent. The Bolar provision is a measure that allows researchers to use the disclosed data of an invention in order to understand it more fully—a measure used to advance science and technology in low income countries. An anti-Bolar provision allows the inventor to keep the data secret until the expiration date of the patent. Keeping data secret until expiration effectively reduces the generic drug industry's capacity to quickly manufacture generics and extends the life of the patent. Such an act actually undermines the original intent of a patent that exchanged inventive data for short-term exclusive marketing. Patents can additionally be taken out on all aspects of a compound—dosages, the compound itself, methods for making it—which creates a 'thicket' of intellectual property rights. Trade secret, copyright and trademarks are also imposed. All are typical strategies for dominating market segments.

Since the last organized meetings, several government sectors have worked out a new draft of the legislation, with some help from the US. No one to my knowledge knows what the draft contains and it has been sitting in the National Assembly since at least 2008. Nigeria was supposed to comply with TRIPs in 2000 and still has yet to do so, to the utter dismay of the US DoC.

CONCLUSION: NON-COMPLIANCE AND DISRUPTIONS OF GOVERNANCE

One of the reasons for creating TRIPs under the WTO was to attach a sanctions mechanism to the already existing GATT dispute resolution so that highly competitive 'copying' industries could be deterred. Plenty of actions were threatened or taken against countries such as Brazil, India, Cambodia, and Thailand since the establishment of TRIPs, all of which manufacture reputable pharmaceuticals that command regional or global circulation. Indeed just about any WTO member state that bans imports or which does not comply with TRIPs and other WTO agreements face trade sanctions. This could be devastating if a country relies upon one or a few principle exports for national revenue. However, sanctioning Nigeria would amount to sanctioning transnational oil companies whose extraction activities make up the bulk of Nigeria's GDP and a good chunk of US oil exports; and so trade sanctions are not imposed upon Nigeria.

As both SAP and TRIPs together were a two-pronged strategy for the U.S. to regain control of its 1970s position in the global economy, different infrastructures to facilitate goods emerged and conflicted. The infrastructure in Nigeria, characterized by legal indeterminacies, emerged out of the logics of devaluation and market reform (SAP), which in turn were woven into routine, everyday life. TRIPs' IP-trade regime was meant to stop the very market logics of copied and pirated goods that the 1970s crisis set into motion, and that SAP later exacerbated. A global system cannot apprehend the protracted ruptures that were in fact generated by earlier and similar logics of state privatization. So what of governance? While TRIPs continues to be debated at the global level, the question of local actors with local stakes may indeed thwart much of these desires for global harmonization of IP-linked trade.

Missing the Nation State

Serving the City: Community-Based Malaria Control in Dar es Salaam

Ann H. Kelly

Introduction

At 6:00 am, in a neighbourhood in the south-east of Dar es Salaam, a Community-Based Resource Personnel (CORP) begins his daily search for sites where the anopheline mosquitoes, the vector of malaria transmission, are likely to lay their eggs. After visiting the Ward office—a district level public authority—where he retrieves a larval dippers, maps and a stack of forms, he walks for three-quarters of an hour into an unplanned settlement, consisting of small houses and garden plots. He follows along a network of hand-dug rain gutters, stopping to dip a makeshift drain for the presence of larvae and marking down the distinct features of the habitat in his notebook. Making his way between and behind the houses, he is greeted by local residents, who let him into his plots to search for any accumulations standing water—rice patties, open containers, the puddles caused by footprints—where mosquito larvae might grow. As the day wears on, his work becomes more difficult: in the second neighbourhood he visits most of the plots there are fenced. Arriving at one gate left open, he knocks but gets no answer. Pushing open the gate, he finds a man holding a knife, who tells him—in no uncertain terms—to get out.

The aim of the Urban Malaria Control Programme (UMCP) is to reduce the incidence of malaria through the elimination of the breeding grounds of anophelines. Designed by a consortium of local, national and international partners, and initiated by the Ilala council—one of three municipalities that comprise Dar es Salaam—the programme aims to integrate mosquito larval control into routine municipal services (Mukabana et al. 2006). Between 2004 and 2009, the UMCP expanded across a substantial portion of the city, an area that includes fifteen wards and roughly 614,000 of the city's 3 million residents. At this scale, the UMCP is not only a research enterprise, but also a public—albeit temporary—service. It has received funding from a variety of sources—the *Bill & Melinda Gates Foundation*, the *United States Agency for International*

Development, and the *Wellcome Trust*—to evaluate the effectiveness of larviciding by conducting regular surveillance of mosquito breeding habitats and mapping the density of adult mosquitoes. These surveys are designed to determine whether the application of larvicide has been comprehensive and to identify areas that have been missed. The UMCP situates malaria control and research within a system of municipal management by delegating the responsibility for larval control to community members (CORPs) appointed by Street Health Committees across the city (Killeen et al. 2006; Vanek et al. 2006; Dongus et al. 2007).

The UMCP's emphasis on generating local capacity and building partnerships between communities, local government and researchers is a central component of international development and public health practice (e.g. World Bank 2001; WHO 2006). Community-based participation is deemed an essential aspect in public health delivery: the assumption is that by being involved in the planning and implementation of interventions citizens can take ownership of the technologies and practices that impact their lives (Hickey/Mohan 2004; Yarrow/Venkatasan forthcoming). In Tanzania, these participatory approaches are further rooted in governmental practice. Following independence, under Julius Nyerere's government, popular participation became a central instrument for socio-economic transformation: "if development is to benefit the people, the people must participate in considering, planning and implementing their development plans" (Nyerere 1967: 41). Much scholarship has interrogated how that political legacy has inflected current understandings of participation (e.g. Samoff 1979; Jennings 2007) and the traction of development programmes premised on community ownership (Green 2007, 2010; Jennings 2007).

This chapter explores how public health governance is articulated through scientific protocols, development practice and the specific political history of Tanzania. Its empirical focus is the encounter between CORPs, scientists, and residents, and the forms of responsibility that emerge when research practices are integrated into the fabric of urban living. The chapter is divided into three sections. It begins by describing the history of larval control from the first large-scale attempts at 'species sanitation' in the early part of the 20th century to latter-day applications of that method in Dar es Salaam. Of particular interest here is the relationship between the technical demands of larval control and the institutional settings in which these activities take place: how, in other words, the task of eliminating the larvae of *Anopheles* mosquitoes is shaped by the relationships between residents, municipal wards, the research institutions active in the city, and the upper echelons of state government. A highly-localized task of detection and management that traverses public and private landscapes, successful larval control is as much a civic as a scientific achievement.

The second section contextualizes that achievement by examining the political culture of Dar es Salaam. Tracking the multiple meanings of participation as an artefact of nation-building, an instrument of development and an emphasis of global health policy (Marsland 2006), we situate the project of larval control within its specific institutional setting. The aim here is not only to understand the scope and potential of enrolling community members in the elimination of mosquito larvae (Dongus et al 2007), but also to better understand the ways in which those capacities are shaped by the institutional forms and administrative practices designed to facilitate them (Green 2010: 1241).

It is within this historical framework that the third section considers the efforts made by the UMCP to transform Dar es Salaam into a 'truth-spot' (Gieyrn 2006), a space of public health intervention and, ultimately, an object of community ownership. This final section details the day-to-day work of the CORP and the multiple roles his work entails—as, at once, a compensated research participant, an informal labourer, and a volunteered public servant—and outlines the constraints and capacities of those multiple and, at times, conflicting roles for the integration of scientific resources into stable institutions (Kelly et al. 2010).

To conclude, the chapter reflects on the shifting alignments and inter-linkages of global science, municipal administration, urban life and pathogen ecologies illuminated by the UMCP. It argues that scrutinizing these contexts—and the spatial political required to manage the proliferation of urban mosquito populations—illuminates the extent to which public health governance in Dar es Salaam has been reconfigured by experimental platforms, and the implications of those changes for civic life in the city.

LARVAL LOGICS

He [Robert Koch] lays particular stress on the opinion of an unnamed 'expert engineer' that the most prolific Anopheles-producing area, the swamp at the mouth of Geresani Creek is undrainable. Let me here remark, by the way, that a survey showed this swamp to be drainable and that when I left Daressalam the creek and swamp were practically free from mosquito larvae, as a result of clearing the creek and ditching, which was done only on a small experimental scale because of the absence of funds.
A.J. Orenstein, 1914: 1932

A.J. Orenstein, an American doctor with extensive experience in public health campaigns, had been hired by the Rand Mining Company to advice on the sanitary conditions of South African mines (Packard 1989: 160-175). His contribution to the reduction of malaria during the construction of the Panama Canal earned him an invitation from the governor of what was then German East Africa, to institute a campaign in Dar es Salaam. He reported his findings in the *Journal of the American Medical Association* in a short article entitled: "Contribution to the Study of the Value of Quininization in the Eradication of Malaria." The piece responds to an article published in the previous issue by Graham Henson, who argued that despite excellent results of anti-mosquito campaigns in places like the Panama Canal, other places, could not expected to eradicate, let a lone, reduce Anopheles, because of poor drainage and climatic conditions. Rather than "wait for the development of our agricultural lands", another method should take precedence—the early diagnosis and rapid treatment of those infected (1914: 1374).

Orenstein's report begins by describing the city's racial geography. "The town," he writes, "is divided into two settlements: the white quarter, situated near the beach and a native quarter further inland" (ibid.: 1932). Though a common tactic of colonial urban planning, Orenstein's disdain for segregation as a policy for disease control is apparent in the comprehensive survey he provides of the city's vector breeding-grounds.[1] His focus rests squarely on the vector; which both bred within and moved across neighborhoods, regardless of the race of their residents. In a similar vein to his research in Panama, which provided an in-depth summary of the specific natural and man-made causes for malarial outbreaks, he details the entomological landscape of Dar es Salaam, linking topographical features and material conditions, marshlands and roof gutters, permanent pools in the native quarter and the sewage tanks installed in European Houses.[2] The report concludes with an experiment. He compares the decrease in parasite levels among "negro pupils of the Dar es Salaam Trades School who live in dormitories and do not come into contact with the outside population, were selected" (1914: 1933) who were treated with quinine over the course of eighteen months, with the infection rate of those living in the vicinity of a Karavanserai Pond, a permanent pool at the centre of the native area that, upon Orenstein's recommendation, was cleared of vegetation and treated with oil every ten days. The study showed a greater reduction in disease for the latter, even without having completely rid the area of Anopheles. [3]

That outcome did not merely demonstrate the public health potential of larval control; it directly contradicted the methods advocated by the famous German bacteriologist, Robert Koch. Following Charles Laveran's discovery

1 | For an elaboration of the role of racial theories in tropical medicine see Anderson 2002.

2 | Orenstein made the detailed case for the impact of construction, migration and urban development in the production of in the breeding success of the mosquitoes and amplifying malarial transmission in *Mosquito Control in Panama*, co-written with Joseph LePrince in 1915 (Sutter 2007: 747).

3 | Orenstein writes: "it is also to be noted that the control of the one breeding area did not by any means eliminate anophelines from the vicinity which the subjects were drawn." (Ibid. 1933).

of plasmodium parasites in the blood-slides of afflicted patients, Koch argued that the best approach to eliminate malaria would be to reduce the infection in humans. For Koch, malaria was, first and foremost, a clinical problem. Through mass treatment of symptomatic patients—particularly semi-immune native children, who, from the point of view of white settlers, represented a dangerous reservoir of infection—transmission could be reduced across the population. Under Koch's direction, Dar es Salaam became the site of the most extensive quinine distribution programme in Africa. Introduced in 1901, the programme involved taking blood slides of all natives working in the white quarter, and giving those found infected a routine dose of chemotherapy.[4] This systematic process, Orenstein points out, focused primarily on servants and artisans, while highly mobile traders, porters and agricultural labours were left untreated.[5] Further, the challenge posed by labour migration to prophylactic treatment is secondary to that introduced by the mobility of Anopheles. After implementing Koch's method for more than a decade, the incidence of malaria in Dar es Salaam had not changed significantly. For Orenstein, in contrast, there was no malaria without Anopheles; his experiment, he argued, clearly demonstrated why this was the case.

Orenstein's report underscores two key conditions of larval control. The first is the necessity of intimate ecological knowledge. In Panama, Orenstein worked under the supervision of William Gorgas, a Surgeon in the U.S. Army who had overseen the elimination of yellow fever in Havana. Gorgas was the pioneer of a method, which came to be known as 'species sanitation', that entailed a complex micro-cartography of intervention—draining marshes, cutting grass by river banks, covering pit latrines and garden wells, oiling ponds, filling ditches with concrete and footprints with sand (Packard 2007: 119-120). Koch's theories fell short, in part, because, Orenstein argued, they relied "on the opinion of an unnamed expert engineer" to contextualize conclusions drawn from the laboratory, as opposed to drawing on direct experience of Dar es Salaam's city streets (Kohler 2002).

But though entomological knowledge was critical to the systematic identification of breeding grounds, their destruction required both social and political capacity. Nowhere do these requirements receive greater emphasis than in Ronald Ross's seminal text, *Mosquito Brigades and How to Organize Them*

4 | The quininization program was implemented by Dr Ollwig, Staff Surgeon in charge of malaria control activities in Dar es Salaam, in 1902. For a detailed discussion of Koch's quininization program, see Curtin 1985: 597-598.

5 | This follows upon observations made by Burton (2003), that to a large extent the African urban populations were neglected prior to World War II: "the urban African was an anomaly in the context of indirect rule, which was predicated on the assumption that an African's identity was necessarily a tribal one" (ibid. 333).

(1902). It was Ross, who famously, during his service with the Indian Medical forces, associated the life cycle of the malaria parasite with the behaviours of the Anopheles mosquito. His strategy, which inspired Gorgas and a generation of public health authorities, outlined in meticulous detail how to coordinate a larval control campaign conducted with limited resources. He stressed the advantages of using local labour, not simply because it was cheap, but because it ensured access into the homes of local residents. No entomological training, no matter how advanced, could prevent the misunderstandings that might arise while searching through someone's trash (1902: 22).

Orenstein also stressed the pragmatic nature of larval control: even his small-scale experimental intervention made a difference. Further, he echoes Ross's emphasis on the necessity of political will and administrative support. At the conclusion of his report, he notes that his efforts "were rendered almost sterile by passive and active resistance, lack of funds, 'red tape' in volumes beyond the comprehension, I fear, of the average American" (1914: 1933). Successful larval control depended on a pervasive and persistent administrative presence; whether in the form of colonial garrisons or paramilitary forces, "a genuine campaign," Ross noted, "[...] must always be a permanent concern of the State" (1911, quoted in Bruce-Chwatt 1977: 1075).

Despite Orenstein's doubts about the commitment of the German colonial administration, by the time his article was printed, a series of sanctions had been passed to reduce mosquito-density in the city. Residents who failed to empty water daily from receptacles—including tin cans and coconut shells—on their properties were issued fines (a minimum of one hundred rupees) and those who could not pay were imprisoned. When Tanzania became a British Protectorate after World War I, these and similar measures began to be applied in earnest. A section of Township Rules entitled the "Extermination of Mosquitoes Ordinance", applicable to all small towns and settlements, elaborated rules for rice and potato cultivation and, demanded that property holders take the necessary steps at their own expense, to prevent mosquito breeding on their land (Clyde 1967: 13). Through the deployment of the Royal Army Medical Corps, the British also carried out a wide range of vector-control strategies, including comprehensive drainage work, stream straightening and livestock surveillance (de Castro et al 2010).

Conducted within the everyday spaces of urban life, larval control inevitably overlapped with sanitation, public education, urban planning and health surveillance. Arguably, it was the very civic character of larval control—its deep entanglement with the municipal fabric of urban life–that made it such an appropriate method for reducing malaria in Dar. Even in the late 1950s and early 1960s, the heyday of the DDT era, focused on altering the fabric of the city, in Dar es Salaam, larval control remained a central method throughout the 1960s and early 1970s. Reduction of malaria incidence was a central piece in Nyerere's plan for national development, a strategy that linked improvements in public health infrastructure to economic growth. With support from the East Africa Malaria and Vector-Control Unit, an organization created to provide inter-regional research (Beck 1970) and enhance Africa's scientific capacity, Nyerere's health initiatives had considerable impact both in Dar es Salaam and nationally. In 1971, the WHO East Africa Aedes Research Unit experimented with an integrated vector control programme in collaboration with the Dar es Salaam City Council. By 1973, the transmission rate of Dar es Salaam reached its lowest point in a century, ironically just at the moment when Tanzania's deepening economic crisis made environmental management programme economically unfeasible. As a result of the pressures of the IMF to rein in the country's budget deficit, spending on health was cut in half, the National Malaria Control Program was discontinued, and chemical treatment of the diseases through pharmaceuticals became *de facto* the sole anti-malaria intervention available. In the 1980s, the density of Anopheles in Dar soared (Yhdego/Majura 1988: 479-480).

It was not until 1988 that the city became once again the site of large malaria control intervention. The Government of Japan, interested in expanding its development aid portfolio, selected Tanzania as its key recipient and sponsored an integrated urban malaria control programme centred on mosquito surveillance. Over the course of eight years, the Japan International Cooperation Agency (JICA) donated resources, equipment and technical expertise amounting to roughly US$21 million. Despite its successes, for instance in rehabilitating drainage infrastructure, the programme never became sustainable (de Castro et al. 2004: 106). In an interview, one of the municipal directors involved in the project attributed this failure to the architecture of the intervention: in accordance with Japanese government policy, Japanese advisors rotated every two years, advising Tanzanian partners on the techniques of vector control but neglecting its more managerial aspects, such as data collection and analysis (Yamagata 1996).

Though not sustainable as a long-term programme of vector control, Japan's intervention produced a finely-grained cartographic profile of the disease. Routine remote sensory images and aerial stereoscopic maps documented the city's ecology and epidemiology, complementing records dating back almost a century. In an intriguing resumption of the work that Orenstein had conducted many decades earlier, the program's in-depth spatial analysis of the urban environment created the conditions to conduct a rigorous larval control campaign. As Marcia Caldas de Castro and colleagues have suggested (2004), the program failed to make use of local administrative resources in implementing the program. "[C]ommunity participation," they note, "turned out to be much more difficult to achieve than was anticipated" (ibid.: 114). The following section considers why this was the case. Through elaborating the political history of Dar es Salaam, it will explore how changes in municipal governance have shaped the civic capacities of the city's residents to participate in disease control.

COUNSELLING WARDS

Dar es Salaam was declared a municipality in 1948. This status coincided with a drastic shift in British colonial policy, from roundly ignoring African urban populations to encouraging their participation in government (Brennan/Burton 2007: 48-49). Up to this point, the city had been generally regarded as a white settlement serviced by a migrant labour force—a misconception that Orenstein's report had already sought to correct. As officials finally came to grips with the rapid pace of urbanization, a series of initiatives were put in place to stabilize employment and orient the development of an African civil society (Burton 2003: 335). One central component of this new colonial scheme was the establishment of Ward Councils to represent the interests of local residents to the Municipal Council. In contrast to the pre-existing communal associations, which officials dismissed as 'tribal', the councils were modern institutions, vehicles for transforming 'tribesman' into civic-minded townsmen (ibid.: 346).[6]

These efforts to involve Africans in municipal government were largely unsuccessful, as Councils were given little or no financial or administrative power (Iliffe 1979: 441). Political mobilization would emerge outside of, and ultimately in reaction to, colonial supervision, first in the form of labour unions and ultimately through the Tanganyika African National Union (TANU). Ultimately the Ward Councils inspired civic consciousness, but not the kind sought by the colonial authorities; as instantiations of the deep inequality between the different racial communities present in the city, they served to catalyze nationalist sentiment (Pratt 1976: 24).

When Julius Nyerere came to power, one of his central goals was bolstering the administrative powers of local government. Eager to distance the newly independent state from the political order of a colonial past, Nyerere abandoned the distinction between bureaucracy and politics and filled district-level positions with TANU chairmen (Picard 1980: 441). Initially, the politicization of the Councils was intended to instil commitment to a socialist cause. Through the philosophy of *Ujamaa,* Nyerere and his government aspired to liberate Tanzania

6 | 'Detribalized' is the term used by British colonial officials to refer to urban Africans, in the 1950s. This shift to a modern and multi-ethnic identity stood in contrast to the political emphasis placed on the notion of tribe by the Germans. While 'tribal elders' or chieftains provided the means to indirectly administrate rural areas, they were also critical actors in the political ecology of towns, as under German law, tribes were responsible for burying their dead (Burton 2003: 389-390).

from chronic underdevelopment by righting the imbalance between rural and urban development.[7] Mass participation and self-reliance were the tools through which Tanzania would be transformed into a modern, egalitarian society, one consistent with traditional African values. Bent on reversing the 'urban bias' of colonial administrations, Nyerere's policies of socialist collectivization implied a general shift away from cities and in favour of the agricultural core of the country –also known as 'villagization' (Pratt 2009 [1976]). As a symbolic gesture of shared purpose, he moved the capital from Dar es Salaam to Dodoma, a less cosmopolitan, but more appropriately 'African' town (Pratt 1999: 148).

To increase financial oversight of developmental processes, Nyerere introduced in 1972 a 'decentralization policy' that replaced local government with a network of regional and district officers (Picard 1980). In theory the system was aimed at coordinating grass-roots programmes, but in practice it served to shift decision-making powers for development from rural districts back to the centre of government. In his detailed analysis of local politics in Moshi during the late 1960s, Joel Samoff commented on the impact of this bureaucratic approach to development:

"The poor articulation of the links between the levels in development planning and the bureaucratic imperative to avoid responsibility where rules and precedents were not clear, function to nurture a tendency to shift decisions to higher levels and thus to limit local participation in development planning." (1973: 97)

Scholars have pointed to the post-colonial recapitulation of the centralist tendencies of the colonial state, a continuity that ultimately eroded the new state's capacity to enrol people in nation-building projects (Burton 2003; Pallotti 2008). In Dar es Salam, decentralization gave the City Council control over the urban councils, whose budget now depended entirely on the treasury. The government's bias against urban areas and the corresponding re-distribution of funding led to a deterioration in urban services and infrastructures, including water and power provision, waste removal, road maintenance and malaria control (Kironde 1995).

Dar's declining conditions led to the reinstitution of urban councils in 1978. But, without financial resources or trained personnel, ward councils and district-level authorities could do little to improve service provision (Kyessi 2005). As the economic crisis became further entrenched and structural adjustment measures were put in place, locally organized groups often took responsibility

7 | The literal meaning of *ujamaa* is family-hood: "for us socialism involves building on the foundation of our past, and building also to our own design...by emphasizing certain characteristics of our traditional organization, and extending them so they can embrace the possibilities of modern technology" (Nyerere 1967: 133).

for the public services that the state no longer could provide (Lewinson 2007). Once rejected as contrary to the spirit of *ujamaa*, informal, unofficial systems of economic activity and infrastructure provision filled the gaps left by the state and mitigated the deterioration of urban life. As Mari Ali Tripp suggests, 'the resiliency of society and its ability to reproduce itself with considerable autonomy from the state is one of the reasons the entire fabric of society did not fall apart during the unprecedented hardship' (Tripp 1997: 5).

In 1996, efforts were again made to formalize civic resources through decentralized planning. Following a National Conference, 'Towards a Shared Vision for Local Government in Tanzania', Dar es Salaam was restructured into a multi-tiered governmental body, with the City Council at its apex, three municipal councils, Ilala, Temeke and Kinondoni functioning as administrative intermediaries, and wards, subwards (*Mtaa*), and Ten-Cell Units (TCU) at its base.[8] While the municipal councils and ward officers are appointed and paid by the city authority, *Mtaa* leaders are elected by residents and work on a voluntary basis. They take responsibility for monitoring land development and organizing residents to perform basic and small-scale public health and maintenance tasks across the Ten Cell Units (TCU). The TCU is also equipped with a chairman, who, like a *Mtaa* leader, is elected by household members living within the cluster and works on a voluntary basis. By virtue of being closest to the 'community' TCU leaders are expected to attract finances from residents and inspire collective action (Gibson/McKean/Ostrom 2000).

The attempts to reduce the role of central government in the post-Nyerere era have been often connected to donor conditionality. While the vocabulary of 'self-reliance' and 'participation' remains, these terms no longer belong exclusively to a nationalist ethic, but rather describe a broader commitment to 'good governance'—i.e. to the efficient completion of specific projects in line with the performance standards of funders (Krause 2010). The distinct roles of employed district officials and volunteer local leaders reflect the assumptions of contemporary development funders that participation is best done through local associations endowed with a significant degree of autonomy (Harrison 2008).

Returning to the question that began this section—the particular challenges of community participation in disease control—several themes emerge from this preliminary analysis. First, our brief sketch of Tanzania's colonial and postcolonial history suggests that 'participation' is a complex and highly resonant

8 | In the Policy Paper on Local Government Reform (October 1998) some of the key principles of reform included: "letting people participate in government at the local level and elect the councils; bringing public services under the control of the people through their local councils; giving local councils political powers over all local affairs; de-linking administrative leaders from former ministries; creating new central-local relations based not on orders but on legislation and negotiations."

term signifying both self-governance and the provision of free labour. Second, an analysis of the Dar's infrastructure indicates that the particular location of civic engagement depends on distinct political formations. For instance, in light of the former role of the wards as vehicles for the central government, one might question the degree to which popular engagement in them overlaps with, or runs counter to, municipal units of administration (Dill 2010).

Returning to the UMCP, the following section considers the effects of this institutional history on the organization of scientific practices at the municipality level. If, as Ronald Ross argued, "a genuine campaign [...] must always be a permanent concern of the State," the question that follows is: How did new formulations of public health and malaria control reconfigure Dar es Salaam's political infrastructure?

Community-Lead Control

In contrast to the program sponsored by the Japanese government in the late 1980s, the current Urban Malaria Control Program (UMCP) delegates both routine mosquito control and surveillance to Community-Owned Resource Persons (CORPs). While trained and paid by the scientific researchers at the Ifakara Health Institute (IHI), CORPs are recruited through neighbourhood health committees and overseen by ward supervisors (Fillinger et al. 2008; Chaki et al. 2009; Geissbühler et al. 2009). The UMCP combines an experimental framework with an operational program, so that lessons may be learned for future interventions. In this sense data-collection does not precede implementation: what is being created is a system of management (Rottenburg 2009: 427). How, then, were scientific and administrative practices aligned to transform Dar es Salaam into a site of knowledge-production and public health intervention?

Because mosquito-breeding sites are bounded and easily located, cities are regarded as the most suitable environments for larval control. But, as we know from Orenstein and Gorgas, effective larval surveillance and monitoring requires comprehensive knowledge of the urban landscape at remarkably low spatial scales (de Castro et al. 2004). In this regard, Dar es Salaam poses considerable challenges. Like many African cities, it is undergoing rapid growth, the vast majority of which is unplanned. Propelled by population increase, lacking in basic infrastructure, and marked by the significance presence of 'rurban' economic activities such as urban farming (Kiunsi et al 2009), Dar's sprawl encompasses a diverse range of habitats, from blocked drains and ditches, to cattle troughs and garden furrows, to tire tracks and pit latrines. In addition to the proliferation of potential breeding grounds, mosquitoes continually and rapidly adapt to the changes in the city. For instance, while it was initially assumed that

Anopheles only breed in clean and clear water, in Dar they are now found in habitats polluted by rotting vegetables or human waste (Sattler et al. 2005).

Advances in Remotely Sensed (RS) imagery, Global Geographical Information Systems (GIS) and Global Positioning Systems (GPS) provide tools to render these dynamic micro-ecologies visible and create models that relate mosquito dispersal to malaria transmission (Killeen et al. 2003). However cartographic problems extend beyond those posed by physical geography. The most recent official map of Dar es Salaam dates from 1995; to a large extent, the administrative boundaries of new settlements or the emerging patterns of land ownership are unknown—at least to local government officials. Recruiting participants through street level committees was, therefore, of critical importance, for only their familiarity with the lay-out and living habits of their neighbourhoods could enable research team to find mosquito-breeding sites, many of which are located within private homes and gardens, or in areas that are difficult to access (Geissbühler et al. 2007).

With the goal of linking lived understandings of the city with the images produced by GPS technology, the UMCP developed a protocol for "participatory mapping". The process began with sketch maps drawn by a CORP—often with the help of household and plot owners—of the Ten Cell Unit area for which he or she was responsible. Mosquitoes provide provided the cartographic anchor of these depictions: the CORPs identified potential breeding sites and habitats and related their positions to features of the plot such as roads, drains, walls or houses (Dongus et al. 2007).

A member of the 'technical team'—typically a scientific member of the IHI –accompanied the CORP to his or her area. Walking along the boundary, the technician calibrated the features of the sketch map to an aerial photograph taken of Dar es Salaam, making regular stops to mark problem-sites and areas yet to be surveyed. These prints were then laminated to protect them during intensive use in the field. Non-permanent pens were distributed to encourage CORPs to adapt the map to their daily experiences and add new data as new observations were made (Vanek et al. 2006; Fillinger et al. 2008).

Of course, knowing where to apply larvicide was only part of the problem. As the vignette that opened this chapter illustrates, some plots are more closely guarded than others. Watchdogs, gates and knife-wielding owners are sometimes enough to dissuade CORPs from approaching a property, let alone asking permission to enter, search for and treat any potential breeding grounds it may contain. Echoing Ronald Ross's recommendations in *Mosquito Brigades*, the UMCP guidelines for the CORPs situate larval control within local norms and relations:

"For the purposes of our program, a plot is defined as a specific physical area with an identifiable owner, occupant, or user [...]. Knowledge of who owns, occupies or uses a certain plot is very important if you are to gain unlimited and regular access in future as this is the person who has the power to say yes or no!" (Fillinger et al. 2008, additional file 1).

In other words, the unit of larval control is the plot, embedded in social systems of regulation and informal land markets beyond the purview of public authorities (Kombe/Kreibich 2001).[9] But while the plot provides the site of intervention, the city—or at least a representative portion of it—is the unit of programmatic analysis. This shift in scale was not only a matter of covering more ground; rather it required integrating the plot into systems of urban governance. This process of bringing the plot into state view involved an iterative network of reportage: summaries, charts, spread sheets and reports circulated between CORPs, Ward Supervisors, the Municipal Coordinators and the City Council on a weekly and monthly basis. The accumulation of paperwork mirrored the escalation of research activity (e.g. modelling ecological variation and mosquito dispersal across scales) that accompanied the move from applying larvicide on individual sites to evaluating the impact of the program on malaria transmission. This system of annotated exchange enabled the assessment of performance and the development of training templates and recommendations for action. It altered not only the scale of the experiment, but also its tempo, producing the capacity to respond to the vicissitudes of mosquito and human activity (Kelly and Beisel 2011).

Yet this administrative hierarchy glossed over some key differences within the pre-existing urban institutional fabric: while street-level workers were considered 'volunteers', the ward supervisors, district coordinators and municipal officers are public servants, employed and paid a salary by the Tanzanian government (cf. Geissler 2011). The grass roots workers, namely CORPs, Mtaa leaders and most ward supervisors that comprise the vast majority of the program's personnel and implement most of the work on the ground, all work on a voluntary, very modestly-remunerated basis. In contrast to this, the municipal and city council officers that manage these teams are salaried government employees while the research partners enjoy even better employment conditions but assume no direct responsibility for the delivery of effective malaria control. Obviously, these disparities are most clearly felt by the CORPs responsible for the labour-intensive, day-to-day execution of the programme activities. Though they receive some compensation for their efforts, the value of these stipends is far less than the salary received by personnel formally employed by participating institutions.

9 | Kombe and Kreibich demonstrate how land-ownership, rights and use are regulated on the level of the neighborhood with the support of *Mtaa* leaders and organised community groups in authenticating and registering land rights, and while they deploy norms and procedures closely linked with the formal sector, they do not have statutory powers or legal mandate to do so.

Moreover, payment through the established legal system for municipal mobilization of casual labour is hinged upon the completion of daily tasks, with no long-term security or provision for illness, bereavement or leave of any description. Though presumably volunteering on a 'part-time' basis, the sheer physical stamina it takes to locate and spray each and every potential breeding ground across even a few houses meant that the CORPs had little time and energy to do any other work. For most, participating in the UMCP was their primary, if not sole, source of income. Compounding the difficulty of negotiating access to private residences without an official mandate, the demands placed on them by the UMCP were experienced by the CORPS as unrealistic and unfair (Chaki et al. 2011; Kelly 2011). One CORP working in Kinondoni Municipality pointed to the temporal limitations of this peculiar form of 'voluntary' participation:

"I have been in the programme for over three years now, yet I have not had leave for even a single day because the programme would not let me do so. Do you think I don't get sick? Do you expect my performance to be the same throughout the year?"

The UMCP's double role as an experimental pilot and a public health (and public employment) programme was also played out, though perhaps less visibly, on higher levels of the administrative hierarchy. Despite efforts to decouple project evaluation from disciplinary action against CORPs, the integrity of the experiment (e.g. its value as a demonstration of the impact of larval control on malaria transmission) and the success of the programme (a reduction in the incidence of malaria) rested on the capabilities of the CORPs to negotiate access to plots and to locate and spray breeding-grounds. An increase in the number of Anopheles in the city could call into question either the quality of scientific training or the stability of municipal infrastructure. That ambiguity in accountability triggered a clash of performance indicators with different financial and political consequences.

However, unlike any number of experiments whose impact on local public health ends with the conclusion of research (c.f. Geissler et al. 2008; Kelly et al. 2010), the Tanzanian government has agreed to fund an expansion of the UMCP across the city. To a certain degree, this enthusiasm can be explained by the project's success: malaria rates have dramatically decreased across the city. Though somewhat surprisingly, that decrease has occurred, regardless of where larval control is taking place. This outcome is problematic from a scientific perspective, as it may suggest other factors, such as changes in housing construction or population density that may be contributing to the decline. However, in light of the relative paucity of knowledge about vector ecology—mosquito dispersal range, lifecycle and behavioural processes—there may be good reasons to believe that larval control has, in fact, played a pivotal role. In any event, the programme, its mobilization of municipal resources, attracted national attention, National Malaria Control Programme to decide to expand the programme by 2013 across Dar es Salaam and into four other Tanzanian cities.

With the UMCP's shift in scale and institutional location, new questions arise as to the how responsibilities for larval control will be distributed and who will pay for it. As the role of IHI wanes and the number of neighbourhoods, wards, households and breeding grounds encompassed by the growth, larval control may undergo a process of "political intensification" (Lezaun 2011).[10] No longer experimental objects, mosquitoes may become evidence of governmental neglect: a preoccupation of residents, not just cadres of experts. In warning against the pitfalls against community participation in vector control Michael W. Service, emphasized that "the expected outcomes of collaborative control efforts by the community need to be explicitly explained to the people" (1993: 231). Moving from pilot plots to urban infrastructures not only introduces new actors, but also different sources of concern.

CONCLUSION: SCALING RESPONSIBILITY

This chapter has drawn together historical and empirical resources to explore how malaria becomes a 'matter of concern'– to use Bruno Latour's terminology (2005)—for Dar es Salaam. Tracking the political ecology of malaria control—the variety of ways in which the material and institutional environment intervene in the creation of public spaces over time—has pointed to the overlapping, yet often distinct, imaginaries of public participation attendant to public service and communal labour, national governance and international research. Participatory planning is now regarded as the *sine qua non* of successful health service delivery, and of development more broadly; without measures to enhance local capacities and ensure community ownership, interventions will fail and services will remain under-utilized or misused (WHO 2006). In Tanzania, popular participation has a politically vivid resonance; as Maia Green writes, here, "participatory forms come to operate as 'boundary objects', effecting the possibilities of translation between disparate communities of meaning" (2010: 1241). The CORPs materialize

10 | In describing how bees and beekeepers have become political actors under EU agricultural 'coexistence' policy for the cultivation of genetically modified crops, Lezaun (2011) describes a twin process of research escalation and political intensification. He defines the later in this way: "the disruption of a series of symbiotic or balanced relationships (and of the political order they support), and the emergence of new collectives (actors that come to operate as a category, rather than as isolated individuals)" (2011: 749). In the case of the UMCP, the process more closely maps on to the emergence of new collectives–such as the CORPs–as the political order, in regards to malaria control has yet to be articulated.

these visions of civic responsibility and scientific integrity; their 'volunteered' participation links experimental and municipal orders.

So what changes to the form and reach of can be anticipated when the UMCP is brought to scale? Clearly, there are critical decisions to be made. As the numbers of anopheles (and with it the incidence of malaria) drop, locating mosquito habitats becomes increasingly more important: one neglected breeding site can suddenly lead to a significant surge in malaria cases. For some of the researchers who had been involved in the UMCP, the solution would be to amplify the efforts to map the urban landscape, focusing efforts on the most productive sites. This approach would necessitate, on the one hand, the active involvement of scientists at IHI, and on the other, a reevaluation of the composition of the CORPs and the form of their recruitment. While, on the whole, CORPS are more successful at locating breeding habitats when they are engaged by local leaders than when the program's staff, there are good reasons to hire fewer but better paid supervisors if the intervention becomes more targeted and spatially less extensive (Chaki et al. 2011). This approach, then, would imply a tendency greater professionalization, with unclear implications for the ethos of local-level responsibility.

The Dar es Salaam city council, however, seems committed to an exhaustive coverage of the city, which could be achieved through a decentralized community-based implementation. In addition to more government autonomy, maintaining the scope of the program could result in a greater local level involvement and potentially, greater coordination may be necessary between larval control and other municipal services, such as sanitation, land development, and urban planning. Those more cynical of the government's motives might point to the *Bti* factory, newly built in Dar es Salaam by the Cubans, and the commitments made to make ample use of its product, as a reason why a potentially more efficient reformulation of the community-based platform of the UMCP is not under consideration. Either way, while the UMCP demonstrated how foreign expertise and funding effectively integrated into municipal governance, the production of publishable scientific data and enhancing the capabilities of national or local authorities operating in the city are not always easy to align.

One consistent observation of public policy professionals is that 'scaling up' a promising public health project is rarely a matter of 'becoming larger' (Bloom/Ainsworth 2010). Shifts in scale imply changes not only in the number but the type of actors involved, and more critically, in the quality of their relations. Expanding the geographical area of application is as much a political as a technical exercise: depending on how Dar es Salaam City Council decides to manage the increasing number of breeding grounds, has implications for who will control the process. What is clear is that through the experimental animation of the CORPs, the UMCP has triggered new occasions for participation and new spaces for the maintenance of urban life.

Stock-outs in global health: Pharmaceutical governance and uncertainties in the global supply of ARVs in Uganda

SUNG-JOON PARK

"No supplies, no programme"
(Basic principle in pharmaceutical supply management)

INTRODUCTION

Judith[1] shows me how to order antiretrovirals (ARVs) for her public hospital located in the center of urban Kampala. Access to antiretroviral therapy (ART) is free of charge at this clinic like almost everywhere else in Uganda. She gives me a blank drug order form to be submitted to the *National Medical Stores* (NMS), which is supposed to supply ARVs[2] and other essential medicines to all public hospitals in the country. I am sitting in her pharmacy. In the back is the store for ARVs, where I fetch the stock-cards with the actual consumption figures for each regimen for the last months. Judith reads out the figures, which are scattered on various pieces of paper. Then I compute the order for each regimen with a calculator. One row for "stock-in-hand", then another row for "consumption", then another row for "quantities received", where I enter "NIL", because the NMS had not delivered any medicines. Then I compute the actual order by subtracting stock-in-hand and then adding two months buffer-stock. The range of regimens is extremely broad. For the fixed-dose combination AZT/3TC/NVP—the recommended standard first-line regimen in Uganda and elsewhere—I multiply months by 60, because each "patient-month" is 60 pills. I multiply the consumption figures by 2 for 2 months' of supplies, and so on and so forth. For AZT/3TC/NVP this yields an order of 739,987 pills, roughly

1 | All names in this text are pseudonyms.

2 | Throughout this chapter the abbreviation "ARV" for "antiretroviral drugs" is used to refer to pharmaceuticals. "ART" for "antiretroviral therapy" is used as an abbreviation for the standardized model of *highly active antiretroviral therapy* (HAART).

12,300 pill bottles. This is the two months' supply for about 6,000 patients. I am not used to these numbers and am constantly worried about punching an incorrect figure into the calculator. But some figures also sound strange to me, for instance, stock-in-hand and previously supplied quantities do not match. Judith says that the NMS has a computer system to rectify errors and compute the right quantities. Later, Judith tells me, she will try to fax the order to NMS or even send a driver to deliver it to NMS in Entebbe.

After I complete the order for about 40 different regimens, I ask Judith if she believes that this order will be "appreciated by NMS". NMS had failed to deliver any ARVs and this order is urgent, because the hospital has been out of stock since November 2009. "They will, they have to". She laughs and says that she would herself go to Entebbe and beg and urge David, the sales manager, to give her the medicines, which she has already done a couple of times before. "They know me", she says, adding "but you never know, let us keep our fingers crossed. I will tell you when the drugs arrive."

The ARVs eventually arrived, though first in the wrong quantities and after a second emergency order with another month's delay. Until NMS trucks had unloaded the boxes at the hospital's pharmacy, nobody had a clear picture of the situation. ARVs were urgent, but their availability was cloaked in uncertainty, because nobody knew when the medicines would arrive. The stock-out of ARVs was not restricted to Judith's hospital. Between 2009 and 2010 pharmaceuticals were out of stock all over Uganda and NMS, the central drug procurement agency, had rationed ARVs and other essential medicines. Respectively, Judith had to ration the medicines at her hospital and borrow from other programmes like many other hospitals during this time.

When the stocks of ARVs became short at Judith's clinic and elsewhere, questions like "When will the ARVs arrive?"; "Who knows where the ARVs are?"; finally "Are the ARVs there?" emerged as central matters of concern in Ugandan mass HIV treatment programmes. These questions also structure the ethnographic analysis of stock-outs in this chapter that traces the situatedness of such concerns as they emerge in the complex entanglement of stable and unstable pharmaceutical supply channels that characterise contemporary global health. Ethnographic inquiries into stock-outs are in this respect not very different from health professionals' efforts to get answers on the uncertainties in the global supply of ARVs by following these objects through multiple channels in the country: contacting the central procurement agency, NMS, private non-profit suppliers like Medical Access, and the Ministry of Health. Equally important were international organisations like USAID, PEPFAR, or the Clinton Foundation for inquiring where the pharmaceuticals are, when they will be delivered, how many ARVs are missing in the country, how many ARVs had been procured, and how many ARVs are still in stock.

In this chapter I approach the stock-out of ARVs to explore how novel forms of pharmaceutical governance emerge in the scaling-up of access to treatment. The shortage of ARVs discussed in this chapter cannot be separated from the way expensive life-saving pharmaceuticals give rise to new regimes of global health that are centred on the global supply of these pharmaceuticals to countries like Uganda, where resources are particularly scarce (Biehl 2006). In this regard, stock-outs emerge against a therapeutic apparatus that comprises a broad range of categories, taxonomies, rules and definitions, which constitute important sites to explore ethnographically how global health operates through these regimes of pharmaceutical governance (Nguyen 2010; Pfeiffer/Chapman 2010).

Stock-outs are situated in this global health network of NGOs, donor agencies, philanthropic organisations, and international health organisations through which access to ART is governed (Janes/Corbett 2009). An ethnographic account of stock-outs differs in important ways from the responses that global health experts and professionals would like to generate in order to put the global scaling-up of access to ART on evidence-based knowledge (see also Geissler/Molyneux 2011; McGoey/Reiss/Wahlberg 2011). Experts and professionals in 'global health pharmacy' often suggest technical solutions, like technical assistance, training of pharmacists to improve reporting systems, or information technologies to increase accuracy and efficiencies in calculating the supply and the demand of ARVs. Some of the reasons for stock-outs described in this chapter are indeed very technical and specific to the Ugandan context, most notably the suspension of Global Fund money to procure ARVs for a couple of years. However, the implications for HIV treatment and the uncertainties that emerge in the erratic supply of ARVs are more generally linked to the orders and disorders in the way donor aid, ARVs, and patients in mass HIV treatment programmes are related to each other in the therapeutic apparatuses of global health in Uganda (Nguyen 2010).

The term therapeutic apparatus, which draws on Foucault's notion of a *dispositif*, is useful to address the broad set of social, political, and biomedical technologies that are cobbled together in ART (Foucault 2001 [1977]; see also Nguyen 2010). This therapeutic apparatus is constituted through the supply of expensive drugs to meet the demand of the large number of patients. Moreover the global supply of ARVs builds on various "calculative practices", which make humans and pharmaceuticals calculable, attribute values, such that they can be counted as human bodies and commodities and related to each other (Callon and Muniesa 2005). As objects, ideas, and models enter into new relations, they materialise new practices, and mobilise other elements in the production of knowledge (Rottenburg 2009: xxxi). Antiretroviral therapy (ART) concatenates objects (pills), ideas ("positive living"), and models ("adherence to treatment").

As the sections below will demonstrate, accurate and reliable knowledge about ARVs deliveries are indeed vital in organising access to ART. In contrast, stock-outs show that comprehensive information and knowledge on medicine deliveries as well as on patient numbers in HIV treatment programmes are hard to come by, because the production of medical data presupposes a material and social order that cannot be taken for granted in the supply side of ART in Uganda. Information is scattered across numerous projects and as interlocutors complained, there is little homogeneity or structure in the supply side of ART, which precludes meaningful answers and information on the availability of ARVs in the country.

In the following sections I discuss three aspects in the analysis of stock-outs in mass HIV treatment programmes. First, an analysis of how ART gives rise to a form of pharmaceutical governance that is centred on ideas in pharmaceutical supply management in global health. In this *infrapolitical* expansion of global health, access to ART and its problems are configured by the global supply of ARVs. Second, this includes the observation of a set of technologies and practices in pharmaceutical supply management to calculate consumption figures, forecasting needs, tracking pharmaceuticals, and monitoring the recruitment of patients and so on. Such practices are better understood as the production of new material and social orders—in the sense of a therapeutic apparatus—which mediates patients' access to ART. These technologies and practices are important sites for understanding how ARVs are made available and accessible as well as in order to capture the uncertainties and contingencies in the production of public health knowledge and information in Uganda. The third aspect is how uncertainties that surround stock-outs pose moral dilemmas to patients and health professionals, which characterises the institutionalisation of ART in Uganda.

The global supply of ARVs and pharmaceutical supply chain management

The shortage of pharmaceuticals has been widely observed—and taken for granted—in healthcare in Uganda and elsewhere (Mburu 1985; Turshen 1999). Neoliberal reforms have in particular contributed to exacerbate the shortage of medicines in health units (Jitta/Whyte/Nshakira 2002; Pfeiffer/Chapman 2010). These shortages are amplified by the emerging therapeutic apparatuses of ART, which undermine these public health systems through "vertical funding" or "disease-specific funding" as various authors describe the exceptionalism of ART (Pfeiffer/Nichter 2008; Whiteside/Smith 2009).

The stock-out of ARVs, however, differs significantly from other types of shortages. Before access to ART became free of charge in Uganda, it was mainly the high costs of treatment that turned access to these life-saving drugs into a moral dilemma, where those who could pay for treatment had priority (Whyte et al. 2006; Nguyen 2004). By contrast, in contemporary mass HIV treatment programmes pharmaceuticals are free of charge and broadly funded through sources like the *President's Emergency Plan for AIDS Relief* (PEPFAR), the Global Fund to Fight AIDS, Malaria TB, UNAIDS and a number of philanthropic foundations, like the Clinton Foundation. Initially, price reductions for ARVs were essential to increase the supply of ARVs. The standardisation of the supply and demand of these expensive pharmaceuticals further enabled the scaling-up of access to treatment from a few hundred to hundreds of thousands of patients. In the Ugandan case, 450 people were known to have access to ART in 1997. By 2002, the numbers had grown to 10,000 people. In 2003 only a handful of clinics were providing access to ART on a cost-recovery basis, mostly in urban Kampala. In 2004, when free access to ART was 'rolled-out'—or 'free ART' as it is simply called in Uganda—treatment numbers reached 45,000. In 2010, more than 200,000 patients were reportedly receiving treatment from one of the many HIV treatment programmes in the country.[3] The 200,000 patients with access to ART are said to constitute 39% of all patients 'in need' of treatment. Today, more than 350 health facilities, including NGOs, faith-based organisations, public and private hospitals, are accredited as HIV treatment programmes in Uganda. The distribution of ARVs is strictly limited to these 350 accredited treatment facilities, and unlike for many other pharmaceuticals ARVs, cannot be bought at one of the numerous private pharmacies in Uganda.

As ART is translated into mass HIV treatment programmes, it too materialises new practices and mobilises new elements in the production of knowledge. The translation of pharmaceuticals into a large-scale intervention increasingly draws on logistical knowledge and expertise in the domain of *pharmaceutical supply management*. Though pharmacy is a much broader medical profession, the high traffic of expensive medicines like ARVs, not to mention TB medicines, antimalarial drugs, and vaccines, have shaped pharmaceutical supply management into a distinctive domain of pharmaceutical expertise in Uganda. The increasing importance of pharmaceutical supply management builds on "the need to know, the desire for information, the push for evidence on which to base further policy and planning" is a powerful driving force in this war as Harper puts it (Harper 2005: 139). The idea that pharmaceutical interventions can deliver life-saving therapies to any place in the world at any time is a powerful imagination. Organisations like PEPFAR do not only provide

3 | These numbers are taken from different sources (Martinez-Jones/Anyama 2002; WHO 2003). The most recent figures are taken from WHO (2010). However, these numbers come from different types of sources, which are often not defined and sometimes even contradictory.

money, but also an encompassing logistical network to transport ARVs from any producer in the world to regional hubs in Accra, Johannesburg, and Nairobi; from there to the various recipient countries and ideally to any health centres, even in the most remote villages.

International donor organisations have not only injected huge amounts of money for treatment but, at the same time, instituted data production tools, audit mechanisms, record keeping practices to track funding and pharmaceuticals as well as treatment protocols and guidelines to expand stable and accountable healthcare infrastructure. Patients, health centres, national and sub-regional warehouses are thus connected in the production and circulation of logistic information to deliver ARVs. It is through these regulations and standards in ART free of charge that capital and pharmaceuticals flow into countries like Uganda and determine patients' eligibility to free access to ART.

These technical elements enable the provision of ART to 3,000-5,000 patients at the largest ART-clinics in Uganda, which manage up to 500-600 patients per clinic day. However, the lack of a stable infrastructure in the public health care system means that the recruitment into and maintenance of patients on free ART is mediated by a patchwork of 'projects' managed by numerous NGOs, bypassing government structures. This proliferation of projects constitutes the landscape of mass HIV treatment programmes, which participate in the "projectification" of healthcare in Uganda (Whyte et al. [forthcoming]; Rottenburg 2009). In this projectification, HIV treatment programmes regularly monitor patients' access to ART using specific "programmatic indicators". These indicators are used to measure a programme's output, which vary considerably between different NGO-projects—depending on the infrastructural specificities in scaling-up access to ART.

But projects are generally very dynamic and fluid: donors withdraw, new donors enter the field, targets are replaced, or new projects are developed, all of which require a constant adjustment of patient indicators to the shifting proportion of people and pharmaceuticals. Thus the above-mentioned overall patient numbers are dispersed and often difficult to come-by, although they are of crucial scientific and political importance in producing evidence on the impact of the substantial amount of health funding on the scaling-up of access to ART.

In contrast, access to ART is characterised by various uncertainties. As a pharmacist commented, "donor money has *disorganised* our system." He continued stating that

"A few years ago, Uganda was so prominent for its AIDS response and there was so much money available, we just turned everything into an ART clinic. 'Take the toilet; turn it into a store'. 'You have a veranda? Transform it into a dispensation area'. 'Here is money'.

And now it has become more competitive. There are so many organisations in the country and we are competing for lesser money and fewer drugs to help our patients."

In order to make sense of these numbers in mass HIV treatment programmes, it is important to understand the complexities in the production of numerical knowledge; the way specific calculative practices establish quantifiable demand for ARVs, and the indeterminacies in the global supply of ARVs that enable such calculative technologies.

INFRASTRUCTURAL MULTIPLICITIES AND THE RULES OF ART

The stock-out of ARVs has to be understood against the background of a therapeutic diversity in mass HIV treatment programmes in Uganda, which result from the complex entanglement of stable and unstable supply channels for ARVs. Depending on the location, size, on the source of funding and most importantly on the availability of ARVs at treatment facilities, access to free ART differs significantly and resonates with a plurality of "the rules of ART" (Meinert/Mogensen/Twebaze 2009). The rules of ART are usually defined by national and international treatment guidelines. However, in practice they are often much more diverse and problematic as the following elaboration of the dynamics, dilemmas, and uncertainties in the stock-out of ARVs show. The rules of ART apply immediately with the registration of patients as "clients" at one of the HIV treatment programmes, whether a public hospital or run by one of the many NGOs in the country. Registration constitutes a decisive step in accessing the range of possible services. Free ART in Uganda differs significantly in what is generally termed "support" provided to patients and their families, like nutritional support, counselling services, particular programmes for Tuberculosis or Malaria, and many more.

Registration in a treatment programme does not immediately lead to therapy. Programmes have a "pool" of clients from which only a minor group of clinically eligible patients is recruited into free ART based on the CD4-count. The CD4-counts are monitored every six months in order to see if patients fall below the official threshold of 350 set by the treatment guidelines. Then eligible patients from the "pool of registered clients" are recruited into the free treatment. However, not all clinics have the same technical means to run a CD4-machine on a regular basis and sometimes use the clinical staging recommended by the WHO. Some clinics send their patients to the nearest clinic with a CD4-machine. Clinics in urban Kampala often run extensive liver and kidney tests before patients are put on treatment, which rarely happens at rural HIV treatment programmes. Some programmes use the most recent threshold of 350, while other programmes stick to a CD4-count of 250 or even 200 as the threshold.

CD4-counts are indicators, which base patients' access to treatment on clinical criteria. Patients below a CD4-count of 350 need to start treatment. However, these indicators are better understood as calculative devices mediating patient numbers and representations of 'demand', which are in turn used to quantify the required supplies for free ART (Callon/Muniesa 2005). These calculative devices are material relations that determine the technical and logistical conditions of scaling-up ART. HIV treatment programmes in Uganda use the term *treatment slots* to calculate the recruitment of new patients into a programme. Statements like "we still have 100 slots for this month", "others still have free slots", or "we exhausted our slots" are common ways to talk about medicines and patients. As my interlocutors explained: "Slots are human beings. Treatment slots are usually set by donors and by the Ministry of Health. In the case of the Ministry of Health in Uganda, they will always say, 'we are ready'. Based on what the clinic reports, they will replenish the stock." Whether clinically eligible patients can be put on treatment depends on the number of "open treatment slots", which in turn depends on the commitment of the Ministry of Health to supply pharmaceuticals for these slots. Ultimately slots determine the threshold for recruiting patients. As an informant explained, "at one time you may find anyone with a CD4-count of 250 is recruited and at another time one of 200 is rejected. So it depends on what is available." Yet, what is available or not in free ART exposes the contingencies and the complexities inherent to the therapeutic apparatus of life-saving pharmaceuticals in the AIDS epidemic.

In the months between 2009 and 2010, public health facilities experienced severe stock-outs, such that ARVs were rationed or patients were turned away without their monthly doses. In contrast to the public sector, where the pharmaceuticals were short in supply, the slots for NGO-run ART-clinics are allocated by various donor agencies, most importantly PEPFAR.

"For a particular period of time, based on the resources we have and what we can handle, they [PEPFAR] are just giving you 900 slots, meaning that you can only recruit up to 900 patients in that year. Your ceiling is 900 and if you have lost some patients you can only replace those ones."

My informants explained to me that the allocation of slots at NGOs by PEPFAR can however be very unpredictable:

"In the middle of the programme, they tell you of additional slots from 'Kalongo' and then you have to rush to recruit more patients. If you have 900 slots and you recruit only 300, then the fear is that next year they may reduce them. Slots can be a double edge. You may be just implementing and suddenly they tell you 'stop recruiting' because they say, we cannot afford to sustain. So the pressure is to get more or it is pressure that you cannot absorb more."

Treatment slots are flexible and reflect the way the complex entanglements in the supply of ARVs structure mass HIV treatment programmes. Slots are devices to translate official guidelines into patient numbers by making pharmaceuticals and human beings calculable. Definitions of treatment slots create technical categories of HIV patients, which establish the rules for recruitment of new patients into treatment and vary considerably according to the source of funding and pharmaceutical supply channels. As Van der Geest, Whyte, and Hardon's work on the social life of medicines suggests, differences in free ART can be understood as an effect of the different biographical life stages medicine can take (Geest/Whyte/Hardon 1996). The same pharmaceuticals can travel through different channels, leaving different paper trails, pass different organisations, and take different geographical routes to reach their patients. As Ian Harper suggests, the different itineraries ultimately constitute different things, reflecting a diversity of rules of ART and multiplicity in ART itself (Harper 2005: 137).

Infrastructural multiplicities and the diversity in the rules in mass HIV treatment programmes are reflected by the way scaling-up and stock-outs of ARVs take place side-by-side. In 2010, *The AIDS Support Organization* (TASO) became the largest non-governmental HIV treatment programme in Uganda by increasing its treatment target from 27,000 to 31,000 patients. These additional numbers referred to the number of patients receiving the standard first-line AZT/3TC/NVP combination, which patients have to take twice a day for the rest of their lives. Any scale-up is thus a difficult calculation of treatment slots, balancing resources and patient numbers. I asked how TASO could add 4,000 additional slots, and whether funding had increased. Simon, the senior pharmacist at TASO, responded

"No, not at all, in fact our funding for drugs has remained stable since we started, we were only *realising savings* through price reductions. We started with 500 patients in 2005. We only ask our funders, if we can increase the number of patients, when we make savings, then we set our new targets."

Saving lives was about making financial savings to procure more pharmaceuticals. "Realising savings"—small and large savings—reflect an organisation of ART where every pill *counts*. Before TASO dispenses ARVs to the patients, the pharmacists remove 2 pills from each bottle, which usually contain the monthly dose of 60 pills. The next refill appointment for patients is usually scheduled after 28 days, which would leave 2-4 pills. The pharmacy retains and accumulates the leftovers in order to recruit additional patients.

As Simon explained, price reductions for the many different regimens that are on the global market have to be regularly computed for any possible savings. Calculative control over treatment numbers, furthermore, builds on a "good working relationship with our supply chain management partner, who regularly solicits for further price reductions from the multinational pharmaceutical companies". A switch from branded to generic regimens, for instance, can produce considerable savings and "lots of slots". Translating savings into possible extra patients requires reliable records as well as close monitoring of the recruitment of new patients using a computerised system to capture accurate information.

TASO's scaling-up of access to treatment was remarkable, because at the time when Simon added 3,000 new treatment slots, most pharmacists and doctors in the country were concerned by heavy stock-outs that put various programmes at the brink of a treatment crisis. During the same period of time, many clinics had stopped the recruitment of new patients or even turned patients away. Jamila's ART-clinic was just a hundred meters away from the TASO headquarters. The clinic, where she worked as a pharmacist, is one of the largest and best-organised clinics in urban Kampala with a total number of 6,500 patients having free access to ART. At one of our occasional meetings in early January 2010, Jamila told me that the supplies had still not arrived. She asked "any news from National Medical Stores? Did they receive stock? Did they release the Global Fund money?" At Jamila's clinic "Duovir –N", the trade name for the recommended standard first-line treatment regimen AZT/3TC/NVP, was almost out of stock and about 5,500 patients were waiting for medicines. In the free ART programme of this clinic, about 1,000 patients were on "PEPFAR drugs", regularly supplied through the private not-for-profit company *Medical Access,* which supplies all treatment programmes funded by CDC with PEPFAR money. The other 5,500 patients were enrolled in the national free treatment programme and receive "MoH drugs", from the Ministry of Health, which were procured and distributed by NMS in Entebbe.

The distinction between "PEPFAR drugs" and "MoH drugs" spoke to the complex entanglements of supply channels in the therapeutic economy of AIDS in Uganda (see Table 1). Both sources supplied Jamila's clinic and the majority of its patients with the same fixed-dose combination AZT/3TC/NVP. But over the previous months, stock-outs had become a major problem at Jamila's clinic, because NMS had not supplied the ordered "Duovir –N". At Jamila's clinic, if NMS does not supply "Duovir –N", she borrows from "PEPFAR-drugs"— the same AZT/3TC/NVP fixed-dose combination –, which will eventually be replaced. Over the last months, when NMS' supply of medicines became extremely irregular, Jamila had been constantly borrowing from the "PEPFAR-drugs", without replacing them.

	"MoH drugs"	"PEPFAR drugs"
Trade name	"Duovir –N"	Any FDA-approved regimen, including "Duovir –N"
Patient numbers	5,500 patients	1,000 patients
Ownership of ART programme	Public Hospital	NGO
Supplier	National Medical Stores	Medical Access Ltd.
Producer	Quality Chemicals in Uganda	Any FDA-prequalified producer in the global pharmaceutical market, like Aurobindo, Matrix, Cipla, etc.
Funding	Government of Uganda	US Government through PEPFAR

Table 1: Difference in ART in regards to the standard first-line regimen AZT/3TC/NVP at Jamila's clinic.

The borrowed "PEPFAR-drugs" were the same, the composition was the same, the therapeutic management was the same, and they might even have the same trade name "Duovir –N". It would have been bought with PEPFAR dollars from manufacturers in Southeast Asia, *Cipla* or *Aurobindo* in India, or *Matrix* in Pakistan, and many others. In contrast, "MoH-drugs" were locally procured by NMS from *Quality Chemicals*, a modern pharmaceutical factory in Luzira, twenty miles South of Kampala. For a long time the producer had not been prequalified by the US *Food and Drug Administration* (FDA) nor by WHO, so that foreign donor aid could not be spent on these pharmaceuticals. The only buyer was the Ugandan government, which committed its budget for ARVs and antimalarial medicines to *Quality Chemicals*[4] for its national free ART programme.

Patients who received the AZT/3TC/NVP fixed-dose combination might have noted some material differences, for instance the packaging or the color of the

4 | *Quality Chemicals* is a *Cipla* subsidiary company and produces the same ARVs. Until mid-2010 it was neither WHO-prequalified nor FDA-approved. Nevertheless, the Ugandan government spent all its ART-budget of about 15 billion Ugandan Shillings to procure pharmaceuticals from this company for a price twice as much as the international price level indicated. Officially, the higher price was justified as the subsidisation of the company.

pills. Perhaps they also would have noticed differences in the names, depending on which particular product had been purchased. Doctors, pharmacists, and counselors would have to explain that these medicines were the same. Pharmacologically speaking, "MoH-drugs" and "PEPFAR-drugs", which were shifted during stock-outs, were equivalent. Yet the differences between them were neither superficial nor insignificant. Rather they revealed underlying logistical, infrastructural, and political specificities that mattered most when it came to stock-outs.

STOCK-OUTS AND THE GLOBAL SUPPLY OF ARVs

Stock-outs emerge within an infrastructural multiplicity of supply channels that make pharmaceuticals in ART into different objects. Although mass HIV treatment programmes have undergone remarkable expansion, they operate within very narrow economic, technical, and infrastructural standardisations. Some of the reasons for the stock-outs were very specific to the Ugandan context. Most notably, the Global Fund had withdrawn its grant in 2005 because of the misappropriation of funds.[5] Although the Ugandan government had established its own national free ART programme, the 'funding-gap' for AIDS treatment left by the Global Fund 'ate' into the overall budget for health in Uganda, which had already been insufficient for many years. As Benjamin and Ruth, both working in central bodies on the supply side of ART, explained:

Benjamin: "When the Government of Uganda was offering USD 30million for ARVs, when we computed it, we saw that we could put 50,000 new patients on treatment. So with USD 30million we can do everything. In other words, if PEPFAR would have maintained their patients and Global Fund would have maintained their patients, it meant we could have the funds of the Government of Uganda for one year to add 25,000 patients, the same amount of patients would be added the next year."
Ruth: "[However] After the Global Fund withdrew its grant. We had to make an emergency procurement to cover at least 50% of what we require for a quarter with some of emergency funds that Global Fund nevertheless gave us. And then, they do not even cover that quarter, namely October, November, and December. ARVs only arrived on Christmas Day. What did NMS distribute in October, November, December—nothing."

---

5 | The diversion of funds and pharmaceuticals has been a major source of the gap in funding health services in Uganda. After Global Fund money disappeared in 2005, the disbursement of all grants had been stalled for several years and subsequently led to budgetary deficiencies in healthcare.

In addition, the Ugandan government had entered into an exclusive contract with the local ARV producer, *Quality Chemicals*, for its national free ART programme, but was paying a much higher price for ARVs to subsidise this company.

Ruth: "With the new prices, where the Government of Uganda buys drugs for USD19 per pack from Quality Chemicals, twice as expensive as elsewhere, it came actually only to [medicines for] 24,000 patients in total."

In principle, the stock of ARVs should have been easily estimated by examining the records of the central drug supply agencies. But stock-outs were extremely difficult to localise. Reports on stock-outs were scattered across different organisations and regions. In fact, during the meetings and workshops, organised by various AIDS organisations, to follow up on the treatment crisis, it became clear that nobody could provide an accurate and comprehensive picture regarding the extent of stock-outs in the country.

Ruth: "We had a lot of PEPFAR coverage in the country. Even within a facility, if the drugs were running out, they were even borrowing from within. Like I understand, up to now PEPFAR money has not even been approved by the US congress. There is no money. They are using the little money that was left over. And yet it was supposed to start on 1 October. I even suspect they use some savings and they can borrow internally from USAID. But now we don't know where the 'PEPFAR drugs' are. *We don't know. Where are they? Who buys them? Where are they stored? We don't know. This is some silly question. But I am telling you we don't know.* I am going to the IRC and I have been seeing some ARVs, but I don't know where they are coming from. JCRC, which supports so many Ministry of Health sites, where do they buy and how do they distribute, we don't know. They are managing their own system. And all are having the same problem with drug shortages. I don't even know whether the PEPFAR supplied sites have better stocks than the non-PEPFAR supported sites. We don't know."

Like other interlocutors she claimed, "these PEPFAR arrangements, they have thoroughly disorganised us." As Ruth explained, because of this uncertainty, organisations and ART clinics had to resolve stock-outs on a day-to-day basis. She explained that central organisations to coordinate the supply of ARVs like the one where she worked "need someone to tell us, at PEPFAR for January and at NMS for January, Efavirenz is enough for the whole month, or for the next three months. We need someone who rings the bell for us and says after February 2010, there will be now Nevirapine in the country."

After various ARV regimens like Aluvia, Duovir –N, and later Efavirenz were stocked-out at several HIV treatment programmes in the country, rumors spread that the standard first-line regimen might again be stocked-out for two months. Informants repeatedly said that Arthur Rutherford, working at one of the donor agencies in Uganda, should know because his organisation was extremely well connected to most organisations in the supply side of ART. But even he did not know exactly what needed to be ordered next before it might again be stocked-out.

Park: "Duovir -N is again running out at NMS, can you tell me if that is correct? I have heard so many different stories in the last week."
Arthur: "Let me see in my emails. I have one from the 24th of May 2010, fairly recent and it says that NMS has 71,000 packs of 'Duovir -N'. This might last for one month. But you know that the consumption numbers are distorted. Further there are about 12,000 packs of Combivir left at NMS, so this is very critical."
Park: "So what is going to happen?"
Arthur: "*I don't know, it is difficult to say.* In theory, there are two big orders in the pipeline. A government order of 150,000 packs of "Duovir -N" and *Quality Chemicals* says they have them in stock at their factory. That money has been earmarked for *Quality Chemicals*, but it seems that the Ministry of Finance has not released the funds. We put a lot of pressure on the government to do it as soon as possible. Then there is another Global Fund order of about 560,000 packs of Duovir -N, but *nobody knows when this will arrive*. 65,000 packs of Efavirenz and 50,000 packs of Nevirapine have been ordered. But we don't know, which one is going to arrive first and when."

These complex and unstable entanglements in mass HIV treatment programmes contrast with claims of access to ART as a fundamental human right. Pharmacists working in pharmaceutical logistics know very well that the quantities of all kinds of essential drugs they allocate to health centers are insufficient: it is "not enough for running a clinic more than two weeks" as an official at NMS explained. Usually, when medicines run out, dispensers write an "S/O" on the prescription forms and send patients to a private pharmacy to buy the medicine, which requires patients and their families to raise money. In contrast, HIV patients cannot be turned away without serious moral difficulties. ART is a life-long therapy and patients are disciplined to adhere to treatment to avoid resistances to the cheap first-line regimens. Patients find it impossible to pay 30,000 Ugandan Shillings a month (about 12USD) for the cheapest fixed-dose-combination. Moreover, ARVs cannot be bought at any pharmacy in Uganda. Stock-outs then might undermine the therapeutic efforts to make patients adherent to the "rules of ART" (Meinert/Mogensen/Twebaze 2009).

Ethical Thresholds

Stock-outs and the uncertainties in the global supply of ARVs raise practical and ethical questions. The pharmacy unit of Jamila's clinic had been running in 'crisis mode' for several months. Since October 2009, NMS had not supplied

ARVs regularly to the clinic. First, "Duovir –N" was out of stock. Then "Aluvia", a more expensive second-line regimen, ran out and the pharmacist had to drive to Entebbe to urge NMS to give her the supplies. In the meantime, NMS delivered "Duovir –N"—"the MoH-drugs"—but less than what the clinic had ordered. Instead of waiting for the next ordering cycle, Jamila immediately prompted a second emergency order, for which the sales officer at NMS "could not blame her". Moreover, Jamila had exhausted the limit for borrowing "PEPFAR-drugs" to keep her patients "on treatment". After several months of stock-outs, she ordered the recruitment of new patients to be slowed. Instead of the recommended threshold of 350, the clinic only started new patients on treatment with a CD4-count below 50. There was nothing much Jamila could do, as she explained, because she had to ensure continued drug supplies for patients who were already on treatment.

At Jamila's clinic, stock-outs turned the recruitment of new patients into a moral dilemma. She did not tell patients the new criteria for getting treatment. Dr Kenneth, the medical doctor in charge of clinical services refused to announce that patients would only be started on treatment if they were severely ill with CD-4 counts less than 50:

"I don't want to frustrate our patients, such that they lose hope. We are not going to formalise the CD4-count of 50. It is scientifically and ethically wrong. What is the difference between 50 and 100? This is an arbitrary definition. This is our *ethical threshold*."

What would be the most ethical conduct when the ARVs were not there and nobody knew when they would arrive? As Dr Kenneth continued to explain, whether 50 or 100, clinically patients are at great risk. Once you start these patients at 50, all kinds of opportunistic infections have to be treated at the same time, which actually increases the costs of treating the patient. Delaying the recruitment of patients might turn out be even more expensive. ARVs and medicines for opportunistic infections, however, were not supplied through the same channels or paid from the same account. This meant that the costs of delaying ART would not have repercussions for the ART budget. Dr Kenneth repeated, as long as the supplies are unstable and unpredictable, 50 was considered to be the clinic's *ethical threshold*. Moreover, as he stated, "it makes my life easier. I don't want to discuss each and every case with the pharmacist, who tells me that we do not have the drugs. We start at 50, whether the drugs are there or not, without any discussion."

Stock-outs reflect the difficulties of reconciling clinical and ethical standard with scarce resources, which Nguyen describes as a form of "triage" in mass HIV treatment programmes (Nguyen 2010). The longer the clinic had to wait for new stock, the fewer patients were enrolled into the free ART. When the stock-level decreased further, the clinic stopped recruitment altogether. Only pregnant women were recruited into free ART through the Prevention of Mother-To-Child Transmission (PMTCT) programme, which could be funded through a different source. Some patients did not bother to have their CD4-count tested, e.g. Henry who had a count as low as 7. He had come to the clinic, because he had lost weight and his appetite and had become weaker over the past months. He was told that his CD4-count was very low, but apparently the clinic could not start him on treatment, because the "drugs are not there". Then Benson, the chairman of the 'clients council', had to take Henry and squeeze him into the free treatment by speaking to the doctors individually and insisting that "friends" like Henry have to be started on ARVs, while other patients had to wait longer until they would receive free ART.

Though reducing the threshold from 350 to 50 and finally to 0 was clinically contra-indicated, it was a necessary precaution for dealing with uncertainties, and even necessary to ensure treatment for all existing 6,500 patients. With regard to patient costs, it did not make sense to wait until patients developed severe opportunistic infections because this would require a range of other medicines making ART even more expensive. With regard to patients' rights, it did not make sense to have a national free treatment programme if only few patients could be provided with treatment. The clinic maintained an ethical threshold in situations of great uncertainty when many patients were waiting for treatment. It did so by adapting treatment guidelines to the constant variation in the number of treatment slots, a variation that reflected the complex calculus of supply and demand in a context of uncertain supply and logistical confusion. Defining ethical thresholds during stock-outs shows how ART produces ethical problems that must be situated in a larger nexus of consistent and inconsistent infrastructural, logistic, and economic circuits on the supply side of ART.

SHARING, BORROWING, AND MORAL DILEMMAS IN ART

Like clinics in urban Kampala the stock-out of ARVs also hit various hospitals in the districts in rural Uganda. The administrative structures in these districts are part of the tiered public health system in Uganda. A main hospital and the district health office can be found in the district capital, which is surrounded by a number of NGOs, with names and acronyms like TASO, CRS, Family Hope, JCRC, Mildmay, and many more. Farther away are several smaller government health units. In addition, NGOs run outreach services to bring treatment and care closer to the villages in order to reduce patient transport expenditures. Here, the coverage of HIV treatment programmes, NGOs, and public health facilities is less dense than in Kampala, where at least a dozen larger clinics are close to each other.

The health centre in Walakuba had registered about 150 patients on treatment. Once a week this health centre schedules an "ART-clinic day" for clients to come for their CD4-counts or to pick up their monthly refills. First it was "Duovir –N", which ran out of stock. Later other antiretrovirals like Efavirenz also ran out. During the stock-out of "Duovir –N" some patients received medicines for a month and then missed to take medicines for another two months. Other patient had to go without medicines for three months. Some could share ARVs with friends, who were registered at HIV treatment programmes like TASO, or might have switched to a different regimen and had some leftovers. Thus some patients had only missed two weeks, but otherwise managed to take the medicine regularly during the three months stock-out. Patients worried when the doctors told them that ARVs were not there. For some patients it was the first time that they had experienced such a stock-out. They recalled that their first thoughts were "are we going to die?" It was not clear, why some patients had received more ARVs, while others had received none throughout the three months. One patient then explained that whenever they had an appointment she would come and pick up a new bottle, and then go home and first finish her old bottle. In this way this patient managed to make "some savings". Other patients, as she explained, stayed at home if they have enough leftovers but when they would come to the health centre the ARVs might not be available. She remarked, "how can you miss to pick the drugs, it is your life".

The pharmacist at this clinic explained that "Duovir –N" was out of stock for only one month. NMS had delivered less than what they had ordered, so at first he had been borrowing ARVs from other health centres, like Buddondo or Bugembe. However, when the ARVs went below the clinic's monthly consumption figures, he decided to retain all ARVs for a month, because it would not be fair to give medicines only to some and not to all.

The clinical officer at this clinic said: "We counsel them to adhere to treatment, and then we are telling them to stop treatment? This is difficult. So this is our challenge. What should we say to the patients? What is clinically right or wrong is difficult to say." Stock-outs in this district, like in Kampala, raised moral dilemmas in rationing ARVs. To resolve these dilemmas nurses and clinical officers had to figure out which ART-clinics and NGOs still had ARVs, so that they could issue a referral letter for these clinics. They had to have a sense of where ARVs could be found throughout the country.

FINAL REMARKS

The production of logistic and pharmaceutical data is a crucial precondition to quantify, supply, and account for pharmaceuticals. But more importantly the steady delivery of pharmaceuticals is itself a crucial precondition to produce reliable data. "No records, no supplies" is written in thick letters on all drug order forms at Ugandan ART clinics. However, proper record-keeping practices are not a guarantee for regular supplies. And "no supplies, no programme", reflects as professionals reiterate, the basic principle in pharmaceutical supply management. If the medicines do not arrive, reports contain distorted consumption figures like higher consumption figures to offset the losses in future supplies. Or, reporting systems collapse because health professionals simply capitulate sending reports to order medicines. Unreliable information and stock-outs are interlinked and exemplify the uncertainties in the supply of ARVs that characterise mass HIV treatment programmes. These uncertainties give rise to moral dilemmas in allocating and rationing medicines, which are, in turn, inextricably linked to the complex entanglements of political, logistic, and infrastructural apparatuses in the global supply of free ART.

Over the last couple of years global health interventions to scale-up access to ART have overly emphasized an effective and accountable supply system for ARVs to govern the scale-up of access to treatment. Among global health experts such interventions are today considered to be too narrow and too inconsistent. Thus infrastructural problems like stock-outs have recently led to a reemphasis of approaches in 'strengthening health systems', which imply a comprehensive view on health and health institutions (e.g. Frenk 2010). The discussion of stock-out in mass HIV treatment programmes in this chapter attempted to offer an understanding of the frictions and fragmentations in the organisation of free access to ART. According to this view, health institutions have to be conceived in a wider sense and against the background of the emergence of encompassing bureaucratic and logistical apparatuses to govern the global supply of medicines like ARVs. These forms of pharmaceutical governance in mass HIV treatment programmes shape ways of knowing, rules and conduct, social and clinical categories through which claims to free access to ART are institutionalised in countries like Uganda. The pharmaceutical governance of people in mass HIV treatment programmes essentially includes the production of crises and dilemmas, which emerge around the scarcity of resources. In this respect, stock-outs reflect some of the crucial aspects in processes of institutionalising free access to ART, which correlate to more fundamental transformations in the economies of power and knowledge through which novel therapeutic orders are created in global health.

Longing for Citizenship

"We are not paid—they just give us": Liberalisation and the longing for biopolitical discipline around an African HIV prevention trial

P. Wenzel Geissler[1]

Introduction

The end of the monolithic biopolitical collective

From the vantage point of the mid-20th century, it seemed as if an almost inevitable connection existed between ideas and practices shaping the well-being of people's bodies, and the larger body of the national collective, represented by its government. The somatic existence of citizens and the larger form of the nation-state jointly demarcated biopolitical space, our later understandings of which were shaped, among others, by Michel Foucault's early writings on scientific knowledge and the clinic. The nature and operation of the nexus between medicine and nation was then open for discussion—ranging from the critical scrutiny by Foucault (but also e.g. Illich 1976), to the positive appreciation of national health as a collective political programme, epitomised in the works of Richard Titmuss (1970). Yet, that such a nexus existed, and that our thinking about the biological as well as the political had to take place within the remit of the national collective, was not put in serious doubt before the end of the 20th

1 | I gratefully acknowledge the assistance of the scientists, research staff, clinicians and participants of the Kisumu HIV trials. Warm thanks to all present and past colleagues in the 'Research communities study', notably Philister Adhiambo Madiega and Gemma Jones, as well as to research students Patricia Kingori and Tracey Chantler. Ruth Prince and Ann Kelly offered invaluable advice on earlier versions. Particular thanks, to the senior colleagues from KEMRI and CDC, who allowed us to study their work. Fieldwork was funded by the Wellcome Trust with support from the Max Planck Institute for Social Anthropology (Research group 'Law, Organisation, Science and Technology').

century. One of the premises of this volume is that this has changed, that the once taken for granted bond between individual and collective body, citizen and nation, has been ruptured, or at least that it no longer is the dominant frame of biopolitics.

The dissolution of the unified collective, the nation, as frame of biopolitical intervention is hard to overlook in Africa. Outside South Africa, national academic institutions have ceased to produce recognised medical science and have passed on this task to "para-statal" institutions that adhere to neoliberal regimes of ownership, property and global standards, and operate largely dependent upon funding, expertise and organizational structures in Europe or North America. Biomedical health care provision is no longer procured, nor indeed often expected, from the state, but provided on a fragmented, partial, emergency-focused basis—as 'projects' and 'interventions'—by non-governmental and transnational agencies and programmes. For the inhabitants of mutating African nation-states, the demise of the national biopolitical collective implies a progressive 'baring of life'; no longer anchored in the entitlements and duties of citizenship in its older nation-state sense, they have to orient themselves within less coherent geographies of rights and responsibilities.

Crucial for those living under these conditions is the search for association, not only to others who in similar conditions pursue aligned interests, or to those in more privileged positions through whom resources or power can be accessed, but to larger wholes that, while never replacing the comprehensive imagined community of the nation, partially substitute it or patch some of the holes in its strained texture. Ethnographic observations of this quest for association have over recent years produced a plethora of (always partial, often 'biological', somatically grounded) 'citizenshipS', with the plural referencing a qualitative shift away from the older totalizing notion of citizenship rooted in enlightenment readings of classic civitas. This inflationary use risks abrogating the claim for citizenship as comprehensive emancipatory reference to (just) society; but notwithstanding whether one calls any quest for collectivization a citizenship or not, this searching movement for larger associational forms is very important for contemporary African lives. It may be expressed in shifting religious groupings that have been observed in cities across Africa for several decades, through attachment to development projects or NGOs, to single-disease vertical treatment programmes or, as I will suggest further on in this essay, through participation in medical experiments.

Transnational clinical trials and post-nation-state biopolitics

Social scientists have observed, over the past decades, a proliferation of transnational medical research—especially clinical trials conducted with funding and expertise residing in institutions in Europe and North America, upon bodies, and in collaboration with medical institutions, in post-socialist and postcolonial nations (e.g. Petryna 2002; Rajan 2006; Cooper 2008; Reubi 2010; see also Turnbull 2003, Leach/Fairhead 2007). These trials differ (to some extent) from clinical trials conducted in the same countries where pharmaceutical industry and leading scientific institutions reside, because they stretch across vast inequalities in health and resources.[2] And they are different from clinical trials conducted within the framework of national health services in that they involve non-nation actors and thereby create different bioscientific territorialities. The most prominent publications about this new regime of clinical research concern south-east Asia and the territories of the former Soviet Union: these areas differ from Africa in terms of their relatively well-organised health and scientific infrastructure and their highly trained, but comparatively cheap, scientific work force, as well as in their disease patterns (resembling those of major Euro-American drug markets), which has made them a main target for pharmaceutical companies' drug trials.

In Africa outside South Africa, this type of for-profit transnational research is still relatively rare although it is likely to grow, for example in relation to anti-cancer treatment (see Livingstone 2012). The dominant transnational formation of bioscientific production in 21st century Africa is not the corporate pharmaceutical drug trial, but the publicly funded collaborative field station or research centre, often with an associated demographic surveillance system, sizable areas, often with several hundred thousand inhabitants, where demographic events as well as morbidity are closely surveyed, in view of providing a sampling frame for controlled clinical trials of health interventions and vaccines (see e.g. Adazu et al. 2005). Such field stations—involving large 'Northern' scientific organisations such as the USA's Centres for Disease Control, the British Wellcome Trust and Medical Research Council, and some of wealthy American universities, in conjunction with African para-statal organisations or health facilities—have over the past three decades emerged all over Africa. Disposing over highly trained and motivated scientific leaders, state of the art laboratories, large and highly trained, flexible workforces, and the mentioned highly capital intensive demographic surveillance systems, these field stations have become the primary sites of bioscientific production on the African continent, and have largely replaced African academic institutions as well as national ministries of health, with whom they sometimes collaborate, as centres of scientific productivity and excellence.

---

2 | While this dimension of inequality is absent in the remaining strong nation and welfare states (e.g. Scandinavia), where most trial participants are recruited from the general pupulation, clinical trials in less egalitarian western societies such as the USA do of course share many of the ethical and political challenges of transnational clinical trials (see e.g. Abadie 2010).

These new large-scale units are exemplary of the biopolitical forms of the post-neoliberal age in Africa. Their relationship to the nation-state is weakened, even though the African partner organisations are often 'para-statal' organisations combining state endorsement with corporate traits, and although they continue to rely on state regulation and state health facilities for subject recruitment and above all for post-trial referral. Usually they are situated close to participant recruitment areas—hence the term *field* station—and distant from centres of national government or higher education, as well as from the global 'centres of excellence' to which they are attached. Due to the high capital input in a context of generalised poverty, these installations tend to be segregated from the surrounding territories—creating enclaves of perfect bioscientific possibility within the wastelands of post-nation-state health care and academia. Biomedical science, rather than progressively extending its reach over a national territory, contracts here into islands; the possibilities and aspirations of the modern rendered as an archipelago. Connections to the national loci of public health governance are sometimes challenging, while worldwide communications, material flows and data exchanges among such enclaves of global bioscience, and between them and the mother institutions in the North are immediate—'hopping' as it were in real time across the globe.[3] As such, the geography of contemporary African clinical trial sites reflects the novel territoriality that anthropologists have described for neoliberalised African resource extraction industries—e.g. multinational mining corporations' and oil industries' 'capital hopping' and 'enclaving' (see Ferguson 2006). They do thus have a distinctly 'neoliberal' flavour to them, without, however, the direct economic causalities, which shape pharmaceutical companies' drug trials.

A second characteristic trait of these installations, intertwined with their spatiality, is their experimental temporality. Their activities are, unlike those of state education or national health care, never explicitly long-term, although, incidentally, many of these sites look back at 20 or 30 years of existence. Instead, they are framed by time-limited funding cycles and temporary contracts, and

3 | Characteristic of these real-time global data neworks are disease specific consortia, such as the HIV Prevention Trials Network (www.hptn.org) or the Malaria Vaccine Initiative (www.malariavaccine.org), which produce 'multi-site' trials, which are centered in some global centre of academic excellence, and recruit participants (often competitively, racing against time) in sites accross the globe, continuously pooling data from study subjects in different parts of the world; many of the most infkuential and important medical research endeavours of our time are organised in this way. Another example of a global network of scientific spots is the International Network for the Demographic Evaluation of Populations and Their Health in Developing Countries (INDEPTH) (www.indepth-network.org), which links health and demographic surveillance areas from around the globe.

by the limited horizons of experimentation, which extend towards previously defined endpoints in time—'outcomes'. With this experimental mode of engagement between research institutions and their congregation comes a particular relationship between knowledge and action, in which interventions (treatment, disease prevention) are conducted as experiments, without certainty about the outcomes; although such 'experimentality' could be said to have existed in earlier, colonial, scientific regimes (e.g. Lachenal, this volume), it becomes a dominant trait of present scientific work in Africa, partly because of the retreat of long-term state interventions based on consolidated evidence (see Rottenburg 2009). Again, these temporal and epistemological conditions are not limited to the production of scientific knowledge, but resemble the politics of 'exception' that anthropologists have described as foundational to contemporary formations of global capitalism (e.g. Ong 2006), without, however implying the same economic determination.

As far as the economics of contemporary African trial sites are concerned, much funding still originates from national governments—albeit not the governments of the nation's where these stations are situated, but that of Northern nations government budgets—and not from private corporations. There is a significant and growing proportion of 'public private partnerships' in which private funding, including that of pharmaceutical industry contributes, and shapes, public scientific enquiry (see Gerrets this volume), but the dominant source of funding remain national government institutions like the US NIH, or the UK MRC, and public charities like the Wellcome Trust. Despite the overall public nature of these institutions, by contrast with the commercial clinical trial settings described for Eastern Europe and south-east Asia, the way these installations are managed and audited, the flexible short-term contracts under which the (predominantly) local workforce is employed, and the structures of transnational management and funding flows, is not entirely dissimilar to transnational corporations. Control over the scientific production process resides with Northern institutions, data is often transferred to and analysed by these, and published by British and American academic journals; processes are managed and supervised by these institutions and their staff, and the existence and continuity of the institutional arrangement depends upon them.

Similar debates about the production and distribution of value created by scientific labour that apply to multinational corporations' outsourced production sites in post-colonial territories, arise then from today's African field stations, although the value produced and transacted around these sites is less directly identifiable as a form of capital. Economic questions about exploitation, accumulation and justice are here often negotiated through the idiom of research 'ethics', which—if sometimes by implicit evasion or explicit exclusion from its purview—engages economic contradictions in the idiom of justice, freedom and social good. It is the active exclusion of value from view that such ethical reflections and regulations often encourage, that provide my starting point for the discussion about experimental value and collective below.

The ethics and politics of bioscientific value

Bioscientific value has recently received attention from anthropologists and bioethicists who—from different institutional and political viewpoints—emphasise the political, economic and practical challenge that this value poses, at this particular juncture, and in economically deprived regions (for ethicists see e.g. Dickert/Grady 1999; Lemmens/Elliott 1999; Anderson/Weijer 2002; for anthropologists see Petryna 2005; Rajan 2006; Hayden 2007; Cooper 2008). The discussion includes very different viewpoints: traditional bioethicists who insist on the 'social value' of scientific knowledge and reject consideration of individual interests and profit, those who propose value-distribution through 'benefit sharing', others who denounce the privatised value of pharmaceutical research and uphold the virtues of the nation-state, and finally those who propose to resolve matters by re-evaluating research participation as paid 'clinical labour'.

What is at stake in all these approaches to the problem of value arising from scientific production under conditions of economic inequality, is the relation between value and collectives (or processes of collectivisation); who creates the value; who is the rightful owner of this value—society, mankind, nation, individuals, or other, intermediate collectives; and how, by whom, and to whom should value be transferred? Value is produced, and disbursed, within and among collectives; but what these collectives are has become much less clear today, compared to when medical science was produced by state institutions through the scientific and bodily labour of national citizens (see Hayden 2007).

This chapter contributes to this discussion about value and collectives, and to the wider problem of post-governmental biopolitics in Africa, by examining the practice of 'transport reimbursement'—small financial payments to trial participants on the occasion of their participation in clinical or data collection procedures. These are part of most medical research settings; I will here discuss them in relation to HIV research conducted in Kisumu, Kenya, in collaborations between KEMRI and its main overseas collaborator, CDC.[4] I draw upon interviews, conversations and observations with research participants and

4 | KEMRI was founded by government act in 1979, as one of several 'para-statal', usually collaboratively funded, scientific institutions. The US government CDC is a main collaborator, conducting research on malaria, HIV and emergent diseases. KEMRI and CDC have since 1979 focused on western Kenya and have jointly built the KEMRI/CDC field research station, which is part of the KEMRI 'Centre for Global Health' which has expanded continuously during the 1990s and is today one of the leading medical research sites in Africa, with world-class laboratories and an annual budget in excess of

staff during long-term ethnographic fieldwork among the 'trial community' (Geissler/Molyneux 2010) of a scientific study evaluating an innovative regime of maternal triple anti-retroviral prophylaxis from late pregnancy through six months of breastfeeding for the prevention of mother-to-child transmission of HIV (PMTCT).[5] The study showed that the relatively inexpensive experimental regime could reduce mother-to-child HIV transmission to less than one fifth of the rate that one would have expected under standard medical procedures in the area; indeed, the rate of transmission at birth was only little higher than what would be the case in developed country medical settings (Thomas et al. 2008). The trial lasted from 2003 to 2009, and involved over 500 women, who were recruited from antenatal care centres upon their diagnosis as HIV positive. The women and their babies were followed for up to two years after delivery. Most of them lived at the beginning of the study in the city of Kisumu, but many moved during the follow-up between city and rural areas, reflecting the instability of many young women's lives in Western Kenya today (see e.g. Geissler/Prince 2010). In spite of the practical difficulties arising from this mobility, the trial lost few participants, because the women, for various reasons, liked to be part of it—which, as I will discuss below, is very important for our understanding of the value of scientific work, and the collectives it engenders.

In this essay, I will show, first, that the financial transactions called 'transport reimbursement' are generally understood not as reimbursement—i.e. zero-sum transactions—but as net value transfers, and that all members of the 'trial community'—study participants and the people they live among, research staff, and scientists—are aware of this discrepancy between the nature of the payments and the term by which they are referred to. The term 'transport reimbursement' attempts to render invisible the value of these transactions, responding to regulatory objections to payments or what bioethicists refer to as 'undue inducement', and as a result, it removes the problem of value from the sphere of legitimate discourse. Speaking about this un-spoken materiality affords us then an opportunity to prise open the transactions of value in transnational clinical trials in order to rethink the political project of public health science, beyond the alternatives of ethics and market, gift and exchange, that shape much of the on-going bioethics debate, especially in Kenya. This will lead us to reflect about the potential collectives and aspired-to futures—emergent 'citizenship(s)' (see Whyte 2009) or the 'publics' in public health—which are referred to as well as

---

USD30 million, hosting approximately 1,500 staff members, funded by CDC and other funders, and employed by KEMRI, and hundred thousands of participants.

5 | Fieldwork was conducted from 2006 to 2010 with the approval of KEMRI, CDC and other collaborators involved in HIV research. I am grateful for the support and trust we received from our colleagues. This article presents the author's reflections and aims to contribute to an open discussion with scientists and ethicists.

produced by clinical trial engagements. Thus the discussion returns us to the political promise and responsibility of public health, as in producing health *and* engendering a collective.

Transport reimbursement

"So what shall I call this?"

Every Friday morning the coordinator of one of the HIV trials conducted in Kisumu, Kenya, meets his staff, including clinicians, laboratory technicians, counsellors and interviewers, employed by the Kenyan Medical Research Institute (KEMRI) in collaboration with the Centres for Disease Control and Prevention (CDC). On this day, about 20 staff members are gathered in the conference room of the custom-built clinical research centre. The principal investigator (PI), who usually attends staff meetings, is absent. One purpose of the meeting is to discuss encounters with specific trial participants. A clinician reports about a pregnant participant who asked for transport to the clinic because she felt unwell and could not walk. After she was taken to the clinic by taxi, she asked for 'transport reimbursement', which she regarded as an entitlement. When the clinician told her that she could only have the taxi fare *or* reimbursement, she responded that she would then come on foot anyway. The case provokes lively discussion, in which the majority of staff members advocate to pay both for the taxi *and* for transport reimbursement.

When the clinician concludes: "She was not really sick. She could walk ...", a female field staff objects: "You can't do this. She is pregnant, she maybe cannot walk! Do you still want her to walk all the way in order to get the reimbursement?" Another male clinician interjects: "We have to look at the ethics. We should not be seen as coercive, and we must not set a precedent." The female colleague retorts: "Now who will see this?" Patiently, the second clinician continues: "Transport reimbursement is supposed to take care of her transport. Now if you give her taxi [fare] and then you still pay her transport reimbursement, this is transport to where? If I still pay her, what shall I then call this?" "*Transport reimbursement*!!" retorts the female staff, supported by laughter and nodding from other staff members. The clinician pauses and resigns, proposing to take the matter up with "the powers that be", the PI. Everybody including the clinicians laughs. No further action is taken on the matter.

On this rare occasion, the problem of 'transport reimbursement' was made explicit, for a moment, before being covered again by terminological rigour combined with mirth and irony. For a moment the gap between names and things was opened, but it was quickly closed again, quite rightly so, because nobody present, nor the "powers that be" can resolve it. I do not want simply to denounce this discrepancy between rules and realities, but take it as a point of departure to reflect about transactions of value in clinical research in HIV trials in Africa. The rhetorical question posed in this exchange: "transport to where?" orientates my enquiry, as I will suggest that one important function of value transfers like transport reimbursement, pharmaceutical treatment, blood specimens or clinical data, intertwined with the more immediate fulfilment of vital needs, is to propose emergent collectives, to evoke futures, engender movement and seek direction—indeed *transport* towards better lives.

"We don't pay..."

Practices and discussions as well as silences around 'transport reimbursement' (TR) concretise the problem of value, faced by transnational research in the current historical and political-economic moment.[6] TR is one of many transfers of material value to individual study participants, which, in the Kenyan context, may include medical treatment and pharmaceuticals, food, bars of soap, bed nets and water containers and other health enhancing commodities.[7] TR is distinguished from these by being monetary, which makes it particularly problematic to bioethicists sharing a broadly 'western' understanding of money as abstract, calculative and individuating (see e.g. Maurer 2006). A bar of soap, a cinema ticket or a project party can here more easily be construed as a gift because none of them is vitally necessary, and the first has additional legitimacy because of its health impact. Such gifts are often referred to in the trial context as 'a thank you', rather than as an 'incentive'. By contrast (general purpose) money is, in this tradition, not suitable as a gift or 'thank you' because it is convertible and invites calculation and notions of economic exchange.

The aversion to money changing hands within a public health context extends—at least in the eyes of many older public health experts—to the wider health care services. Only after considerable national and international scholarly debates could so-called "user fees" for government health services be introduced within the broader framework of neoliberal "structural adjustment"; today, Kenyans have to pay contributions to almost all medical services provided by government facilities; and although these fees are relatively low, they do set

6 | Since in most economically deprived settings, receipts for transport are hard to get (or all too easy to obtain), TR is often based on fixed rates specific to a site or a particular trial. Rates vary between collaborative sites and sometimes between research groups and projects in one site, usually ranging from 2-5£ (higher amounts being paid in trials based at referral hospitals covering large areas, and for participants who for various reasons travel long distance).

7 | Even cinema tickets, underlining the attempts to retain the notion of the gift and the effort to keep transactions separate from any actual needs and survival.

limits to the care available to poorer people, they opened, some argue, the door to inofficial payments and corruption in health facilities, and they did away with the idea of health care as a service that the nation bestowed upon its citizens (see e.g. Mwabu et al. 1995). It is this liberalised world of illness and health, which provides the context for local understandings of value transactions in clinical research.

As money may easily be confused with 'payment', regulatory ethics guidelines applied in Kenya insist that monetary transactions should be a mere prevention of cost;[8] the sum of transport fare and reimbursement is assumed to be zero; no personal gain should be incurred.

Like in most transnational research sites in Africa that adhere to 'Good Clinical Practice' (GCP) and international ethics guidelines, net monetary benefits for participants—'incentives' or even 'payments'—would here be considered 'undue inducement' contrary to the spirit of voluntariness, and they would not be given approval by the Institutional Review Boards (IRB) that assess project ethics. Likewise, IRB approval can be denied if the proposed TR, which increasingly has to be specified on the research protocol and information materials and consent forms, is considered too high, constituting 'coercion' of poor participants. Official documents emphasise therefore the link between reimbursement and travel, relating reimbursement rates either to transport fares or to distance, but not usually to other equivalents such as time spent, effort undertaken, leave alone risk incurred. In accordance with these conventions and with written study documents, if TR is discussed among trial staff and especially with participants, any mentioning of 'payment', as in 'how much do you pay your participants?' is likely to be rebuked by a 'we don't pay'.

Reimbursement and voluntarism are flip sides of one coin: the notion of reimbursement safeguards the freedom of voluntariness, in the sense of individual choice. The significance of using 'reimbursement' instead of 'payment' is underlined in the terminology applied to another kind of bodily research participation in entomological research conducted by KEMRI around Kisumu: young men recruited to catch mosquitoes off their bodies (human landing catch), and those who sleep in tent-traps to catch mosquitoes, can only be recruited as 'volunteers' and be given 'reimbursement' for that time as well as the risk of malaria infection (reduced by chemoprophylaxis); their remuneration must not be referred to as 'payment', and rather than employment contracts, they sign consent forms. By contrast, young men recruited from the same village communities to set mosquito traps or empty them are employed as casual

8 | In other regularly contexts (e.g. USA) payments are acceptable, even to pull participants, as long as they do not induce unreasonable risk taking (undue inducement), but even where such payments are formally allowed, they often draw public moral debate, such as around the 2006 British Parexel incident (e.g. Wadman 2006).

workers and paid exactly the same amount as volunteers for a specified number of hours. The terminological rigour is important here, so as not to create the ethically problematic situation in which one pays for bodily risk. Lending one's body to science remains here linked to voluntarism and citizenship, to avoid the potential accusation of exploitation, which does not seem to arise from ordinary labour relations. Apart from terms, however, the two kinds of research work and pay are identical.

To maintain the moral value of autonomy, and to protect participants from the force of resource-rich research institutions, transfers of material value, notably money, to them are avoided or kept minimal. While this is the argument behind ethics rejections of 'inducement', one could argue that the notion of 'voluntariness', understood as autonomous choice without material entanglements, is anyway less than straightforward under conditions of extreme poverty—in the words of one scientist 'a bit of a middle/upper class luxury'—and that one should instead explore concepts such as 'responsibility' or, in medical terms 'care', as a frame for ethical scientific engagement. I will return to this.

Reimbursement in western Kenya

TR is a relatively recent development. When I conducted epidemiological research in Western Kenya in the early 90s, study participants in rural areas did not expect monetary transactions around their research participation. Indeed, the government scientists and technologists with whom I worked at the time where strongly opposed to the idea, both on the grounds that they regarded people's participation in research as a citizen's duty (reciprocated by their own efforts at government disease control), and because they feared that independent research by Kenyan government agencies without external funding would be made impossible if Kenyan citizens would expect individual payments for blood, stool or urine specimen delivery. In other words, at the time the collective nation-state frame of medical research and public health intervention was still taken for granted; from this followed not only that participants were not paid, but also that their consent, as citizens, was taken largely for granted by the government researchers, and no individual written consent was sought.[9]

9 | The organisation that I worked with at the time, and which had dominated medical field research in Kenya for many decades, was probably relatively more conservative in its civic values and 'developmentalist' nation-state imaginary than others who began operating in the area at the time, and who eventually took over at the helm of medical research. The anachronism of some of their procedures in a changed scientific world, in which good science was no longer nation-state public health, but 'Good Clinical Practice', became very clear when a large collaborative project of the former (government) organisation was closed down in 2000 after an external review by North

Since that time, new agencies have become leading in Kenyan medical research, and the social contract that the older generation then still envisioned as basis of public health science has been eroded; instead, along with standard consent procedures, TR has become an obligatory part of medical research and potential research participants are keenly aware that research participation entails some monetary transactions.

Among the reasons for transport reimbursement becoming ubiquitous in Western Kenya are changes in the conduct of transnational medical research, its relation to the national health system, and the wider political economy, from epidemiological field research to the model of clinical trials run according to global regulatory frameworks—and the attendant transnational transfer of procedures and models, as well as growing prominence of Euro-American institutions in research collaborations. While up to the early 1990s collaborative medical research projects in Kenya had minimal expatriate staff and operated usually within facilities provided by the Ministry of Health, using government transport and permanently employed civil servant staff, today's medical research programmes in Western Kenya are widely known by the name of their overseas collaborative partners, and recognised by their custom built research centres and laboratories (often erected within or next to public facilities but recognisably different from them) and their highly visible modern transport fleet. Staff—on temporary short term contracts funded by the external collaborator—and research participants today tend to identify with the overseas collaborator (as in 'I'm with ...') rather than with national government and citizenship.

While medical research in the past used to be integrated more tightly with government health care provision and often directly linked to public health campaigns, the social benefit of today's transnational clinical trials is often less immediate and visible to participants—mediated through a long loop via academic centres of excellence in the USA, and international policy bodies such as WHO, making short-term benefits a more salient and contested issue. Moreover, the exponential growth of medical research and aid activities in Western Kenya—one of Africa's key HIV intervention zones—has during the last decade led to a very different local economy, marked by new income opportunities and raised expectations of monetary gain among the general populations (see also Prince, this volume). In areas like this, models and relationships derived from medical research have extended across society, and transport reimbursement—tied to the notion of 'voluntary' action—has gained currency far beyond the limited purview of medical research. Thus, in HIV care and treatment, which in this area are again spearheaded by KEMRI and CDC,

---

American reviewers, who found the ethics procedures lacking. This was, then, the definite endpoint, in Kenya, of medical research premised on and legitimesed by the taken for granted social contract between citizen and nation.

large numbers of 'volunteers' assist donor funded patient support centres with recruiting, counselling and testing, and tracing patients who defaulted, as peer educators and by transporting blood samples and managing patient records. Volunteers may in such facilities well outnumber regular employees, and the status of the volunteer—often envisaged as a step between HIV self-help or 'peer' assistance, and more formal employment in the HIV-NGO sector—has become emblematic of especially younger people's lives in Western Kenya. As volunteers, they are not paid for their labour, but given 'reimbursement' or 'tokens'. This economy of voluntarism and reimbursement opens up new possibilities of engagement, learning and civic identity to young people, but it also creates possibilities of exploitation and abuse by institutions and by formally employed actors.

Do we have a Standard Operating Procedure?

The fact that transport reimbursement still is a relatively new phenomenon is reflected in the flexibility of the practices around it. Thus, in the HIV prevention trial we followed, the project protocol from 2003 contains no details about TR. The fact sheet for prospective participants states under "benefits" that: "Neither you nor your baby will be paid for being in this study. But you will receive money to pay for your transport," and, under the heading of "costs", that: "there is no cost to you or your baby for the study drugs, study clinic visits, physical exams, transport to study clinic visits, lab tests for the study, or for your delivery at the hospital." An attached sub-study protocol specifies: "Participants will be reimbursed transport according to standard ... guidelines already described in the main study protocol. For their time, sub-study participants, like all KEMRI/CDC participants will receive a bar of soap." The main protocol does not specify amounts, presumably based on the assumption that actual transport expenses will be refunded. The distinction made here between monetary reimbursement and soap as appreciation of time underscores the careful hedging of monetary transfers as presumed zero sum transactions, separate from gifts and not to be confused with exchanges.

When the PI, after the end of the study, tried to find us some documentation of reimbursement rules and asked his staff for the 'standard operating procedure' (SOP), no such document existed, although trial practices had been regulated in great detail by specific SOP's. The staff member who had been in charge of reimbursements explained retrospectively: "We did not have an SOP for transport reimbursement. The initial figure of 100 KSh was arrived at from [a preceding] study [in the same site]. After a while due to the amount of time mothers spent in the clinic it was agreed that we increase the figure by 200 KSh to compensate for the time they took in the clinic" (K29; e-mail, May 4th 2010). This change of rates, motivated partly be the realisation that some women travelled longer distances, and partly by the long time the study procedures took, was recorded in staff meeting minutes, which were the only official written document concerning TR rates for this study: "scheduled visits participants will receive Ksh.300 [up] from Ksh.100" and, "participants will start receiving Ksh.300 on enrolment" (Minutes K, August 2006). These decisions were taken by research staff and the PI based on practical experience and personal judgement, joint deliberation and improvisation in a setting where even the most mundane research procedures were fixed in written SOPs. Part of the motivation behind the threefold increase of the rate was to provide some payment over and above the actual transport fare (which at the time was about 50 KSh for most distances within Kisumu), as underlined by the provision, in the same minutes, that for "those who come from far Ksh.200 will be added on the rates they receive." Moreover, the additional 200 shillings were only to be paid for visits to the clinic relevant to the study, whereas "unscheduled visits" due to sickness were only compensated by the old rate of 100 shillings, based on the assumption that those who attend the clinic for health reasons already receive a benefit and do not need further incentive. As the PI recalled: "There was quite a bit of abuse going on with sick visits... we figured we were already providing care for the sick visit, so perhaps we could compensate a little bit less for transport" (C26.3).

Between 2003 and 2009, transport reimbursements were regularly paid to over 500 participants. The amount paid was based on the considerations discussed by the study team, which were not recorded as they arose in everyday practice. The PI recalled the discussions with study staff:

"Well, ...it is fair to say for someone who walked, it covered more than their transport, literally their transport reimbursement. [...], there was another rationale there ... we were setting it perhaps at the minimum wage? Which was about 250, so we were slightly above minimum wage. I think just to compensate...they may be there for a long time, so ...they might have been, could have been, working, ... to compensate. And we did, for women who came a long way and brought a receipt, we compensated even over and above [the actual rate]." (C26.3).

This PI was particularly thoughtful and open about his considerations, and the potential ethical issues involved—"I mean its a fine balance, you know, to sort of compensate people for their time, sitting in a matatu [minibus]... without being coercive." (C26.3)—and he repeatedly encouraged us to study TR, which he, like other colleagues, found a slightly awkward concept. Similar themes emerged in conversation with other PI's and study coordinators, who were struggling with the task of setting an adequate rate, aware of ethical norms of non-payment as well as participants' needs and the requirements of trial management. Some said they had used an assumed minimum wage as a standard, others had added a token onto documented transport fees, others again had copied other research groups. Underneath the seeming obviousness of the concept of 'reimbursement' many other considerations were at play and informally negotiated. These included questions of justice and ethics, and personal commitment to provide some help for poor study subjects, but also budgetary constraints, competition with other groups for participants, and concerns with recruitment rates and participant retention. The resulting negotiations between researchers and research staff were somewhat improvised, and with little input from participants.

Stabilisation

At the time when our study came to an end, transport reimbursement became stabilised in an official document. This was provoked by an oversight: a research student moving from the urban research zone to a rural area had used the common TR rate in the city (300 Kenyan shillings) on her ethics application for a new project in the rural area (reflecting growing awareness of the issue, by 2008 the KEMRI ethics committee required the stipulation of transport reimbursement rates in every protocol). Upon arrival on the new research site she realised that the rural rate was lower (120 Kenyan shillings), and other researchers on site understandably urged her to adjust her rate in order to avoid competition. When this change was submitted, with reference to 'standard guidelines', as an amendment to the ethics committee, the committee comprehensibly wished to see those guidelines. In collaboration with senior colleagues, the research student produced official 'reimbursement guidelines' which formally stated the different rates for, respectively, the urban and the rural research site. It also ended ambiguities concerning the meaning of transport reimbursement—such as the reference to the time spent in the clinic, noted above—by stating: "Reimbursement is understood as meeting travel costs participants incur to attend study visits", and specifying further that based on a "mapping exercise of rural districts" it had been determined "how much a participant would spend to travel to a facility" arriving at the lower rural rate, and that "travel costs are higher in peri-urban and urban Kisumu and participants usually travel longer distances to reach the research facilities" within the city, justifying the urban rate of 300 shillings.[10]

10 | Interestingly, the rural rate of 120 Kenyan shillings that had been determined through careful deliberations by the rural research teams prior to the formalisation of reimbursement rates, had, according to one rural study coordinator, been derived from comparison with approximate daily labour rates in agricultural production. While, as we saw above, the urban rates had been produced by adding 200 shillings–to appreciate time and effort–onto an earlier rate inherited from a previous project, the rural rates

VALUE APPRECIATED, ACKNOWLEDGED AND HIDDEN AGAIN

Receiving reimbursements: 'But I am paid'

Much as the notion of payment, and of monetary value, is avoided in official trial documents, study participants perceive these transfers not as mere reimbursements. That they value the additional cash is unsurprising in a place where, for most people, a day's manual labour would earn 100-200 KSh—an amount that could pay for one substantial family meal—in a situation of generalised unemployment, rising food prices and unstable food production, where opportunities to earn even such modest amounts are scarce.

Participants expect, at least after some time in a project, reimbursement attached to every trial activity, usually even if they had no actual transport expenses or when a research team had come to visit them to collect data or conduct an interview. All participants expected some amount over and above their actual expenses—"they don't give you the exact transport, you are just given, so it really helps." (KP8)—and many were aware of the 200 shillings excess that had emerged from the deliberations above. The amount of cash that the participants took home varied slightly, depending upon the number of clinic visits and the actual transport expenses; but all mothers appreciated the money, and praised CDC's 'generosity' (lit. 'wide hand', *bade lach* (KP18)), embodied by the PI, whom they referred to as the 'owner/father of the clinic' (*wuon* clinic) or the leader of the study (*jatend* [study]), and the attentive and generous KEMRI staff. The idiom of generosity and the emphasis on the paternal figure inserts trial participation into a wider frame of patronage as local idiom of entitlement and responsibility. I will return to his relational and collectivising effects of the payments below.

Even medical care and pharmaceuticals, probably the most important transfer of material value around trials and definitely more significant than TR, was discussed by participants in monetary terms, when the prices of medical procedures such as deliveries, in public and private hospitals, were converted into costs. Several participants remarked upon the fact that the study not only liberated them of the cost of consultations and drugs—"Even if I'm a little sick, they give me good medicine which can cost a lot of money if I go to buy it and this relieves (lit. 'frees') me (*giketa thuolo*)" (KP8)—but even used "original drugs [brand packaged], not just drugs that are being sold ..." (KP 14). While these conversions of care into money underline the participants' awareness of

---

had been directly derived from comparison with labour rates. The result of the mapping exercise stabilised the more complex, contextualised considerations of research teams in city and rural area, and translated earlier deliberations about compensation for time and effort into reimbursement for transport fees.

value and the inseparability of value and care, their desire to be treated with 'original' drugs also indicates, again, that there is more than money to these considerations. The care bestowed by the study is also associated with higher reliability, and with wider, more robust, global medical connections, for example to leading multinational pharmaceutical companies or the technical standards of ISO certified research laboratories: if one's HIV test is done by the world's largest and most influential public health agency, by staff trained by a world leading old school of tropical medicine, or if one's drugs are produced by a known multinational pharma-company and licensed by the FDA, one's bodily state and well-being is, if ephemerally, connected to much larger wholes, which—despite the fears and concerns that power always also provokes in the powerless—engender expectations and trust that the nation-state health system can no longer instil in its citizens. Thus, while value calculations permeate social engagements of the trial, this does not prevent them from being linked to wider notions of belonging and care. I will come back to that.

Covering vital needs

The cash obtained through trial participation is quickly converted into life sustaining food—"something to swallow because, you know, we were breastfeeding, [...] so this money helped us a lot; we could have at least something to eat" (KP10). Invariably, the women describe how they would use the 'reimbursement' for food, to eat, to obtain particularly "good food [such as fruit] to boost up your blood/foetus" (KP4), or, more commonly to feed their children and to share with others: "the money that we were given, these 200, was helping us all. When I leave Kisumu I carry something. Doesn't it help everybody? You can buy something for the baby, and you can cook something in your house, and people share; so people are happy" (KP15). While daily food needs were the priority, some participants increased the value of their reimbursement by investing it, as they travelled between home and clinic: "the remaining fare [TR] made me join business; when I come to them I can go back with three or two pairs of shoes. I sell them higher than I bought them. The ones from this side have a bit of profit" (KP15).

The small amounts of reimbursement money contributed to the women's, and their children's, lives in an economy of survival, where the means to satisfy one's vital needs have to be found anew, day after day. Many of them described not having access to cash and often not knowing in the morning how to buy supper. Many lived in rented accommodation (single rooms) which cost around 5-700 Kenyan shillings a month, and described a family meal as consisting of vegetables for 20 shillings cooked with tomatoes for 10 shillings, accompanied by maize porridge (in 2009, maize flour cost 120 shillings for 2 kgs) which gives an indication of their regular cash flows, that transport reimbursements added to. The scarcity of money in these women's lives, often controlled by husbands and relatives, was underlined by their quest for health care: "when the child becomes sick, or when I am sick, I am in problems. I don't have money, I will not be treated. But then [with the study] I was just treated even if I don't have money" (KP9). "Sometimes the baby is sick, you carry the baby for treatment; in the hospital you are prescribed expensive drugs but you cannot afford them at that time, so you leave the baby until the sickness becomes worse, and only then you get money to go and buy" (KP18).

Those who had moved out of the city since the beginning of the study to live with relatives experienced particular difficulties in obtaining even the money (at times less than hundred shillings) needed to take a child to hospital in town. They had to borrow from neighbours and relatives, promising them to repay upon their return—which, incidentally, was comparatively easy for those who were known to 'be with KEMRI/CDC', since the association made them more creditworthy; often they walked, even for hours. For poor HIV positive mothers, the possibility of reaching the city or a hospital is about survival: "If a child is sick or if I am sick, even when I am far, I can call them to come for me or I just go and they will pay the transport" (KP12). "[When I was told the study was over] I said 'what am I going to do?' I had got used to Kisumu: when I'm sick I just looked for fare to go to Kisumu, and they treated me, or my child" (KP15). To have an institution pay for your transport when the need arises—"If you really need to go, it is always easy to borrow from a neighbour, because in the evening, he knows, you can repay [because he knows you are with CDC]" (KP10)—means here more than just a bus ticket; here again, trial participation is about remaining connected, to escape geographical and often social isolation, and to live.

Being cared for

Striking in the women's accounts was the lack of social networks and help that they could rely upon in times of need: vain attempts to secure funding for medical bills from husbands or relatives, and narratives of sick husbands unable to contribute—"it was at night and my husband refused to give out money so that I go to hospital so what could I do, I just gave birth" (KP9)—and not least stories about lack of trust between the women and husbands, relatives and neighbours, whom they hid their HIV status from. While some participants lived in supportive marriage and kin relationships, many others gave a picture of a lonely struggle for their own, and their children's, survival, where study participation provided vital associations: "if I had not joined [the study], the way I later became sick, nobody would have treated me. I would have stayed in the house until I was yellow and there was nobody there to take me to the hospital" (KP8).

Under conditions of isolation (economically, and in kinship and gender terms, compounded by HIV status and stigma) it is not surprising that the women described their participation in an HIV research project in extremely positive terms: "they really care about the children. These [study] children of theirs, they really liked them' (KP4); "they were happy people, they loved people, they loved us so much" (KP21); "They were taking good care of us. [...] transportation, [...] food, tea when you are hungry, there were nice to us" (KP6). Money, conviviality and attachment were intertwined: "like, sometimes I left my house before taking breakfast, so when they gave [breakfast] I say it is a good place because they consider others. Sometimes I could use my transport to come from home, and they gave it back to me; I said it is a good place, these people are really there to help me and I was happy with them" (KP1).

The experience of caring personal relations was also underlined by the prevailing idiom of kin- and friendship ('our baby', 'my sister' etc.); and the boundary between reimbursements and gifts was further blurred by the fact that staff members regularly extended the official reimbursements with small personal gifts of money or in kind. Thus, most follow-up staff who visited participants in their homes reported that they occasionally had given mothers small sums of money to buy food for their children, or brought them used clothes or flour. 'Being with' a study created a collective—if temporary, unstable, fragmented—out of mutual claims and responsibilities, as well as affect.

Material transfers came along with less tangible experiences of positive staff attitudes and new relations: "they gave me ... encouragement, they are talking to you ...they don't just talk to you like that" (KP15); "I was getting different teachings [...that] make your heart strong: my husband had left me then, but I said that we are many, I am not alone." (KP17). In particular, many mothers praised the knowledge they had gained—"knowledge on how I will continue living in good health, what I can do when I have a baby, the health of the child..." (KP9)—"a way of reasoning how one can live, with HIV" (KP12); "exposure", as some of them called it, to new ways of thinking and living, enforced by a sense of encouragement and of being cared for, being included into a larger collective. All women wished for greater continuity in the relations with the research project, and expressed regret that 'their' trial had ended, and said that they would be happy to join another research project. They summarised these experiences in terms of relief, if only temporarily, from the burden of everyday survival: "I saw a lot of lightness [due to the fact that I am cared for]" (KP18); "They really set me free" (KP8).[11]

11 | When, during a dissemination meeting that fed back trial results to the women, our own anthropological study was mentioned, almost all women were keen to join this new 'project', even though it fell short of some expectations.

This does not mean that everything was perfect. While most mothers appreciated the good healthcare, some were unhappy with how they were treated. Among the many who were proud that they had prevented their children from being HIV positive were others who had lost their children or had to cope with HIV positive babies. Some disagreed with particular staff members, and about 50 women out of 500 left the trial because of misgivings, or because they did not see the point. Twelve women had died of AIDS during the trial either because they had been recruited in an advanced stage, or because they could not adhere to treatment. Almost all remained desperately poor after the trial and continued to struggle for their daily needs and for health care from insufficient public institutions. What these quotes do suggest, however, is that material transfers, knowledge, conviviality, relatedness and belonging were intertwined in their experience. Economy and epistemology on the one hand, and morality and sociality on the other, were here not separate, even antagonistic domains, but mutually dependent and reinforcing each other. 'Being with' the study and the institution conducting it—'being with CDC or KEMRI', as people in Kisumu often say about trial participants as well as staff—implies a broad sense of attachment. Even if this sort of belonging may not always be achieved or lasting, it appears that people who participate in trials seek a broader sense of association, beyond attaining immediate personal material fulfilment of needs. Material value, everyday needs, the desire for knowledge, trust and care, are mixed in trial participation in ways that make the liberal idea of individual autonomy and voluntariness questionable. Instead, monetary transactions and other transfers of material value are experienced as part of wider connections and collectives, larger possibilities and hopes.

The failure of the gift?

A misnomer

Trials transfer value, including money, to participants; this value transfer is appreciated by recipients, and recognised by everybody involved; and yet it is excluded from the public space of the trial. It is, in the words of more than one of the researchers and staff we spoke to, an 'open secret'. This is morally and politically problematic. It can seem dishonest on a personal level, and may inhibit open debate, preventing questions of value and justice from being raised, and from becoming part of public debate about public health.[12] As it stands,

12 | One space in which such negotiations could have occurred were the 'community advisory boards' (CAB) that were set up by the HIV research group with distinguished 'community representatives', and which served to facilitate 'community engagements',

TR looks like a compensation for trial participants' value-creating efforts, which is set more or less arbitrarily by the trial management—analogous to a wage determined by the owner of the production process at will.

Given the fact that everybody involved seems to have accepted that value is transferred in TR it would seem appropriate to abandon this performance of valuelessness. There isn't much point to calling payments 'transport reimbursement' any more. But then, how ought one instead understand the transfers of value in clinical trials, epitomised by 'transport reimbursement', instead of concealing them. This 'ought' is not only a matter of representation—how does one correctly *represent* the reality of value transfers—but at least as much a problem of deontology—how *should* one speak about the value of public health research, if one takes seriously the women's biopolitical longing to be part of the trial, and aims to contribute to public (just, equitable) health in a healthy public sphere?[13]

Gift or commodity?

The centrality of value in clinical trials stands in contrast to earlier bioethicists' insistence that considerations of value and profit—any nexus between trial participation and the fulfilment of needs—is antithetical to ethical research

participant recruitment, and the negotiations of potential problems. However, during the years of this fieldwork the only occasions when transport reimbursement was discussed by the advisory board was in relation to the board members' own transport reimbursement, which eventually was set at a higher rate than that of research participants, presumably somehow related to the higher income of these employed or professional advisers. These different transport reimbursement rates again underline that something other than reimbursement is at play, in this case the different value of people, while the absence of other negotiations of reimbursement from community advisory board deliberations demonstrate the non-public nature of the reimbursement problem (and might raise the question whether the advisory board represents the interests of participants or of the research organisation).

13 | In a recent, methodologically very different, economic study carried out among Zambian HIV volunteers, experiments showed similarly, that money was at best part of social engagements and not the prime driver of voluntary health work (Ashraf et al. 2011). Monetary incentives were here less efficient to provide motivation than 'social' rewards and recognition. While the authors explained this–limited by their rational actor paradigm–as pointing to 'intrinsic motivation' and 'social comparison' (rather than mere financial rewards) as prime drivers of action, they also note in an aside that the 'reputable organization' for whom the volunteers worked, might have influenced their willingness to contribute. From our perspective, this dimension of belonging to a larger whole would deserve greater weight.

practice (see e.g. Titmuss 1970). This dissociation of ethical medicine from its political-economic context has been debated among progressive academic bioethicists for a while, most notably in reflections on 'benefit sharing' around medical research (see e.g. Hayden 2007). Yet, in the Kenyan context, ethics review boards as well as scientists and institutions take as yet little notice of these ongoing discussions (see discussion in Lairumbi et al. 2011); and in practice they remain focused on protecting individual autonomy and voluntariness, which they see threatened by implications of need and interest. Ethics appears here as antithetical to economics. To remain ethical, material transfers attendant on bodily participation in research must conform to a specific idea of the gift—what anthropologists have referred to as the hypothetical concept of the 'free gift', a 'gift for nothing', valueless, non-calculating, pure, and without expectation of return. Such gift should have no ties attached, not to other people, not across time, nor to one's bodily needs and desires.

From the observations about TR, above, one could then be led to conclude that this gift has simply failed as foundation for ethical medical science. Indeed, it seems futile to deny the omnipresence of value and calculation throughout human subject engagements with trials. If the gift has failed, its supposed opposite, the commodity rears its head. If people don't deal with research in terms of gifts, well, then transactions are probably commoditised—that is they should be recognised as exchanges of value in different currencies, including bodily substance, risk, time and money. This is a logical move, which some ethicists propose in an effort to realign medical ethics and a particular economic notion of freedom. The crudest conclusion from this shift would be to consider research participants' bodily materials as commodities—selling blood samples, organs etc.—but this conflicts with the near universal idea of the inalienability of the body.

Instead, one could move to consider participation in trials as free 'labour' (which can be bought and sold), and transactions of value, such as 'reimbursement', as payments or wages. In recent literature this idea of 'clinical labour' (Cooper 2008) comes in two different versions. One, proposed by some bioethicists, is economically liberal, aligning clinical labour with other unskilled labour in economically poor, low-wage settings, at a fixed low rate—talking about the 'price of a research subject' (Dickert/Grady 1999)—accepting the commercialisation of research and the place of unskilled labour in late capitalism as givens. Trial participants are here, like labourers, free to choose selling their time and bodily substance. The second one, developed by anthropologists and sociologists of medical research, comes to a similar conclusion out of broadly Marxist reasoning. By critiquing the misrepresentations that the concept of the free gift produces, and replacing them with a materialist understanding, the hope is that the correct recognition of 'clinical labour' would unleash social transformation analogous to older labour movements. The former proposition wants to adjust norms to the economic status quo, while the latter proposes, within a progressive deontology, to find origins of political-economic transformation in the given material reality. While the political intentions of both arguments are somewhat different, both seem to accept that the gift has failed, and the market—variously understood as invisible hand, or as generative of transformative contradictions—has taken over.

If matters are discussed, and resolved, within this frame, the linkage between bodily participation in public health research and similar medical practices and the older biopolitical collective exemplified by the developmental nation-state fades from view; the market appears as the only possibility in a post-governmental age. In the remainder of the chapter I consider the possibilities and limitations of this move in view of the evidence, above as well as in the literature on 'trial communities', that clinical trials in Africa (and similar settings) continue to engender associations and visions of collectives, against the backdrop of the relative weakness of the older nation-state forms of collectivity. I will conclude by considering what the gift, which according to anthropologists never was free, may still have to offer to our rendering of medical research and public health.

Emergent labour markets?

The notion of 'clinical labour', noted above, does open some political possibilities. In some situations, participants' bargaining power could allow for negotiations about the fair remuneration for their efforts. One of these situations is in the middle of long term trials, when each participant carries the value of the previous investment into examinations, treatments and other procedures; at this stage, participants are, as trial staff are the first to acknowledge, 'too valuable to lose', and trial managers and researchers invest considerable additional funds into maintaining participants or finding them and bringing them to the clinic (yet, participants seem to rarely notice the relative power they hold at this point, partly because they have started worrying about the end-of-the-trial). Another situation of potential bargaining power is when a research organisation has established a long term research site with high investment of capital, infrastructure and training; in such trial sites, which are increasingly common all over Africa, negotiations with (potential) participants are increasingly high on the agenda—often under the heading of 'community engagement' and 'public engagement' (see Molyneux et al. 2005). Finally, participants hold bargaining power where different research groups or projects operate in the same area and compete for participants. Here we see some form of incipient struggle, in which we can discern the shapes of an emergent clinical labour market.

If, within one area, different research groups offer different TR rates to the same potential trial population, this is quickly picked up by potential participants and discussed in terms of payment. Competition becomes particularly sharp when different trials are looking for participants with specific, rarer conditions or particular risks, in the same population. This situation is less uncommon than one would think, partly because transnational clinical trials are increasingly concentrated in large-scale, long-term research sites with favourable epidemiological conditions and global standard laboratories and facilities, and partly because scientific and policy developments, as well as drug market trends, can lead to waves of certain kinds of studies at a given time. If, for example, in HIV research and intervention, male circumcision is en vogue, young men have an edge; if HIV resistance genomics are hot, prostitutes in cities with state of the art laboratories are needed; and if drugs for pre-exposure prophylaxis (PREP) are to be tested, HIV negative members of 'high risk groups' such as prostitutes, youths or widows are needed; for such studies, HIV discordant couples, in which one partner is positive and one not, and in which both infective and uninfected partner can be enrolled in the same trial (giving either the positive or the negative part antiretroviral treatment to prevent transmission between them) are in particularly high demand.

The market analogy of these situations is recognised by trial managers who may express concern with the differences between different research collaborations' TR payments and the competitive effects on recruitment and trial success. As managers, they are constrained both by institutional agreements and study protocols, and by budgets, and find themselves thus squeezed between the need of recruiting numbers within a limited time, and the need to cap production costs—like any manager in moments of labour scarcity. In such situations, participants might enter into actions that bear analogy to incipient labour struggles. One of the more rudimentary forms of contestation is 'double enrolment' in more than one trial at the same time. This poses a scientific problem as it may affect a trial's validity, and a grave medical and ethical concern, as it might affect the health of the participant, especially where pharmaceuticals and invasive procedures are involved. Another form of contestation can be found in rumours about the 'exploitation' of research subjects and the alleged profits of the researchers—the so called 'guinea pig' rumours, which can express discontent and make claims for better remuneration (Geissler/Pool 2006; Leach/Fairhead 2007; Graboyes 2010; see White 2000). Thus, in 2004, a main national broadsheet carried large articles in which inhabitants of Kemri/CDC's demographic surveillance system accused the institution of major abuses; CDC responded, exposing the cited witnesses as disgruntled ex-employees, and by setting up a dedicated and well-funded "community engagement" section, with the "responsibility ... to generate community support and acceptance for KEMRI/CDC activities and to mobilize the community for informed participation". If local resistance and claims were put forward in more organised forms, demands for compensation, or just higher TR, might be pushed forward by local groups like 'community based organisations', which often play an important role in trial recruitment itself, or even by local administrators and chiefs, on behalf of their constituency. Such situations may offer opportunities to mobilise critical research subject advocacy in Africa, which so far have often failed because they did not account for African participants' fundamental desire to be part, through trials, of larger regimes of reliability and care.

In spite of these incipient political possibilities, so far research institutions and groups respond effectively—though mostly unwittingly—to preclude the possibility of such challenges. One important strategy is, not unlike missionary societies of the past, to stake out territorial claims, which are more or less informally negotiated with and acknowledged by different groups. Thus, in western Kenya, one large zone covering several districts is the principal area of KEMRI/CDC research (as well as, until recently, KEMRI/CDC managed, GAP funded HGIV care and treatment), a neighbouring district is covered, in terms of research and HIV care, by the US Department of Defence, beside this area is (with a slight, not unproblematic overlap) a zone 'run' by AMPATH, the 'Academic Model Providing Access to Healthcare', a Kenyan bridgehead of major US Medical Schools combining research and care provision, and parts of Kisumu city by FACES, 'Family AIDS Care and Education Services', a similar outfit initiated by another main US medical school running numerous collaborative trials etc. This territorial organisation ensures relatively uncomplicated recruitment in one's given study area—although for rare participant types like discordant couples, these might have to travel some distance to attend a particular trial—and avoids competitive participant claims. Also, the massive investments made during the past decade by the leading transnational research groups, universities and funders in local infrastructure, allow groups to lay claim to areas and their populations and preclude competition. If a territorial agreement cannot be reached, the very different resources and power of research groups or organisations can lead to effective struggles over territories, and weaker groups tend to withdraw from areas worked on by stronger ones.

An important mechanism in this context is demographic surveillance data collection, i.e. establishing longitudinal databases of the population in particular areas as well as their morbidity, which constitutes the backbone of randomised controlled trials in many parts of Africa. Such demographic surveillance systems, which come at very high cost and greatly enhance the value of a study population, constitute a novel form of governance over a specific territory (usually in the range of 100-300.000 inhabitants, in some cases much more) which is much more long-term than the usual clinical trial; as such they tend to prevent incursions by non-collaborating research groups, and thus competition for participants. While demographic surveillance areas indubitably stake a claim in an area, they also provide a form of governance and attendant forms of citizenship, which can be utilised both for improved health care provision, as is the case in many surveillance areas, and as a framework for wider negotiations about clinical trials, their benefits, and other health care related matters. They are thus both a potential mechanism of control and of representation, of discipline and democracy.

If competition cannot be avoided and different groups work on similar issues in one area, double enrolment can be prevented using Photo ID cards and fingerprint readers, and sharing the attendant person-codes and data between different projects and research organisations. This strategy is increasingly used by clinical trials management in areas without reliable person registration and documents, and high concentration of research. And finally, if different clinical trials by several groups have to share the same population, the inevitable competitive instincts between groups and their scientific leaders must be overcome and agreement reached over TR rates and the level of other participant benefits.[14]

Freedom?

As these examples show, the political promise of reframing research participation as labour is still limited given the unequal distribution of power, and the unlimited pool of (bare-)life labour. More important doubts also arise on a more analytical level. The older bioethicists who insist on participation being a free gift, and those who advocate the liberation of 'clinical labour' could be opposed (and pose at times) as 'idealist' and 'materialist'. However they share certain premises regarding the nature of money and monetary exchange.

First, they seem to agree that moral and economic considerations belong to separate spheres and should not be conflated, each of them giving, respectively, priority to morality or political economy. Promiscuity between the two is a threat, much as in Marx' understanding as acid that dissolves the social. Money materialises the abstract, amoral, calculating quality of economic rationality that must be kept away from moral reasoning, lest sociality will suffer. This understanding of money as amoral, even immoral, and anti-social, does not seem to be as obvious to the women quoted above, who appreciated precisely the moral value of monetary support as much as the material manifestations of care. The distinction between money and morality has for long been analysed

14 | In this case, if groups actually negotiate to cap reimbursements and benefits at one level in order to curb competition, TR is treated almost openly like labour-wage within a labour market, running very much against the formal denial of TR being a payment. This paradox is possible, because the two processes happen on the different, disjointed levels of the protocol and its GCP commitments, and of trial managers and local implementers; and because the two operations are separated, in the everyday of trial planning and operations, by the veil of discursive rigour, denial and ironic detachment.

as a crude simplification by social anthropologists who showed that monetary exchanges and moral action are commonly intertwined, and that the neat separation between morality and economy may indeed be part of a particularly cultural formation, or even of an ideology of capitalism, while people all over the world, including those in core capitalist institutions, tend to mix and connect economic and moral domains (see e.g. Shipton 1989; Parry/Bloch 1989; Maurer 2006; see also Mauss 1923). In other words, the common-sense association of money with individuation and rational calculus, which continues to underlie much medical ethical discourse, might not be helpful to understand the workings of value, and values, in a clinical trial.[15]

The notion of money as abstract and individuating is linked to another premise shared by advocates of purist bioethics and of clinical labour alike: the idea of freedom and autonomy as basis of good science. For both, the gift is free, that is an (individual) gesture without calculus, value and expectation of direct return, performed by free, individual actors out of individual moral (or spiritual) motivation. This idea of gifting is in their vision opposed to an alternative vision of individual action as commodity exchange, premised upon self-interest, calculation and the maximisation of pleasure or utility. Liberty and autonomy are here the central nodes around which both the free gift, and free labour are constructed.

What is absent from both these renderings of value transactions is the notion of a collective—a 'social'—be it as an existing reality that facilitates and underwrites value transfers, in the way in which the nation-state did in mid-20th century ideas about voluntary blood donation (e.g. Titmuss 1970), or as project entailed by these transfers, a future evoked by transacting value, such as in the communities engendered by 'benefit sharing' in relation to bioprospecting and intellectual property (see Hayden 2007). The possibility of value transactions, not as individual acts but as *produced by and productive of* collective forms does not occur either in the imaginary of free gifting, or in the alternative proposition of free labour. It is assumed that the act of giving and receiving material value is a momentary engagement between individuals, existing in the present. These

15 | In the scientific context examined here, a related common assumption about money deserves mention. By engendering an interest in personal profit, money might endanger not only moral reasoning, but also the (supposedly amoral) validity of scientific knowledge which, in theory, arises from impartial investigation premised upon universal social values. Economy and epistemology are here opposites, just like morality and economy. While this argument deserves consideration where funding for medical research and the commodification of its results are concerned, this opposition does not seem to hold for the women above, for whom 'being with' the trial produced simultaneously knowledge of medical facts as well as health care possibilities, and opportunities for modest material gain.

assumptions about the (a)sociality and (a)temporality of clinical trial transactions reflect only one, narrow understanding of the gift, which may be symptomatic of the current historical, political-economic condition, which some sociologists also described as the 'death of the social' (Rose 1996).

While it may be practically advisable to acknowledge the vital value transacted in TR (and thus to get rid of the misnomer of 'transport reimbursement'), this does not lead to the replacement of the pure gift with a pure commodity or free labour. By way of conclusion, I want to argue in favour of retaining, somewhat doggedly, the notion of the gift to science.

End: Gift as collective

When I propose that we hold on to the notion of the gift to designate trial value transfers, it is not in the sense of a pure, free gift, but as a gift in a classic anthropological sense (supported by the trial participants' experiences detailed above). Gifts imply, firstly, social relationships, attachments, and the collectives that arise from such associations; and secondly, they are deployed over time involving memories of past actions as much as anticipations of futures. The gift understood as such is thus a pointer towards futures collectives and possibilities, as early anthropologists had argued and as has been reiterated with different emphasis for more than a century of anthropological writing (e.g. Malinowski 1922; Mauss 1923; see e.g. Strathern 1988).

In a completely different social and historical context from that of classic ethnographic accounts, but somewhat closer to our clinical trial site, the link between gifting and collective forms was explored by Richard Titmuss in his work on blood donation in mid-twentieth century Britain (Titmuss 1971, in Oakely and Barker 2004)). In Titmuss' version, the collective in question is the nation-state, and, he argues, it is because this collective is already in place that people are able to give 'gifts to strangers' (1970). What Titmuss' analysis is less interested in, is that gift-value transfers also contribute to bringing collectives into being. The post-war British National Health Service, Titmuss' prime subject of analysis, was not only premised upon the nation but also contributed to the creation of the specific mid-twentieth-century British nationhood. For Titmuss, the nation-state in its post second world war welfare version was a quasi-natural frame of reference and the question of how collectives such as this come into being was of less interest than what they can make one do.[16] By contrast, if we think about practices such as blood donation—or transnational clinical trials—

16 | While the foundation of the NHS was premised upon a nation state that had just emerged solidified from the collective effort of the World War, the question of how, in turn, health services can help making the nation was a more obvious issue in Titmuss

today, the nation-state no longer provides such an obvious framing. Indeed, as Cecilia Busby has warned us, the nostalgic evocation of past collectives such as 'the nation' can be problematic and indeed dangerous in a situation where the nation-state has decayed or where it no longer pursues public wellbeing (2006). Such, we might argue, is the case in some contemporary African nations.[17]

If I suggest here that we recognise the ability of gifting to create collectives and open futures, I do not want to evoke 'traditional' cultural collectives of the Levy-Bruhl'ian kind (*pace* certain African bioethicists 'Ubuntu'-inclinations); neither do I believe that we can 'return' post-neoliberal Kenya to Titmuss' (and Keynes') 1948 welfare Britain. But at the very least we should expand—maybe inspired by these older imaginaries—our ethnographic sensitivities to the possible collectives and aspirations that are implied and evoked when trial participants choose to give their time and bodily substance, and to accept material transfers of value, including money.

Citzenship as experiment

Partly in response to the less stable and obvious nature of government and national collective today, compared to Titmuss' times, the past decade has seen an abundance of fruitful anthropological explorations of increasingly manifold, fluid and fragmented 'citizenship(s)', including, importantly 'biological citizenship' (Rose/Novas 2005). The latter concept, and its more comprehensive predecessor 'biosociality' (Rabinow 1996), would seem particularly relevant here (see especially Biehl 2004; Nguyen 2004). The social ties described above could, derived from this literature, be described as 'experimental citizenship'. Such terms would reflect some of the participating women's claims and desires: the material transfers provided by the trial substitute in part for the welfare and health care they would be entitled to as national citizens, and in turn most of them struggle to be 'good citizens' of the trial and of KEMRI/CDC. 'Experimental citizenship' would also reflect the peculiar nature of this kind of association: it is citizenship on time, on trial, more a search for citizenship, than a comprehensive and lasting attachment as national citizenship would claim to be.

On the other hand, describing the tentative associations produced within the trial as (yet) another form of 'citizenship' risks devaluing the larger promise held out by the older, more comprehensive political project, conceived in enlightenment readings of an even older civitas. The inflationary use of multiple citizenshipS makes it difficult to measure the shortcomings of emergent and

efforts to help shaping the health services of the newly independent nation Tanzania (see Titmuss 1964).

17 | Busby reminds us that the relationship between imaginaries of association and political economic realities needs to be continually assessed (2006).

fragile forms of association that arise, in part, in response to the collapse of nation-state citizenship; the latter seems now just like one of many of its kind, rather than a universal standard and aspiration. Thus, although trial participation might entail a search for a lost citizenship, and although it indeed is an experimental social formation, the multiplication of citizenships is marred by the same problem as the anthropological proliferation of 'modernities' in the 1990s: that of discounting people's aspirations for a more encompassing, universalist and enduring form of societal association (see Ferguson 2006).

The women quoted in this essay evoke the 'hospitality' and conviviality of trial relations, they describe trust and care, and they make reference to the larger institutions of scientific knowledge of health care and of government that they imagine behind their clinical trial. These allusions to 'being with' something larger than individual and local do not map onto one another, nor add up to one coherent whole. Some are limited to the trial in question and its caring staff; others refer to the Kenyan and US government institutions behind it; others again evoke the certified standards of drugs and diagnostics sourced from Europe or the US; and all of them are aware of the ephemeral temporality of any of these associations, and yet, they yearn for a stability (that in turn is referenced in memories and remains of past national projects). These associations cannot match the high-modern 'imagined community' of the nation-state. But although these imagined and experienced collectives are limited and temporary, they reveal the Kenyan trial participants' longing for biopolitical inclusion. In the absence of effective care or control, leave alone biomedical discipline, even fragments of larger wholes are objects of desire: the chip card for trial participants, the GIS based surveillance, the finger print scan, even the regular blood specimen collection, become not threatening targets of potential anti-biopolitical resistance, but signify towards imaginary—sometimes remembered—modes of inclusion and citizenship.

Similar observations to those above were made by other ethnographers who attended to the experience of African participants in transnational public health research and found that they pursued long-term relations and new kinds of belonging in their engagements with clinical trials, rather than seeking mere material benefits or means of survival under conditions of deprivation (and far from resisting the threat of biopolitical domination) (see especially Leach/Fairhead 2007; Molyneux et al. 2005; Geissler et al. 2007). This does not mean that a Kenyan woman gifting bodily specimens and accepting reimbursements necessarily has a clear picture of the collectives and affiliations she aims to attach herself to, and in this regard her situation may be different from mid-20th century nation-state citizens. Maybe the collectives that she seeks to associate herself to do not yet exist in a specific form. It is through her attachments that she pursues them and that they gradually, and partially, take shape. As ethnographers—as well as scientists in public health, I would argue—we should attend to this search for 'transport', mentioned earlier in this chapter, for movement and transformation—of knowledge and of the world that is made known—beyond the existing conditions of life and of economic, political and social deprivation.

In Africa after the demise of the monolithic biopolitical nation-state, our primary challenge then may not be to discern and critique (or delineate resistance to) the classic biopolitical regimes of surveillance and discipline—which have become almost extinct species, confined to the reservations of demographic surveillance systems and HIV treatment programmes—but to attend to the longing and nostalgia that these older, once threatening orders evoke today. The shadow, not of the dark, imposing underside of modernity as in 1970s antimodernism, but the rather more faint shadow of a distant modern constellation, which from the vantage point of contemporary African ex-citizens of biopolitical nationhood, appears again as an utopia.[18]

18 | In terms of concrete responses to this situation, then, the proposition by de Cernival to extend health care in clinical trials to everybody, within and outside the trial, points towards a political debate about the collectivising aims of public health research (de Cernival 2008). Although theoretically closely linked to the liberal 'clinical labour' proposition, above, this seems to me a politically more promising route.

Sleeping Sickness and the Limits of 'Biological Citizenship'

PETER REDFIELD

"Best Science for the Most Neglected"
DRUGS FOR NEGLECTED DISEASES INITIATIVE BROCHURE, 2004

Can one be a "citizen" of a neglected disease? For anyone positioned outside a particular strand of academic discussion relating health and politics, the question might appear counterintuitive, if not oddly contradictory. Nonetheless, at a historical moment when appeals to "global health" resonate powerfully through state and private philanthropy, when pharmaceutical products constitute a normal (and at times vital) component of daily routine, and when rhetorics of victimization and trauma underscore claims to compensation, political status appears increasingly attached to bodily condition. Indeed, recent work focused on problems of governance, bodies and transnational forms has proposed a clutch of variations on the theme of citizenship to identify medical politics of the present. Thus we might consider an individual to be—in acutely pragmatic terms—a "biological" citizen in the aftermath of the Chernobyl disaster in Ukraine, or a "therapeutic" one when surviving on imported anti-retroviral medications in West Africa (see Petryna 2002; Nguyen 2004 and 2010;Biehl 2007; Ecks 2008). What, however, about a less publicized threat, positioned at the edge of both biomedical and political concern?

In the essay that follows I will situate this question by examining a particular condition, human African trypanosomiasis (HAT) or sleeping sickness.[1] Once a classic colonial anxiety, sleeping sickness now finds representation in global health circles as a "neglected" disease, meaning that it primarily afflicts poor, marginal populations and consequently receives little attention or research investment. By comparing recent NGO efforts to combat the disease with

---

1 | Sleeping sickness appears in several forms, affecting both humans and nonhumans in different ways as outlined below. For most of this essay I will refer to the condition by its more evocative colloquial name rather than HAT.

earlier responses to it under British administration in Uganda, I seek to highlight the manner in which contemporary health initiatives may reflect an altered configuration of governance. I make two general claims: first that global health engenders, at best, a "distant" form of citizenship, constructed out of humanitarian concern rather than territorial projects of nation state or empire. Consequently it lies closer to the figure of the human than to that of a rights bearing subject. Second, I wish to suggest, and illustrate, how disease particularities matter when seeking to investigate and generalize about contemporary intersections between life and politics. Now positioned at one end of a spectrum of attention and neglect, sleeping sickness embodies the essence of a global humanitarianism practiced at a molecular level.

By pursuing sleeping sickness through the question of citizenship I thus seek to trace a limit to an otherwise productive trope, one that might in turn reveal another topography of emergent forms. In *The Politics of Life Itself*, perhaps the most general statement of the significance of life to contemporary political forms, Nikolas Rose devotes a chapter to the theme of biological citizenship. There he concludes that "new kinds of biological citizens—with new subjectivities, new politics and new ethics—are forming around contemporary developments in biomedicine," identifying this development with "a new space of hope and fear [...] around genetic and somatic individuality" (Rose 2007: 154). Rose is careful to specify that his analysis applies to what he terms "advanced liberal democracies"—settings like Britain, Germany or the United States where individuals lead lives suffused with biomedical care, legal regulation and market exchange. He further notes that in "residual social states" demand might focus on government support rather than entrepreneurial self-fashioning. Yet amid the epochal language inspired by epic new technologies, it is easy to forget other emerging futures, such as new scenarios surrounding even an old disease. Precisely because the term citizen is seductive and fertile, it merits not only extension, but also recognition of the limits of its translation.

Keeping with a theoretical lineage that I share, I follow Rose in referencing Michel Foucault's classic concept of "biopower" and examining an assemblage of actors concerned with fostering the life of a given population (see e.g. Foucault 2003; Rabinow/Rose 2006). The perspective of a particular, marginal condition like sleeping sickness, however, suggests a rather different biopolitical vision—or set of visions—than either Foucault's account of early modern Europe or Rose's depiction of its genealogical descendants. As a vector driven disease confined to Africa, sleeping sickness inhabits a different historical sequence, one of colonial rule followed by postcolonial states and an aid regime. Citizenship here, then, bears a different relationship to other elements of associative vocabulary, including "subject" and "human."[2] As I shall suggest, the latter is of particular consequence with regard to sleeping sickness. Notably, the contemporary humanitarian form of global health, constructed around a secular value of human life and typified by such entities as the Gates Foundation and the transnational NGO Médecins Sans Frontières, suggests a politics driven by moral claims. Thus political standing relative to global health—its "citizenship project" as it were—involves reference not only states and sovereigns, but also the longer arc of humanitarian concern for "suffering at a distance."[3] The boundary lines of such a project do not conform to those of nation states, and involve a lineage of pity as much as rights.

My argument in brief is that international efforts to combat sleeping sickness increasingly claim the intrinsic value of human life. The human subject they imply is thus less the citizen of a nation state or the object of imperial rule, than the constituent of humanitarian concern. Since the sovereign responsible for the care of this subject's health appears incapable of protecting it, that health becomes the affair of other entities, including international and non-profit organizations, research scientists and pharmaceutical suppliers. In contrast to earlier biopolitical formations, life here stands at a remove from milieu. Citizenship in this context, I will suggest, may likewise stand at a remove from the liberal subject it implies, a distance measured in the space and time of "neglect." For advocates of global health, then, those suffering from sleeping sickness are emblematically human and yet only distantly and secondarily citizens. Their political weight appears at a remove, glimpsed through moral discourse asserting a right to receive the benefits of biomedicine (as practiced at the level of protocol standards and drug research), and through the abstracted, collective interest of the afflicted as a "stakeholder group." My goal in deploying the citizenship metaphor in this context is not to denounce humanitarian efforts to combat neglected diseases (a categorically noble effort from any perspective valuing human health) but rather to examine their political effects and parameters. Biomedical responses to sleeping sickness suggest a spiralling history, first from a hierarchical focus on biological pathogens to a more comprehensive ecological effort to cleanse territory, the breakdown of that control and a subsequent humanitarian focus on pharmaceutical agents. In the last case the biopolitical formation only constitutes a polity in a minimal and dispersed sense—citizenship "at a distance."

Over the following pages I offer three sketches of sleeping sickness. Two describe the disease from the contemporary perspective of a key medical

2 | See, e.g. debates surrounding Mahmood Mamdani's *Citizen and Subject: Contemporary Africa and the Legacy of Later Colonialism.*

3 | Phrasings borrowed from Rose 2007 and Boltanski 1999 [1993]. For more on the history of humanitarianism see e.g. Calhoun 2009; Redfield/Bornstein forthcoming.

humanitarian NGO, both at the level of a local project and the larger, global pharmaceutical effort to which it contributed. The other outlines the historical discovery and response to the disease under colonial rule. All three involve biomedical sensibilities and are set in the region now known as Uganda. By positioning each within a biopolitical frame, I suggest differences within their commonalities, ones that both distinguish the projects involved and reflect back on the concepts used to analyse them. In a fourth section I return to the conceit of citizenship to consider the problem of neglect in global health, along with the form of humanitarian science it inspires. While this approach emphasizes distinctions for analytical clarity, I do not intend to imply complete epochal shifts; a more complete accounting would recognize overlaps, inconsistencies and continuing negotiations.[4] The goal here is simply to recognize political forms beyond nation state, and thus productively complicate the figure of citizenship.

SKETCH 1: A SITUATED CHALLENGE

First, a cursory ethnographic account. In the summer of 2003 I visited a sleeping sickness project in north-western Uganda.[5] Founded over a decade and a half earlier by the humanitarian group Médecins Sans Frontières (Doctors Without Borders or, in native acronym, MSF), the project had shifted and altered course several times. By the point of my arrival MSF had officially handed clinical operations over to the Ugandan Ministry of Health, and only supported the last phase of a research study run by its epidemiological subsidiary, Epicentre. Although my visit was brief, as my first foray to an MSF field site it left a lasting impression and coloured subsequent encounters elsewhere. A pathos of loss associated with closure hung in the air; people pointed out where MSF previously had rented a house, staffed a clinic, adopted a dog. The sleeping sickness team went about its work with stoic determination, tinged with foreboding. Those now on the government's rolls complained about not being paid, while the rump Epicentre team repeatedly explained to health workers and patients alike why they were still screening but not directly enrolling or treating new subjects.

4 | For an example of historical complexity at the local level see Lwoba/Ombongi/Geissler/Malowany 2011.

5 | The material I draw on here stems from a larger ethnographic and historical study of MSF, with the bulk of research conducted between 2002-2006 in a number of sites in Europe and Uganda. Although actually a federation of 19 semi-autonomous national sections, for the purposes of this essay I will refer to the organization in the singular (this particular project in Uganda belonged to MSF-France, which also played a lead role promoting DNDi within the organization). See e.g. Redfield 2005 and 2006.

As the only non-Ugandan in the vehicle, I attracted shouts of children when we drove through remote hamlets, while the gaze of curiosity of their elders mingled with expectation: surely the white man in the white car would be in charge. The team's actual leader, an energetic Ugandan nurse I'll call Grace, stoically negotiated the tensions of being a younger woman instructing older men. Originally from the area herself she was intimately familiar with local languages and regional culture, a fact that she found a mixed blessing. She was glad at least to be working one district over from where most of her kin and classmates resided. Indeed, she eventually confided that her goal was one day to work for an NGO elsewhere—ideally far from a rural hospital in north-western Uganda—since she found there were problems with operating locally:

"I know the people here and they know me. They expect me to be just like them and to listen to their problems. At the same time the NGO wants you to perform a certain way. In town there would be nurses who were ahead of me; if I were in charge of them they wouldn't like it. It's much easier if you're from somewhere else and they don't know you."

Due to this background it had been difficult at first for her to take control of the remaining program. The staff, used to international leadership and doubting the ability of a young Ugandan woman, failed to show up on time and ignored direction, to the extent that one driver had to be fired. By now Grace had garnered sufficient respect to exert authority, but still found it a constant effort. Following this explanation I better understood her manner in wards and public settings like screenings, which I—used to a consumer oriented model of health care, alternately obsequious or indifferent—found startlingly authoritarian. She spoke in commanding tones and frequently in English, the national language of education. Her dress was inevitably "smart" in the British idiom. Like many Ugandans employed by MSF and other NGOS in positions of professional responsibility, she looked the part, in marked contrast to the casual, camping aesthetic favoured by international volunteers.

One morning we visited the stockroom of the local hospital to which Epicentre directed most sleeping sickness cases. Supply was clearly a problem: many shelves were bare and dusty, or had only one or two boxes or bottles on them, reminding me of stores I had seen in remote parts of Eastern Europe prior to 1989. Much of the visible supply sat in boxes marked MSF from their last delivery, which Grace anticipated would run out by the end of the year. A woman who worked there told us about their continuing problems with the authorized distributor, exemplified by a crisis over surgical gloves that the hospital's director resolved by buying a supply privately. Leaving the stockroom we ran into him, and he elaborated on the problem of sustainability as it pertained to the sleeping sickness program:

"At the moment we don't have special funding for this, but rely on what the ministry sends. Active screening and transport are expensive, so now we're just encouraging people to come in like with other diseases. We're trying to make sure we don't stop where MSF stopped, but try to continue where we can. But our limitations are national limitations."

While pleased to have trained personnel available, the director remained doubtful about the continued availability of drugs for treatment of the condition. At this regional level the question of drug access translated into basic problems of expense and unreliable transport. For him, sleeping sickness was simply another iteration of a general theme of inadequate supply.

Grace spent a good part of her day exhorting others to fulfil their duties. "With MSF it was like the police working," she told me, with a hint of wistfulness. "Almost all were treated; there was no reason not to. MSF would go and pick them [up]...with MSF there were no excuses not to get treated." The network of Sleeping Sickness Assistants had clear areas and well-defined responsibilities, and consequently followed up each case. In addition to free transport, those admitted received a food supplement courtesy of the World Food Program: beans, cooking oil, maize flour and sugar. The NGO also sponsored community education programs, not only about the disease but also about the need to support prevention efforts such as tsetse fly traps issued by the government.[6] Since poor people remained likely to encounter flies in the course of daily subsistence activities—digging, fishing, herding cattle—they needed to leave traps in place, and not use their materials for other purposes. Moreover, if infected they should report promptly for treatment; although familiar with sleeping sickness in its debilitating later form, people remained reluctant to submit themselves to painful and expensive care until it proved unavoidable. Such a pattern was typical for all local health care, Grace noted, but with sleeping sickness such delay could prove fatal.

Now, however, everything was in decline. Individual actors might make efforts, such as one clinic struggling to maintain food supplements for example, if only flour and beans. The sleeping sickness staff continued to run screenings, check on cases and educate hospital staff and patients alike. ("Antibodies are the soldiers of the body!" Grace barked at a line of school children at one stop, "Ask your teacher.") However, even maintaining proper statistics remained an uphill struggle. Grace's team had a continuing disagreement with the district health administration over whose responsibility it was to calculate the local prevalence rate. After speaking at length with an official on the phone, Grace fumed that

6 | As the presence of these traps indicate, MSF's program did not run in strict isolation, but rather comprised a new, lively element amid layers of semi-active and historical programs.

no one read the reports she sent. Someone in the district office needed to go through the register book and district population records and calculate, not just call her at the last minute wanting a number for lobbying purposes. That was their job. The current information was hardly representative, she explained, showing me a paper that listed the hospital we had visited as having no cases, even though we had just seen some. If she gave officials a number they would quote it immediately, and should it prove wrong her credibility would be shot. A neighbouring district listed a prevalence rate of 12-15%, but no one believed that—it would be an epidemic!

My brief encounter with Grace's sleeping sickness team partly resonated with Foucault's classic formulation of biopower in dawn of liberal Europe. The disease clearly mobilized strategies related to the governance of life, generating a community of expertise, which in turn fostered strategies for a population to work on its own health. And yet in this context it would be a stretch to define such governance in terms of state action. Under NGO management and financing the experience of care resembled something like that of a liberal welfare state, minimalist, perhaps, but nonetheless comprehensive. Absent such subvention, however, the regular government apparatus offered few services, and even these functioned only intermittently. Uganda, even in its north-western reaches, hardly represented a "failed state"—indeed, by MSF's standards it was a relatively present and active one, requiring significant negotiation in such areas as customs controls and medical protocols. But likewise it was far less "biopolitical" than any contemporary European polity, in the sense of actively fostering life. Without intervention by other entities, some populations would likely be allowed to die. This prospect stemmed less from any exceptional action on the part of the state, than from quite ordinary facts of limited resources and logistical obstacles in a relatively poor, relatively populous country with eroded infrastructure. As a sleeping sickness patient one's national claims to benefits of citizenship remained distinctly limited. At the same time Ugandan professionals faced significant challenges in performing expertise appropriate to the work of governance. Grace experienced her local ties through the burden of received racial and gender norms, alongside the weight of expectations born of kin and tribal affiliation. For her (like many other Ugandans associated with the project), the state was an undependable figure at both national and regional levels, its agents alternately suspected of inattention, incompetence or corruption.[7] NGO administration represented the prospect of effective procedures as well as reliable payment, a norm that clearly depended on ties to elsewhere. True biopolitics lay over the horizon.

7 | For discussion of tensions surrounding the contemporary African state see e.g. Ferguson 2006.

SKETCH 2: A COLONIAL MIRROR?

Given that sleeping sickness carries the colonial resonance of a pith helmet, the condition begs comparative examination through time. Here I will briefly review some of the history of biomedical efforts to respond to the disease and their relation to governance of life.[8] In its concern and techniques MSF's medical project might mirror earlier interventions, but it suggests a different political geography than the configuration of high imperial rule, where concerns over security and labour dictated attention to milieu and population movements.

Between 1900 and 1905 an epidemic of sleeping sickness swept through Uganda, then a British protectorate. Perhaps a quarter of a million people died, arousing concern among colonial authorities. The Royal Society dispatched a research team to investigate, and in October of 1902 they identified a "fish-like parasite" in a blood sample, matching the trypanosome discovery made in Ghana less than a year before (Lyons 1992). Although accounts of a distinctive "African lethargy" had appeared centuries earlier, sometimes credited with emptying whole villages, this was the critical moment in the biomedical definition of the disease. Having linked the pathology with a parasitic infection, researchers subsequently identified the tsetse fly as the insect vector of transmission.

Initially unsure of the disease's potential to spread, the British government feared infection flowing up the Nile to India and struggled to come up with appropriate administrative measures in response. Other European powers watched warily and followed suit, partly for propagandistic reasons. To Uganda's west in the Belgian Congo, King Leopold saw the benefits of improving the image of his ruthless colonial venture with a public health service and invited the Liverpool School to send an expedition. At the same time some early researchers recognized that that sleeping sickness had achieved epidemic form precisely because of imperial expansion, and the disruptive effects of population migrations and invasive expeditions (ibid.: 72-75).

Over the ensuing years further scientific research revealed an increasingly complex picture of sleeping sickness. The form initially identified in the Ugandan epidemic, *Trypanosoma brucei gambiense*, acquired a sibling in 1910 with the identification of *Trypanosoma brucei rhodesiense* in Northern Rhodesia.[9] Although similar in their ultimate effects on human health, the two differed in the precise nature of their vectors (different species of tsetse flies), their favoured climatic conditions (moist riverbanks vs. arid savannahs), their primary reservoir

8 | A more comprehensive historical presentation would incorporate additional threads, such as sleeping sickness control by the later colonial and postcolonial state, and the MSF's ties to French colonial medicine. See Lachenal/Taithe 2009.

9 | Precisely which form produced the Ugandan epidemic is now less clear (see Fèvre et al. 2004).

hosts (human vs. animal) and the speed of their onslaught (a matter of months or years vs. weeks). The human form of this disease divided Africa rather neatly west to east, with Uganda on the fault line between "chronic" Gambian and "acute" Rhodesian varieties. In addition, other trypanosomes infected livestock, also to devastating effect. From the perspective of colonial administrators all forms constituted a threat to their project of rule. In medical terms the human varieties were hard to detect without screening, particularly the slower acting *gambiense* strain. If left untreated, however, in both varieties the infection would ultimately move beyond the lymph nodes and cross the blood-brain barrier. Sleeping sickness thus proved a fearsomely fatal disease. Researchers gradually came to realize that its prevalence, however, depended on a relatively delicate balance between parasite, fly vector, environment and human host. Only under certain conditions—e.g. temperature range, intervals of feeding—could the parasite properly develop in the fly's gut and subsequently infect its human host. By and large, the collapse of stable settlement offered ideal opportunities for the spread of the pathogen. At the same time it could not spread indefinitely, or range far from its regional habitat (Hoppe 2003; see also Lyons 1992; Ford 1971). Both Europe and India, it turned out, were safe from this African scourge. Most Africans were safe as well, so long as they inhabited stably settled and well-cleared land. Ecologically constricted and yet potentially mortal, sleeping sickness proved a quintessentially colonial condition.

Along with the British, Belgian, French, Portuguese and German colonial administrations all developed and maintained efforts to control and combat the disease, sharing information and techniques. These approaches took two forms, one "medical" and the other "biological"—what would now be termed ecological (Hoppe 2003). In addition to research the first involved screening examinations to identify infected patients and the administration of drugs to treat them. By contrast the second sought to destroy the fly vector, eliminating its habitat and removing people from its vicinity. Generally speaking, the British emphasized ecological measures more than other colonial powers, seeking to restrict the movements of both human and fly populations. While the British might focus on limiting trypanosome carrying tsetse flies and the Germans and French on developing medicines, at moments of outbreak all sought quarantine and social control, embarking on sanitation campaigns to protect public health (ibid).[10]

10 | In a review of Hoppe's book, Imperato suggests the difference stems in part from the fact that the British in East Africa dealt with the *rhodesiense* form. While simplified, the point merits further investigation, as a suggestion by both author and reviewer that the temporary disappearance of sleeping sickness in the 1960s and 70s might stem from a decline of surveillance by newly independent African states (Imperato 2005; see also Hoppe 2003; Tilley 2004).

The motivation of these colonial interventions, however, was not simply humanitarian, or primarily concerned with human suffering. Rather, these actions retained a resolutely economic and social perspective, focusing on disease outbreaks as a structural threat. To quote Megan Vaughn:

"In the first half of the twentieth century any contact which the majority of Africans had with colonial medicine was likely to have been in the form of a 'great campaign'. Epidemics of smallpox, of meningitis, of plague, and of sleeping sickness posed a constant threat to the economic (and political) viability of the early colonial state. The rise of tropical medical research was an outcome not merely of the elevation of germ theory, but of the continuing threat posed by epidemic disease to the entire colonial enterprise." (Vaughn 1991: 37)

By definition, the political economy of empire concerned itself with place, investing expectations in defined territories. The results were indeed productive, if not always in the economic sense. Research associated with these colonial health interventions contributed to early understandings of disease ecology (Tilley 2004; see also Anderson 2004). Thus while key compounds to combat sleeping sickness emerged during the era of colonial governance (e.g. the venerable drug melarsoprol), they did so amid a broader effort to remake humans and their landscape. The project of saving lives blurred with that of transforming them, to the calculable benefit of a larger enterprise. As a talk for the United Fruit Company once baldly put it: "the future of imperialism lay with the microscope" (cited in Lyons 1992: 69, 267).

The colonial experience of sleeping sickness, then, suggests something of a biopolitical regime—however fragmentary and incomplete—but one that remained inseparable from the work of ordering territory. Combating a problem likely exacerbated by the very disruptions they fostered, European administrators encouraged the development of expertise related to this condition under the name of "tropical" medicine.[11] This expertise subsequently generated truth about human life and health and directed interventions in their name. The subjects produced may have been colonial rather than liberal, i.e. potential rather than actual citizens, possessing few if any rights and requiring paternalistic oversight. The objects of concern may have remained the crude disruptions of epidemic disease, rather than finer grained measures of a population's health. Nonetheless, sleeping sickness inspired strategies to govern life on the part of colonial authorities, ones moreover that would prove remarkably durable. In this sense colonial efforts to combat the disease recall something of Foucault's

11 | For once not a misnomer, given the regional restriction of sleeping sickness, unlike other "tropical" conditions with broader geographic range and frequently associated with poverty, e.g. cholera, malaria etc. (Lyons 1992: 68; see also Worboys 1994).

classic sketch of biopower. In contrast to the European case, however, here strategies of governance continued to prioritize epidemics, and focused on colonial rather than national populations.[12] These were hardly the emerging states of Rose's "advanced liberal democracies," however much they remained linked through colonial rule.

SKETCH 3: A GLOBAL CONCERN

Returning to the ethnographic present, I will now widen the focus and lengthen the timeline for my particular case. Despite Grace's reluctance to produce numbers on demand, the shepherding of statistics was her primary role at the time of my visit. Epicentre's studies sought to analyse the effectiveness of different protocols used by MSF's project in the treatment of sleeping sickness. The efforts of the remaining team ensured that two decades of clinical work would translate into scientific medicine, not only enhancing MSF's expertise with the condition but also encouraging a renewed commitment to pharmaceutical development related to it. Analysed and eventually published, some of the data would make a strong case for alternative therapies to melarsoprol, the highly unpleasant and hazardous compound derived from arsenic used to treat the deadly second stage of the disease (MSF 2006; Checchi et al. 2007). More generally, it would also contribute to MSF's worldwide endeavour to improve access to essential medicines and foster research on "neglected" diseases. To explain this latter significance, I need to backtrack and pursue the larger story of this emerging humanitarian concern.

In 1986-7, when MSF first began its sleeping sickness project in Uganda, the organization was still relatively small and almost entirely focused on projects providing basic health care in crisis settings, usually to refugee populations. The group had already experienced a series of acrimonious splits since its founding in 1971, and recent controversy in the form of the very public eviction of the original French branch from Ethiopia. In response MSF initiated an array of initiatives during the late 1980s to enhance its professionalism, developing a standardized logistical system and incorporating public health and epidemiological knowledge. To that end a member who had studied at Johns Hopkins University (and worked at the Centres for Disease Control in the United States) helped set up Epicentre. Although nominally independent, it would primarily serve MSF's interests by producing rapid, targeted studies on demand.

In Uganda, where the French section had been running refugee projects in the northwest of the country, the political situation slowly stabilized after a

12 | Foucault describes the shift in Europe between a concern for epidemics to "endemics" (Foucault 2003: 199; see also Rabinow/Rose 2006: 199).

period of turmoil following the fall of Idi Amin. As the refugee project wound down, the group decided to launch the sleeping sickness venture, due both to a noticeable rise in prevalence, and to the contingent fact that a key doctor involved had written his medical thesis on the disease. Long considered endemic to the area, sleeping sickness re-emerged as a problem during the period of upheaval in the early 1980s, due to the movement of refugees in both directions across the Uganda and Sudan border, the collapse of control programs and health infrastructure and the decline in land cultivation. Tsetse flies, it turned out, thrived on civil war (Priotto/Kaboyo 2002).

The resulting project would evolve in a series of different sites in the same general region, and incorporate a research element alongside its clinical practice. In this regard it contrasted with MSF's "classic" emergency missions, and at times resembled efforts at community health development, a form of engagement from which the organization (and especially the French section in question) generally distanced itself. For this particular project the NGO saw itself working in partnership with the Ugandan Ministry of Health, providing one part of a more comprehensive effort to combat the disease. By training a network of personnel it would also aid the larger cause of rebuilding the country's health infrastructure. The project ended up lasting a remarkably long time, shifting locations in response to its own success in lowering local prevalence rates. It also evolved to gradually emphasize research. By focusing on this specific disease, MSF became increasingly aware that the prevailing medical protocol was a problem. Not only did melarsoprol fail to work in over a quarter of the cases, it also ended up killing some 5% or more of those treated (Priotto/Kaboyo 2002). In addition, few alternatives had appeared in the pharmaceutical pipeline. As a vector driven disease confined to marginal habitats, sleeping sickness almost exclusively afflicted poor populations; consequently it offered little prospect for profit and was of little interest to commercial drug companies. Labouring in the fields of frontline medicine, MSF thus discovered a fundamental weakness in the infrastructure of international health.

The sleeping sickness program proved emblematic. By approaching its work more epidemiologically and treating key diseases over time, MSF began to recognize recurring patterns of failure associated with drug resistance in its mission sites, and the importance of affecting official protocols. At the same time its essential drug supply proved increasingly uncertain. Within some quarters of the organization (particularly the ancestral French section), concern was rising over the perennial problem of unequal access to medicines, as well as a general lack of drugs to combat unprofitable conditions. Another pivotal step towards MSF's pharmaceutical epiphany had occurred in the early 1990s. Combating meningitis in Sudan MSF found that its usual treatment, oily chloramphenicol, did not translate into the former British Empire, where protocols inherited from the colonial era favoured ampicillin instead. To justify the French preference Epicentre conducted a study demonstrating the French treatment's effectiveness, while NGOs lobbied the World Health Organization to include oily chloramphenicol on its list of essential medicines. At the very moment of triumph in 1995, however, the manufacturer of the drug abruptly decided to cease production after finding its profit margin too minimal. The scramble to find an alternative supply confirmed the significance of drug issues, while bringing the group in closer contact with generic manufacturers and the assistance of the International Dispensary Association.[13] Over the ensuing years MSF sponsored a conference and subsequently formed a working group to address the issue. By the late 1990s MSF had dropped its earlier resistance to HIV/AIDS work and increasingly involved itself in campaigns to combat that spreading pandemic. In 1999—on the eve of receiving the Nobel Peace Prize—MSF launched a "Campaign for Access to Essential Medicines," denouncing global inequities in biomedical supplies, and demanding new measures to address the problem. The subsequent award of the prize, together with the publicity and funds it generated, helped fuel the rapid growth of MSF's advocacy work over the ensuing years.

From its inception the Access Campaign included an even more significant departure for the MSF movement: a collaborative effort to directly fund and coordinate the research and development of drugs for "neglected" diseases. Surveying the greater terrain of human afflictions from a global perspective, MSF distinguished four categories of conditions relative to the pharmaceutical market (MSF 2001). The first was that of "global diseases," maladies such as cancer or cardiovascular disorders that affect all populations, including wealthy ones where profits could be made. Unsurprisingly, the focus of pharmaceutical corporations rested here. MSF's second category was that of "neglected diseases," maladies such as malaria and tuberculosis that might occasionally strike people who live in wealthy countries, but largely affect poorer ones. Such conditions remained generally marginal to pharmaceutical profits and hence research. The third category was that of "most neglected diseases," vector driven maladies such as sleeping sickness and leishmaniasis that exclusively afflict the marginal poor. Offering little opportunity for profit, these conditions received almost no corporate attention. The fourth and final category was that of conditions "other than purely medical," defects such as wrinkles, cellulite or baldness that obsess wealthy populations and thus have constituted a growing area of commercial drug research (ibid).

Facing this constellation of diseases only partially addressed by commercial drug development, MSF eventually decided to join with several partner organizations and launch an effort known as the Drugs for Neglected Diseases

13 | I owe this account to the excellent interview conducted by Johanna Rankin in her unpublished honours thesis (Rankin 2005 esp.: 93-96 and interview in Appendix A).

Initiative (DNDi).[14] Incorporated as legal entity in Geneva in July of 2003, DNDi began the task of identifying both shorter and longer-term projects that would modify or enlarge the arsenal of medications available to combat neglected diseases, especially the most neglected. Rather than plunging directly into comprehensive research and development itself, the initiative sought to operate as a virtual drug development organization, eliciting, supporting and coordinating a portfolio of projects within existing infrastructures. The goal was to circumvent the marketplace by focusing on medical need and treating drugs as "public goods."

Throughout the development of MSF's Access Campaign and DNDi, the group's on-going project on sleeping sickness played a prototypical role. Indeed, as an MSF administrator told me in Paris in 2003, "sleeping sickness really was the Access Campaign before it existed." As it continued to expand its research portfolio to include other diseases like malaria, Epicentre established a field station in Uganda. Some key figures within MSF spent formative years in the country, becoming familiar with the mission. At the same time the drug eflornithine also became a topic of public controversy. Originally developed as a cancer treatment, eflornithine emerged as a key alternative to melarsoprol in treating the later stage of sleeping sickness. However, its manufacturer, Aventis, discontinued production in 1995 after finding the drug nonprofitable. Following lobbying by MSF and WHO (as well as a famously fortuitous discovery that the compound could also treat unwanted facial hair in postmenopausal women) manufacture resumed in 2001. The terms of the agreement guaranteed availability of a supply designated for the treatment of sleeping sickness, at least for the short term.[15] This minor victory—like the larger struggle over AIDS drugs around the same time—suggested the potential of a pharmaceutically focused humanitarianism. Beyond suffering individuals and endangered collectives, MSF could defend life in the form of "neglected diseases" and the resources needed to combat them.

Who, however, would speak for a dispersed, impoverished population of sleeping sickness patients at the level of pharmaceutical research? Unlike with AIDS, there was no ready group of vocal community advocates, demanding to be heard. While in Geneva in the fall of 2004, I paid a visit to the offices of DNDi. Little more than a year old at that point, the organization still exhibited signs of

---

14 | In addition to MSF, founding partners in DNDi included the Oswaldo Cruz Foundation in Brazil, The Indian Council of Medical Research, the Institut Pasteur in France, the Malaysian Ministry of Health and the Kenyan Medical Research Institute. The new organization also worked in association with the UN-World Bank-WHO program known as TDR (Research and Training in Tropical Diseases). For further details see the DNDi website (www.dndi.org).

15 | MSF press release, May 3, 2001, "Supply of Sleeping Sickness Drugs Confirmed."

hurried growth, if far less frenzied than in most MSF settings. The atmosphere struck me as distinctly more sedate and corporate, befitting the pharmaceutical focus and institutional timeline. A cheerful young woman responsible for communications gave me a briefing, outlining their early prospects and future plans. One key question, she noted, was how to compose their advisory board. DNDi was keen to include a patient representative. Although the organization felt it had a pyramid of networks to draw upon, having one person to report to the board would be ideal for consultations in the context of meetings. Identifying an appropriate individual to play this role, however, was proving difficult:

"We're shooting for the moon, finding someone who can represent three diseases and three continents. The patient's voice needs to be heard. For example one leishmanias drug is available but prohibitively expensive. Also hospitalization is expensive. People don't think of these things when developing drugs. We need to identify one person on each continent to discuss such issues. We obviously want Nelson Mandela, Koffi Anan and Jesus Christ rolled into one. We need a Superman or Superwoman [...] someone who can speak a world language, but also comes from a local one. It's a challenge to find such a person, to put it politely."

At the same time, the organization did not have an industry representative on its board. "It's the shadow of MSF," she explained, "it's given us enormous credibility, but also flak we have to endure." Recognizing the deep-seated mistrust between their parent NGO and the entity it conceived of as "Big Pharma," she felt tension would die down in the context of DNDi discussions, where the goal of nonprofit drug development could dovetail with industrial desires to exhibit corporate citizenship. Still, she noted, there remained an essential difference between profit-making and what she termed "obscene profits." For MSF "how much is enough" was not rhetorical question but a moral boundary.

DNDi (along with similar recent efforts to foster nonprofit drug development for unprofitable diseases) suggests still another, narrowed and distanced variation on the larger theme of biopolitics.[16] Here intergovernmental and

16 | A number of recent initiatives have focused philanthropic and humanitarian energy on providing the world's poor with greater access to pharmaceutical products. Joining older entities like the TDR (Special Programme for Research and Training in Tropical Disease, established by the WHO and other international entities in Geneva in 1975), and the IDA (International Dispensary Association, begun by pharmacists in Amsterdam in 1972), this newer wave of acronyms focuses on developing treatments for specific diseases afflicting poor populations through mobilizing "public private partnerships." The Bill and Melinda Gates Foundation has played a central funding role, providing substantial support to the MMV (Medicines for Malaria Venture, started in Geneva, 1999), OWH, (One World Health, San Francisco, 2000), the TB Alliance (Global Alliance

nongovernmental actors play a central role in fostering life for given populations, constituted through infection with a particular disease rather than by territory. The focus of these projects rests directly on ensuring access to effective remedies for this specific condition, not on a more comprehensive effort to improve general hygiene or alter community life around it. At the same time the overall vision connects life and politics as a matter of course. If a state or interstate agency fails to fulfil biopolitical expectations, that failure is now understood in relation to the particular form of the state more than to the normative project of health governance. Thus a disease that does not enjoy attention by state and interstate entities acquires the revealing designation of being "neglected." By further addressing market failures that produce medical neglect, non-profit drug initiatives acquire a moral tone, seeking—as of DNDi's slogans has it—to produce the "best science for the most neglected." This secular echo of Christian reprioritization inspires a highly specific and attenuated array of interventions. It involves states as secondary partners rather than targets, enrols corporations as well as chiding them, and defines populations in medically differentiated terms. As a biopolitical project, then, it remains a restricted endeavour, a meeting ground for diffused experts and good will, not the engine of an expanding, bounded state.

The work of non-profit pharmaceutical development does suggest an identity project of sorts, but one detached from any particular national context and restricted to a population constituted by a disease. Moreover, this project derives neither from popular pressure, nor from state imposition. Instead it takes shape amid an assemblage of international actors and moral sentiment—sideways and at a distance, as it were, rather than bottom up or top down. The desire to enrol representative subjects remains a part of the endeavour, if somewhat as an afterthought. Even when framing survival as a molecular issue, DNDi still seeks to assure some measure of self-representation of patient interests. The degree to which this proved challenging in practice, however, only underscores the displacement involved. Only a "Superman or Superwoman" could properly articulate "the patient's voice" for a neglected disease.[17]

---

for TB Drug Development, run between New York, Brussels and Cape Town, 2000), the DNDi (Drugs for Neglected Diseases Initiative, established in Geneva 2003), and a looser consortium of researchers led by UNC-Chapel Hill (2000).

17 | In 2005 DNDi announced that a woman from Ghana had joined their board as a patient representative. See DNDi Newsletter Number 12, November 2005. http://www.dndi.org/newsletters/12/news.htm

GLOBAL HEALTH, DISTANCE AND THE LIMITS OF CITIZENSHIP

Thus far I have suggested variations on the theme of biopolitics as they appear relative to different projects responding to sleeping sickness. I now wish to examine the contemporary topic of neglect more closely, by elaborating on "distance" relative to citizenship and the moral politics of global health.[18] In his book *Distant Suffering*, Luc Boltanski takes up and extends Hannah Arendt's observations about the "politics of pity." Pity, for Arendt, ignores questions of justice, concentrating instead on the fact of suffering. It does so, however, at a remove and en masse, unlike say, the grief of a parent for a child or the compassion displayed between particular, situated individuals. By generalizing suffering in this way, pity opens a problem of distance for the public it constitutes, one it seeks to resolve through eloquence and sentiment (Boltanski 1990 [1961]; see also Arendt 1990 [1961]). Boltanski is particularly concerned with this "dimension" of distance and its effects on the capacity of a moral spectator for action. He frames his meditation on media and political theory through reference to a classic scenario of contemporary suffering: the drama of "humanitarian emergency" as scripted by international broadcast over the last decades of the 20th century. This is precisely the terrain upon which MSF emerged following spectacles of suffering in Biafra and Bangladesh, and to which it has represented a continuing form of medical response.

In its emergency mode, MSF has certainly embodied something like a politics of pity (albeit stripped of the ruthlessness of Robespierre), being intimately aligned with media spectacle and tightly focused on the present. Like all humanitarian organizations it defines its engagement in ethical terms, through a fundamental concern for human suffering and a refusal of justifications for it. Once properly channelled through a project, this moral logic goes, human feeling might bridge distance with action, allowing something like individuated compassion to emerge. Relative to other groups MSF is outspoken and relatively concerned with political effects. Nonetheless, it is important to note that MSF does not offer political remedies. The NGO may provide temporary, limited governance related to health, but from the organization's perspective political responsibility lies emphatically elsewhere, with nation states and intergovernmental organizations. MSF's volunteers and donors—even its national staff in their professional capacity—remain at a political distance from general problems of any given territory. With the end of an emergency the structures of their minimal governance of life evaporate, re-condensing in the next crisis.

---

18 | I have found essays by Jeremy Greene, Andrew Lakoff and Tobias Rees quite helpful thinking beyond about "global health" as a contemporary formation, and thank the authors for sharing them. See Lakoff 2010: 59-79.

MSF's move to advocate for pharmaceutical equity and sponsor DNDi, however, suggests a slightly altered configuration of humanitarianism, one attuned to market failure as well as political disruption and cast on a longer timeline. The primary referent is less that of visible disaster than of slower moving structural inequities, the stark inequities that belie humanitarian assertions about the value of life (see Fassin 2007). This configuration may still define suffering as an exceptional state, but not necessarily as an emergency in the medical sense, where procedures are standardized and every moment counts. Rather, it fits into a larger assemblage of global health, advocating policy initiatives and sponsoring laboratory research. Appropriately for an era of "biocapital" and "twenty-first century biomedicine" it also implies a measure of standing based on medical condition and research (Rajan 2006; Rose 2007). Mobilizing a global conception of humanity, this citizenship applies an international scale. Its political frame is not a nation state or empire, but something far more dispersed, appearing in far-flung meeting rooms and pharmaceutical compounds. The political weight of this humanitarian configuration and the degree of its local purchase vary, however, depending on the nature of the condition addressed.

Beneath its unified array of brochures asserting the human need for essential medicines, MSF's Access Campaign bridges a number of tensions between different diseases. These tensions emerged in debates within DNDi over what constituted a truly "neglected" disease. Would HIV-AIDS, or even malaria count, despite the considerable attention and media exposure each inspired? However coherent as a moral project—eloquently defined around the worth of human life—the humanitarian strain of global health is hardly a singular or unified enterprise in practice. Cholera, Ebola and HIV-AIDS, for example, inspire different responses at both technical and political levels, producing different constituencies and possibilities. Cholera, a classic health concern in refugee settings and relatively simple target for biomedical hygiene, helped prompt MSF to create a mobile kit system of emergency logistics (see Redfield 2008). Ebola, a comparatively new condition with uncertain risks, has commanded the attention of international media, security planners and the CDC as well as MSF. And HIV-AIDS, of course, has famously produced a vast array of social movements and organizations, fuelling the larger pharmaceutical out of which MSF's Access Campaign arose. The fact that all three conditions appear in Uganda, or within this particular NGO's portfolio, does little to erase significant distinctions between them.

To illustrate this last point I will expand slightly on the comparison between HIV-AIDS and sleeping sickness. Just down the road from its atrophied sleeping sickness project, MSF had opened an AIDS clinic to offer free anti-retroviral treatment to selected patients in the region. In contrast with the Epicentre study, this venture burgeoned with new patients and an expansive sense of the future. Part of the organization's decision to roll out such programs worldwide beginning in 2000, the clinic also reflected a wider sea change related to ARV treatment at the time.[19] Fuelled by the stark contrast between prospects for rich and poor patients with the same disease, a moral campaign by heterogeneous group of actors—including MSF—helped lower drug prices and suggested new norms, both of treatment and global health (See, e.g. Whyte/van der Geest/Hardon 2002; Petryna/Lakoff/Kleinman 2006). The moment marked a conversion for the organization as well. Although sponsoring a few projects earlier in the 1990s (including an local NGO involving traditional healers in Uganda), MSF had largely kept its distance from AIDS work prior to the advent of ARVs, feeling both that the disease received ample attention and fell outside their technical expertise. Once treatment became available, however, pressure mounted inside and outside the organization and a different logic took sway: surely the threat of pandemic disease merited equal attention to the threat of disaster.

Like sleeping sickness, AIDS was not an emergency in MSF's terms; to combat it the organization would need to develop new techniques, conduct research and alter its practice and timeline, accepting a far longer commitment than its classic norm. Both also led to a focus on pharmaceuticals, including the protocols governing their delivery and the infrastructure that permitted their availability. A crucial distinction, however, lay in the scope of transmission for the two diseases and the sense of vulnerability each might inspire. Although far from evenly distributed, the risk of HIV infection stretched worldwide, into rich as well as poor settings. Claims by or on behalf of AIDS patients mobilized a broad constituency; the condition was not distant from the experience of middle class spectators and many shared a potential need for the same medication. Thus any citizenship projects AIDS might inspire would include measures of shared risk and potential profit. Sleeping sickness, by contrast, constituted a regional problem from the perspective of global health, and even in Uganda primarily concerned a marginal population. Its constituency therefore has remained narrow, only exacerbated by the fact that in its later stages the disease's very symptoms impair the ability of patients to represent themselves. Thus any citizenship projects sleeping sickness might inspire depend more strictly on moral sentiment and claims made on behalf of others, in this instance via common humanity and the value of life.

For MSF the essential break between the AIDS and sleeping sickness surfaced when DNDi emerged as a distinct entity. As my contact at the organization helpfully pointed out, people might talk about AIDS, TB and malaria as underserved,

19 | The Arua clinic began offering ARVs in 2002, and in a recent count had well over 4000 under treatment, part of the 100,000 MSF supports worldwide in 2009. See (http://doctorswithoutborders.org/news/issue.cfm?id=2392)

neglected conditions. Nonetheless, degrees of "neglect" varied significantly, she noted: "The most neglected diseases, however, no one is interested in them at all. That's why there's no AIDS in [our] portfolio."[20] After all, by 2004 AIDS clearly aroused considerable interest. By contrast, a century after British colonial medicine feverishly deployed its microscopes "no one" cared about sleeping sickness. In launching a project to address this oversight, then, humanitarianism could rediscover the disease precisely in the distance of its neglect, and the moral claim of those afflicted to pharmaceutical production. The result might be biopolitical in a general sense and operate in the shadow of biocapital. But it would be unlikely to contribute much to the formation of a states or the dissolution of markets. Rather, it would remain a matter of more modest ethical claims.

Conclusion

To ask whether or not one can be a "citizen" of a neglected disease leads less to any definitive answer than to a reformulation of the question. Taken seriously, it recalls the work of translation involved in resituating theory, the extent to which displacement reorients terms by revealing their assumptions and limits. Citizenship implies a particular form of polity as well as standing within it. Neglect implies normative expectations of treatment as well as the failure to provide it. And the specificities of a condition like sleeping sickness suggest that with it biological citizenship reaches a limit, becoming a suggestive point on the horizon of possibility rather than a substantive condition. In an era oriented by the global pandemic of AIDS, it is particularly important to recall that some diseases present more opportunities for political recognition than others. When sleeping sickness threatened control over territory, it was a political problem of empire, one that subsequently framed the inheritance of postcolonial states. Now thought to endanger only marginal regions of poor countries, it has become an ethical problem of humanitarian action, the concern of NGOs as much as governments.

Alongside the citizen, then, we should place two other conceptual figures: the subject and the human. The former proves particularly relevant at the contemporary moment, when governance projects related to health have supplanted territorial projects of rule. The human, after all, is a figure of ethical as well as political claims. It lends itself to moral enterprise under secular worldviews. The form of "citizenship" it offers extends beyond a given milieu or particular nation state, being primarily an assertion of universal rights and

20 | DNDi's portfolio at the time concentrated on three parasitic conditions (sleeping sickness, kala azar and Chagas disease), as well as some work on malaria. For current projects see http://www.dndi.org/.

dignity. It is, in this fundamental sense, a distant condition. The cases sketched in this essay suggest shifting aspects of such distance: its value in performing expertise, its practical application in the practice of colonial rule, and its thinness with respect to political representation.

To conclude, then, I return to a classic appraisal of the fateful line between citizen and human. In the wake of the Second World War, Hannah Arendt famously compared the promised rights of man with actual rights of citizenship, and found the former sorely wanting. Real political status, she suggested, depended on membership in a polity; without it one was human only in abstract terms, and consequently lacking the essential capacity for public life. The dilemma of stateless people, Arendt trenchantly observed, derived less from the loss of particular rights than from the loss of a state. Only citizenship held out any hope of meaningful representation, and through it any claim for equality. Reprising Burke's scepticism about the abstract guarantees of the Rights of Man, she noted caustically that when put to the test "[t]he world found nothing sacred in the abstract nakedness of being human" (Arendt 1973: 299). Despite the general prescience of her observations regarding statelessness, we might amend her words for an era of humanitarian intervention and global health. Now the abstract nakedness of distant others suggests moral value in the form of a drug—providing, of course, they have a parasitic disease.

References

Abadie, Roberto (2010): *The professional guinea pig: big pharma and the risky world of human subjects*, Durham: Duke University Press.

Abatucci, Dr. (1910): "Le milieu africain considéré au point de vue de ses effets sur le système nerveux de l'Européen", in: *Annales d'hygiène et de médecine coloniales* 13, pp. 328–335.

ACT UP New York (2009) www.actupny.org/documents/montreal.html (accessed 13.11.2009).

Adazu, Kubaje / Lindblade, Kim A. et al. (2005): "Health and demographic surveillance in rural western Kenya: a platform for evaluating interventions to reduce morbidity and mortality from infectious diseases", in: *Am J Trop Med Hyg* 73(6), pp. 1151–1158.

Agamben, Giorgio (1998): Homo Sacer: Sovereign power and bare life, Stanford, CA: Stanford University Press.

Agyepong, Irene Akua (1992): "Malaria: ethnomedical perceptions and practice in an Adangbe farming community and implications for control", in: *Soc Sci Med* 35(2), pp. 131–137.

Airhihenbuwa, Collins O. / Obregon, Rafael (2000): "A critical assessment of theories/models used in health communication for HIV/AIDS", in: *J Health Commun* 5(Suppl), pp. 5–15.

Ake, Claude (1996): Democracy and Development in Africa. Washington DC: Brookings Institute.

Alaii, Jane A., et al (2003): "Factors affecting use of permethrin-treated bed nets during a randomized controlled trial in western Kenya", in: Am J Trop Med Hyg 68(4 Suppl), pp. 137–141.

Amrith, Sunil (2006): *Decolonizing international health: India and Southeast Asia, 1930–65*, Basingstoke, UK: Palgrave Macmillan.

Anderson, James. A. / Weijer Charles (2002): "The research subject as wage earner", *Theoretical Medicine and Bioethics* 23(4), pp. 359–376.

Anderson, Jane (2009): *Law, knowledge, culture: The production of indigenous knowledge in intellectual property law*, Cheltanham: Edward Elgar Publications.

Anderson, Warwick (2002): "Going through the motions: American public health and colonial 'mimicry'", in: *American Literary History* 14, pp. 686–719.

Anderson, Warwick (2004): "Natural histories of infectious disease: Ecological vision in twentieth-century biomedical science", in: *Osiris* 19, pp. 39–61.

Anderson, Warwick (2006): *Colonial pathologies: American tropical medicine, race and hygiene in the Philippines*, Durham, NC: Duke University Press.

Annan, Kofi (2001): Secretary-general proposes global fund for fight against HIV/AIDS and other infectious diseases at African leaders summit, New York: United Nations Press Office.

Apter, Andrew (2005): *The pan-african nation: Oil and the spectacle of culture in Nigeria*, Chicago: University of Chicago Press.

Arendt, Hannah (1958): *The human condition*, Chicago: University of Chicago Press.

Arendt, Hannah (1973): *The origins of totalitarianism*, New York: Harcourt Brace Jovanovich.

Arendt, Hannah (1990 [1961]): *On revolution*, NY: Penguin Books,

Asein, John Ohi (1994): "Consumer literacy and confusing similarity of pictorial trademarks in Nigeria", in: *The Trademark Reporter* 84, pp. 64–78.

Ashforth, Adam (2002): "An epidemic of witchcraft? The implications of AIDS for the post-apartheid state", in: *African Studies* 61(1), pp. 121–143.

Ashraf, Nava / Bandiera, Oriana et al. (2011): *No margin, no mission? A field experiment on incentives for pro-social task*, Harvard Business School Working Paper 12-008. Cambridge, Mass.: Harvard Business School.

Atkins, Kim (ed.) (2005): *Self and subjectivity*, Oxford and Malden, MA: Blackwell.

Bado, Jean-Paul (1996): *Les grandes endémies en Afrique, 1900–1960: lèpre, trypanosomiase humaine et onchocerchose*, Paris: Karthala.

Balandier, Georges (1957): *Afrique ambiguë*, Paris: Plon.

Bancel, Nicolas / Denis, Daniel / Fates, Youssef, eds. (2003): *De l'Indochine à l'Algérie. La jeunesse en mouvements des deux côtés du miroir colonial, 1940–1962*, Paris: La Découverte.

Baronov, David (2008): *The African transformation of Western medicine and the dynamics of global cultural exchange*, Philadelphia: Temple University Press.

Barrett, Ronald, et al. (1998): "Emerging and re-emerging infectious diseases: The third epidemiological transition", in: *Annual Review of Anthropology* 27, pp. 247–271.

Bayart, Jean-François / Ellis, Stephen / Hibou, Béatrice (1999): *The criminalization of the state in Africa*, Bloomington: Indiana University Press.

Beck, Ann (1970): *A history of the British medical administration of East Africa, 1900–1950*, Cambridge, MA: Harvard University Press.

Beck, Ann (1977): "Medicine and society in Tanganyika 1890–1930: A historical inquiry", in: *Transactions of the American Philosophical Society* 67(3), pp. 5–59.

Beck, Ann (1981): *Medicine, tradition, and development in Kenya and Tanzania, 1920–1970*, Waltham, Mass.: Crossroads Press.

Beckerleg, Susan (1994): "Medical pluralism and Islam in Swahili communities in Kenya", in: *Med. Anthropol. Q.* 8(3), pp. 299–213.

Beckmann, Nadine / Bujra, Janet (2011): "The 'politics of the queue': PLHA politicization and AIDS activism in Tanzania" in: *Development and Change* 41(6), pp. 1041–1061.

Beti, Mongo (1956): *Le pauvre Christ de Bomba*, Paris: Robert Laffont.

Biehl, Joao (2002): "Biotechnology and the new politics of life and death in Brazil: the AIDS model", in: *Princet J Bioeth* 5, pp. 59–74.

Biehl, Joao (2004): "The Activist State: global pharmaceuticals, AIDS and citizenship in Brazil", *Social Text* 22(3), pp. 105–132.

Biehl, Joao (2006): "Pharmaceutical governance", in: Adriana Petryna / Andrew Lakoff / Arthur Kleinman (eds), *Global pharmaceuticals: ethics, markets, practices*, Durham: Duke University Press, pp. 206–239.

Biehl, João (2007): Will to live: AIDS therapies and the politics of survival, Princeton / Oxford: Princeton University Press.

Bilharz, Joy A. (2005): "Paradigms lost: Cultural and legal implications of sexual ambiguity", in: *Forum on Public Policy* 1(3), pp. 247–288. http://www.forumonpublicpolicy.com/vol1.no3.gender/bilharz.pdf last accessed 02.10.2011.

Bloom, Gerald / Ainsworth, Peroline (2010): *Beyond scaling up: Pathways to universal access to health services*, STEPS Centre.

Boateng, Boatema (2011): *The copyright thing doesn't work here: Adinkra and Kente Cloth and intellectual property in Ghana*, Minneapolis, MN: University of Minnesota Press.

Boesten, Jelke (2011): "Navigating the AIDS industry: being poor and positive in Tanzania", in: *Development and Change* 42(3), pp. 781–803.

Boltanski, Luc (1999 [1993]): *Distant suffering: Morality, media and politics*, Cambridge: Cambridge University Press

Bonah, Christian (2007): *Histoire de l'expérimentation humaine en France. Discours et pratiques, 1900–1940*, Paris: Les Belles Lettres.

Bonnecase, Vincent (2008): *Pauvreté au Sahel: la construction des savoirs sur les conditions de vie au Burkina Faso, au Mali et au Niger (1945–1974)*. Unpublished dissertation Paris.

Bonneuil, Christophe (1997): *Mettre en ordre et discipliner les tropiques: les sciences du végétal dans l'Empire français, 1870–1940*. Unpublished dissertation, Paris.

Bonneuil, Christophe (1999): "Pénétrer l'indigène: Arachide, paysans, agronomes et administrateurs coloniaux au Sénégal", in: *Études rurales* 151–152, pp. 199–223.

Bonneuil, Christophe (2001): "Development as experiment", in: *Osiris* 2(15), pp. 258–281.

Bornstein, Kate (1994): *Gender outlaw: On men, women, and the rest of us*, New York: Vintage Books.

Boswell, Holly (1998): "The transgender paradigm shift toward free expression", in: Dallas Denny (ed.), *Current concepts in transgender identity*, New York: Garland Press, pp. 55–62.

Bovaird, Tony (2004): "Public–Private Partnerships: From contested concepts to prevalent practice", in: *International Review of Administrative Sciences* 70(2), pp. 199–215.

Braun, Lundy / Hammonds, Evelyn (2008): "Race, populations, and genomics: Africa as laboratory", in: *Social Science and Medicine* 67(10), pp. 1580–1588.

Brennan, James R., and Andrew Burton. (2007): "The emerging metropolis: a short history of Dar es Salaam, circa 1862–2005", in: James R. Brennan/ Andrew Burton/Yusuf Lawi (eds), *Dar es Salaam: Histories from an emerging African metropolis*, Dar es Salaam/Nairobi: Mkuki na Nyota/BIEA, pp. 13–75.

Brinkerhoff, Derick W (2004): "Partnerships between international donors and non-governmental development organizations: Opportunities and constraints", in: *International Review of Administrative Sciences* 70(2), pp. 253–270.

Brinkerhoff, Jennifer M. (2002): "Government-nonprofit partnership: A defining framework" in: *Public Administration & Development* 22(1), pp. 19–30.

Brouwers, Ria (2011): *When 'civics' go 'governance': On the role and relevance of civic organisations in the policy arena in Sub-Saharan Africa*, The Hague: International Institute for Social Studies, Erasmus University.

Brown, Peter J (1986): "Socioeconomic and demographic effects of malaria eradication: a comparison of Sri Lanka and Sardinia", in: *Soc Sci Med* 22(8), pp. 847–859.

Bruce-Chwatt, Leonard J. (1969): "Malaria eradication at the crossroads", in: *Bull N Y Acad Med* 45(10), pp. 999–1012.

Bruce-Chwatt, Leonard Jan (1977): "Ronald Ross, William Gorgas, and malaria eradication." *American Journal of Tropical Medicine & Hygiene* 26: 1071–1079.

Bruchhausen, Walter (2003): "Practising hygiene and fighting the natives' diseases. Public and child health in German East Africa and Tanganyika territory, 1900–1960", in: *DYNAMIS*. Acta Hisp. Med. Sci. Hist. Illus 23, pp. 85–113.

Brush, Stephen (1993): "Indigenous knowledge of biological resources and intellectual property rights: The Role of Anthropology", in: *American Anthropologist* 95(3), pp 653–671.

Burr, Vivien (1995): *An introduction to social constructionism*, London: Routledge.

Burton, Andrew (2003): "Townsmen in the making: Social engineering and citizenship in Dar es Salaam, c.1945–1960", in: *The International Journal of African Historical Studies* 36, pp. 331–365.

Busby, Harriet (2006): "Biobanks, bioethics and concepts of donated blood in the UK", in: *Sociology of Health & Illness* 28(6), pp. 850–865.

Buse, Kent / Harmer Andrew M. (2007): "Seven habits of highly effective global public-private health partnerships: practice and potential", in: *Soc Sci Med* 64(2), pp. 259–271.

Buse, Kent / Walt Gill (2000): "Global public-private partnerships: Part I—A new development in health?" in: *Bull World Health Organ* 78(4), pp. 549–561.

Butler, Judith (1990): *Gender trouble: Feminism and the subversion of identity*, New York/London: Routledge.

Calhoun, Craig (2009): "The imperative to reduce suffering: charity, progress and emergencies in the field of humanitarian Action", in: Michel Barnett/ Thomas. G. Weiss (eds.), *Humanitarianism in question: Politics, power, ethics*, Ithaca: Cornell University Press, pp. 73–97.

Califia-Rice, Patrick (2000): "Family values: Two dads with a difference—Neither of us was born male", in: *Village Voice*. Tuesday, June 20th. http://www.villagevoice.com/2000-06-20/news/family-values/ last accessed 02.10.2011.

Callahan, Michael (1999): *Mandates and empire: The League of Nations and Africa, 1914–1931*, Brighton, UK: Sussex Academic Press.

Callahan, Michael (2004): *A sacred trust: The League of Nations and Africa, 1929–1946*, Brighton, UK: Sussex Academic Press.

Callon, Michel / Muniesa, Fabian (2005): "Peripheral visions: Economic markets as calculative collective devices", in: *Organization Studies* 26(8), pp. 1229–1250.

Cantier, Jacques (2004): "Un enjeu essentiel. Vichy et les jeunes dans l'Empire français", in: Jacques Cantier/Eric Jennings (eds), *L'Empire colonial sous Vichy*, Paris: Odile Jacob, pp. 91–115.

CAOM—Centre des Archives d'Outre-Mer, Aix-en-Provence (1924): *Proposition locale tendant à attribuer l'exercice des pouvoirs disciplinaires aux médecins chargés de lutte contre la maladie du sommeil*. CAOM: SG Togo-Cameroun, carton XXX, dossier 261.

Carter, Eric D. (2008): "State visions, landscape, and disease: Discovering malaria in Argentina, 1890–1920", in: *Geoforum* 39(1), 278–293.

Castleman, Tony / Seumo-Fossil, Elenore / Cogill, Bruce (2004): "Food and nutritional implications of antiretroviral therapy in resource limited settings", in: *FANTA* (Food and Nutrition Technical Assistance), Technical Note, revised May 2004. http://www.fantaproject.org/downloads/pdfs/tn7_ARVs.pdf

Catlaw, Thomas J. (2008): "Constitution as executive order: The administrative state and the political ontology of 'We the People'", in: *Administration and Society* 37(4), pp. 445–482.

CDLP (NoDate): http://www.cldp.doc.gov/cs/root/about_us/cldp_programs, last accessed 02.11.2009.

Chaki, Prosper et al. (2009): "Achieving high coverage of larval-stage mosquito surveillance: challenges for a community-based mosquito control programme in urban Dar es Salaam, Tanzania", in: *Malaria Journal* 8, pp. 311.

Chaki, Prosper et al. (2011): "Community-owned resource persons for malaria vector control: enabling factors and challenges in an operational programme in Dar es Salaam, United Republic of Tanzania", in: *Human Resources for Health* 9, pp. 21 (28 September 2011).

Chalfin, Brenda (2010): *Neoliberal frontiers: An ethnography of sovereignty in West Africa*, Chicago: University of Chicago Press.

Chamayou, Grégoire (2008): *Les corps vils. Expérimenter sur les humains aux XVIIIe et XIXe siècles*, Paris: La Découverte.

Checchi F. / Piola P. / Ayikoru H. / Thomas F. / Legros D. et al. (2007): "Nifurtimox plus eflornithine for late-stage sleeping sickness in Uganda: A case series", in: *PLoS Negl Trop Dis* 1(2), pp. e64.

Chef de Région (1942): Circulaire du Chef de région, 8 avril 1942. ANY: APA 10.999.

CIOMS (Council for International Organizations of Medical Sciences) (2002): *International ethical guidelines for biomedical research involving human subjects*, Geneva, WHO.

Clyde, David F. (1962): *History of the medical services of Tanganyika*, Dar es Salaam: Govt. Press.

Clyde, David F. (1967): *Malaria in Tanzania*, London: Oxford University Press.

Clyde, David F. / Mzoo, F. M. / Mluba, S. (1964): "Therapeutic trials of chloroquine silicate in Tanganyika", in: *Bull World Health Organ* 30, pp. 135–136.

Cohen, David W. / Odhiambo, Eisha S. A. (1989): *Siaya. The historical anthropology of an African landscape*, Nairobi: Heineman Kenya.

Colman, William G. (1989): *State and local government and public-private partnerships: a policy-issues handbook*, New York: Greenwood Press.

Comaroff, Jean (1981): "Healing and cultural transformation—the Tswana of Southern-Africa", in: *Social Science & Medicine* Part B-Medical Anthropology 15(3B), pp. 367–378.

Comaroff, Jean (2007): "Beyond bare life: AIDS (bio)politics and the neoliberal order", in: *Public Culture* 19(1), pp. 197–219

Comaroff, Jean / Comaroff, John L. (2000): "Millenial capitalism: First thoughts on a second coming", in: *Public Culture* 12(2), pp. 291–343.

Commission de la Maladie du Sommeil (1941): *Séance du 28 mai 1941. Compte-rendu de la lutte contre la Trypanosomiase [pour l'année 1939]*. Arch. IMTSSA: 252.

Conklin, Alice (1997): *A mission to civilize: The Republican idea of empire in France and West Africa, 1895–1930*, Stanford, CA: Stanford University Press.

Coombe, Rosemary. (2003): "Fear, hope and longing for the future of authorship and a revitalized public domain in global regimes of intellectual property" in: *DePaul Law Review* 52, pp. 1171–1193.

Cooper, Frederick / Packard, Randall M. (1997): *International development and the social sciences: Essays on the history and politics of knowledge*, Berkeley: University of California Press.

Cooper, Melinda (2008): *Life as surplus. Biotechnology and capitalism in the neoliberal era*, Seattle and London, University of Washington Press.

Coquery-Vidrovitch, Catherine (1979): "Colonisation ou impérialisme: la politique africaine de la France entre les deux guerres", in: *Le Mouvement social* 107, pp. 51–76.

Correa, Carlos (2000): *Intellectual Property Rights, the WTO and Developing Countries. The TRIPS Agreement and Policy Options*, London and New York: Zed Books.

Creese, Andrew / Floyd, Katherine/Alban, Anita/Guinness, Lorna (2002): "Cost-effectiveness of HIV/AIDS interventions in Africa: a systematic review of evidence" in: *The Lancet* 359 (9318), pp. 1635–1642.

Crenshaw, Kimberlé W. (1989): "Demarginalizing the intersection of race and sex: A black feminist critique of antidiscrimination doctrine, feminist theory and antiracist politics", in: *University of Chicago Legal Forum*, 1989, pp. 139–167.

Crichton, Derk (1993): "Gender reassignment surgery for male primary transsexuals", in: *South African Medical Journal* 83(5), pp. 347–349.

Cueto, M. (2004): "Social medicine and 'leprosy' in the Peruvian Amazon", in: *The Americas* 61(1), pp. 55–80.

Cullet, Philippe (2005): "Patents and medicines: The relationships between TRIPS and the human right to health", in: *International Affairs* 79(1), pp. 139–160.

Curtin, Philip D. (1961): "'The White Man's Grave': Image and Reality, 1780–1850", in: *Journal of British Studies* 1(1), pp. 94–110.

Curtin, Philip D. (1985): "Medical Knowledge and Urban Planning in Tropical Africa", in: *American Historical Review* 90, pp. 594–613.

Daughton, J.P. (2006): *An empire divided: Religion, republicanism, and the making of French colonialism, 1880–1914*, Oxford/New York: Oxford University Press.

David, Jean Joseph (1940): *Région Médicale du Haut-Nyong. Plan d'action de 1940* (accepted in February-April 1940). ANY: APA 10.999.

David, Jean Joseph (1942): *Région Médicale du Haut-Nyong. Rapport de gestion.* ANY: APA 10.999.

De Castro, Marcia Caldas et al. (2004): "Integrated Urban Malaria Control: A Case Study in Dar Es Salaam, Tanzania", in: *The American Journal of Tropical Medicine and Hygiene* 71, 2: 103–117.

De Castro, Marcia Caldas et al. (2010): "The importance of drains for the larval development of lymphatic filariasis and malaria vectors in Dar es Salaam, United Republic of Tanzania", in: *PLoS Negl Trop Dis* 4 (5): e693. doi:10.1371/journal.pntd.0000693 de Cernival, Marie (2008): "L'éthique de la recherche ou la liberté d'en sortir. (Ethics of research: the freedom to withdraw)", in: *Bulletin de la Societe de Pathologie Exotique* 101(1), pp. 98–101.

De l'Estoile, Benoît (2004): *L'Afrique comme laboratoire. Expériences réformatrices et révolution anthropologique dans l'empire colonial britannique (1920–1950).* Unpublished dissertation, Paris.

de Savigny, Don, et al. (2004): "Care-seeking patterns for fatal malaria in Tanzania", in: *Malar J* 3, pp. 27.

Degremont, Antoine A., et al. (1987): "Longitudinal study on the health status of children in a rural Tanzanian community: comparison of community-based clinical examinations, the diseases seen at village health posts and the perception of health problems by the population", in: *Acta Trop* 44(2), pp. 175–190.

Dickert, Neal / Grady, Christine (1999): "What's the price of a research subject? Approaches to payment for research participation", in: *N Engl J Med* 341(3), pp. 198–203.

Dilger, Hansjörg (2005): *Leben mit Aids: Krankheit, Tod und Soziale Beziehungen in Afrika. Eine Ethnographie*, Frankfurt: Campus.

Dilger, Hansjörg (2008): "'We are all going to die': kinship, belonging, and the morality of HIV/AIDS-related illnesses and deaths in rural Tanzania", in: *Anthropological Quarterly* 81(1), pp. 207–232.

Dill, Bill (2010): "Community-based organizations (CBOs) and norms of participation in Tanzania: Working against the grain", in: *African Studies Review* 53(2), pp. 23–48.

Dongus, Stefan et al. (2007): Participatory mapping of target areas to enable operational larval source management to suppress malaria vector mosquitoes in Dar es Salaam, Tanzania", in: *International Journal of Health Geographics*, Biomed Central 6, pp. 37.

Dorlin, Elsa (2006): *La matrice de la race. Généalogie coloniale et sexuelle de la nation française*, Paris: La Découverte.

Dorsey, Michael K. (2003): "Political ecology of bioprospecting in Amazonian Ecuador: History, political economy and knowledge", in: Brechin, et.al. (eds), *Contested Nature: Power, protected areas and the dispossessed, Promoting international biodiversity conservation with social justice in the 21st century*, New York: SUNY Press.

Dozon, Jean-Pierre (1985): "Quand les pastoriens traquaient la maladie du sommeil", in: *Sciences sociales et santé* III-3/4, pp. 27–56.

Dozon, Jean-Pierre (1991): "Pasteurisme, médecine militaire et colonisation", in: Michel Morange (ed.), *L'Institut Pasteur. Contributions à son histoire*, Paris: La Découverte, pp. 269–278.

Dozon, Jean-Pierre (2008): *L'Afrique à dieu et à diable. États, ethnies, religions*, Paris: Ellipses.

Drahos, Peter (1995): "Global property rights in information: The story of TRIPS at the GATT", in: *Prometheus* 13, pp. 6–19.
Drahos, Peter / Braitewaith, John (2007): "Information feudalism: Who owns the knowledge economy?" in: Ekpere, Johnson (ed.), *The Organization of African Unity Initiative and the African common position on TRIPs*, Lagos, Nigeria: OAU/STRC.
Dumett, Raymond (1971): "The rubber trade of the Gold Coast and Asante in the nineteenth century: African innovation and market responsiveness", in: *Journal of African History* 12(1), pp. 79–101.
Dumett, Raymond (1985): "Africa's strategic minerals during the Second World War", in: *Journal of African History* 26(4), pp. 381–408.
Dunson, Marvin, III. (2001): "Sex, gender, and transgender: The present and future of employment discrimination law", in: *Berkeley Journal of Employment and Labor Law* 22(2), pp. 465–506.
Dutta-Bergman, Mohan J. (2005): "Theory and practice in health communication campaigns: A critical interrogation", in: *Health Communication* 18(2), pp. 103–122.
Eckart, Wolfgang (1997): *Medizin und Kolonialimperialismus. Deutschland 1884–1945*, Paderborn: F. Schöningh.
Eckart, Wolfgang (2002): "The colony as laboratory: German sleeping sickness campaigns in German East Africa and in Togo, 1900–1914", in: *History and Philosophy of the Life Sciences* 24(1), pp. 69–89.
Ecks, Stefan (2005): "Pharmaceutical citizenship: antidepressant marketing and the promise of demarginalization in India", in: *Anthropology and Medicine* 12(3), pp. 239–254.
Ecks, Stefan (2008): "Global pharmaceutical markets and corporate citizenship: The case of Novartis' anti-cancer drug glivec", in: *BioSocieties* 3(2), pp. 165–81.
Edelman, Marc (2001): "Social movements: Changing paradigms and forms of politics", in: *Annual Review of Anthropology* 30, pp. 285–317.
Edmond, Rod (2006): *Leprosy and empire: A medical and cultural history*, Cambridge, UK: Cambridge University Press.
Edwards, Michael / Hulme, David (1995): "Too close for comfort? The impact of official aid on nongovernmental organizations", in: *World Development* 24(6), pp. 961–973.
Ekpere, Johnson (2001): *"The OAU model law and Africa's common position on the TRIPs review process"*. Unpublished paper presented at the Eastern and Southern Africa Multi-Stakeholders Dialogue on Trade, Intellectual Property Rights, and Genetic Resources (Nairobi, July). Available online at www.isctd.org.
Ekpere, Johnson (2003): "African model law on the rights of local communities, farmers and breeders, and for the regulation of access to biological resources", in: Kent Nnadozie/Robert Lettington/Carl Bruch/Susan Bass (eds), *African*

perspectives on genetic resources: A handbook on laws, policies and institutions, Washington DC: Environmental Law Institute, pp. 275–286.

Ekpere, Johnson (No Date): *The Organization of African Unity Initiative and the African common position on TRIPs*, Lagos, Nigeria: OAU/STRC.

Epstein, Helen (2007): *The invisible cure: Africa, the West and the fight against AIDS*, New York: Farrar, Straus & Girroux.

Epstein, Steven (1995): "The construction of lay expertise: AIDS activism and the forging of credibility in the reform of clinics trials", in: *Science, Technology and Human Values* 20(4), pp. 408–437.

Epstein, Steven (1996): *Impure science: AIDS, activism, and the politics of knowledge*, Berkeley: University of California Press.

Epstein, Steven (2008): "Patient groups and health movements", in E.J. Hackett et al. (eds),*The handbook of science and technology studies*, 3rd Edition, Cambridge: MIT Press, pp. 499–539.

Escobar, Arthur (1995): *Encountering development: The making and unmaking of the Third World*, Princeton, NJ: Princeton University Press.

Eskridge, William N., Jr / Hunter, Nan D. (1997): *Sexuality, gender, and the law*, Westbury, NY: The Foundation Press.

Essomba, Philippe Blaise (2004): *Le Cameroun: les rivalités d'intérêts franco-allemandes de 1919 à 1932*, Strasbourg, FR: Presses Universitaires de Strasbourg.

European Parliament (2011): European Parliament resolution of 28 September 2011 on human rights, sexual orientation and gender identity at the United Nations. http://www.europarl.europa.eu/sides/getDoc.do?pubRef=-//EP//TEXT+TA+P7-TA-2011-0427+0+DOC+XML+V0//EN&language=EN, last accessed 02.10.2011.

Evans-Pritchard, Edward E. (1937): *Witchcraft, oracles, and magic among the Azande*, Oxford: Clarendon Press.

Fabian, Johannes (2000): *Out of our minds: Reason and madness in the exploration of Central Africa*: The Ad. E. Jensen lectures at the Frobenius Institut, University of Frankfurt, Berkeley, CA: University of California Press.

Farinaud, Dr. Colonel (1944): *Rapport Annuel. Année 1943*. Service de Santé. Cameroun Français. A.—Partie administrative. Arch. IMTSSA: Boite 111.

Farinaud, Dr. Colonel (1945): *Rapport Annuel. Année 1944*. Service de Santé. Cameroun Français. A.—Partie administrative. Arch. IMTSSA: Boite 111.

Farinaud, Dr. Colonel (1946): *Rapport Annuel. Année 1945*. Service de Santé. Cameroun Français. Arch. IMTSSA: Boite 111.

Farinaud, Dr. Colonel (1947): *Rapport Annuel. Année 1946*. Service de Santé. Cameroun Français. Arch. IMTSSA: Boite 111.

Farmer, Paul (1992): *AIDS and accusation: Haiti and the geography of blame*, Berkeley: University of California Press.

Fassin, Didier (2001): "Au coeur de la cité salubre. La santé publique entre les mots et les choses", in: Jean-Pierre Dozon/Didier Fassin (eds.), *Critique de la santé publique. Une approche anthropologique*, Paris: Balland, pp. 47–73.

Fassin, Didier (2007): "Humanitarianism as a Politics of Life", in: *Public Culture* 19(3), pp. 499–520.

Fassin, Didier (2007): *When bodies remember: experiences and politics of AIDS in South Africa*, Berkeley: University of California Press.

Fassin, Didier (2009): "Another politics of life is possible", in: *Theory Culture Society* 26(5), pp. 44–60.

Fausto-Sterling, Anne (2000): *Sexing the body. Gender politics and the construction of sexuality*, New York: Basic Books.

Feierman, Steven (1981): "Therapy as a system-in-action in northeastern Tanzania", in: *Soc Sci Med* 15(3), pp. 353–360.

Feierman, Steven / Janzen, John M. (1992): *The social basis of health and healing in Africa*, Berkeley: University of California Press.

Feldman-Savelsberg, Pamela / Ndonko, Flavien T. / Schmidt-Ehry, Bergis (2000): "Sterilizing vaccines or the politics of the womb: retrospective study of a rumor in Cameroon", in: *Med Anthropol Q* 14(2), pp. 159–179.

Ferguson, James (1990): *The antipolitics machine: Development, depoliticization and bureaucratic power in Lesotho*, Cambridge: University of Cambridge Press.

Ferguson, James (2006): *Global Shadows. Africa in the Neoliberal World Order*, Durham: Duke University Press.

Ferguson, James / Gupta, Akhil (2002): "Spatializing States: Toward an Ethnography of Neoliberal Governmentality", in: *American Ethnologist* 29(4), pp. 981–1002.

Fèvre, E.M. / Coleman, P.G. / Welburn, S.C. / Maudlin, I. (2004): "Reanalyzing the 1900–1920 sleeping sickness epidemic in Uganda", in: *Emerging Infectious Diseases* 10(4), pp. 567–573.

Fillinger, Ulrike et al. (2008): "A tool-box for operational mosquito larval control: Preliminary results and early lessons from the Urban Malaria Control Programme in Dar es Salaam, Tanzania", in: *Malaria Journal* 7, pp. 20.

Fintz, Matthieu (2004): *Moustiques et gouvernement du paludisme en Afrique. De la conservation de la nature à l'organisation des biens de lutte.* Unpublished dissertation, Strasbourg.

Ford, John (1971): *The role of trypanosomiases in African ecology*, Oxford: Claredon Press.

Ford, Nathan (2003): "Public health and company wealth", in: *BMJ* 326, pp. 1296.

Foster, George M. (1976): "Disease etiologies in Non-Western Medical Systems", in: *Am Anthropol.* 78, pp. 773–782.

Foster, S. (1995): "Treatment of malaria outside the formal health services", in: *J Trop Med Hyg* 98(1), pp. 29–34.

Foster, Susan D. (1994): "Care and treatment of HIV disease in developing countries from a socio-economic perspective", in: *AIDS* 8(S1), pp. 341–347.

Foucault, Michel (1975): Michel Foucault, Entretien avec Roger-Pol Droit (1975) http://foucault.info/documents/foucault.entretien1975.fr.html

Foucault, Michel (1975): *Surveiller et punir. Naissance de la prison*, Paris: Gallimard.

Foucault, Michel (1976): *Histoire de la sexualité.* Volume 1: La volonté de savoir, Paris: Gallimard.

Foucault, Michel (1977): *Discipline and punish: The birth of the prison*, London: Penguin.

Foucault, Michel (1978): *The history of sexuality*, Volume 1: An introduction, London: Penguin.

Foucault, Michel (1980): "Truth and power", in Colin Gordon (ed.), *Power/knowledge*, NewYork: Pantheon.

Foucault, Michel (1982): "The subject and power", in: *Critical Inquiry* 8(4), pp. 777–795.

Foucault, Michel (1988): "Technologies of the self", in: Luther H. Martin/Huck Gutman/Patrick H. Hutton (eds), *Technologies of the self: a seminar with Michel Foucault*, Amherst: University of Massachusetts Press.

Foucault, Michel (1989): "Sex, power and the politics of identity", in Sylvère Lotringer (ed.), *Foucault live: Collected interviews, 1961–1984*, New York: Semiotext(e).

Foucault, Michel (1990): *The history of sexuality: An introduction*, Volume 1, New York: Vintage Books Edition.

Foucault, Michel (1994): "Des espaces autres (conférence au Cercle d'Études architecturales, 14 mars 1967)", in: *Dits et écrits 1954–1988*, Paris: Gallimard pp. 46–49.

Foucault, Michel (1997): *"Il faut défendre la société": cours au Collége de France (1975–1976)*, Paris: Seuil/Gallimard.

Foucault, Michel (2000): "Power: Essential works of Michel Foucault 1954–1984", in: James D. Faubion (ed.), *Essential works of Michel Foucault 1954–1984*, Volume 3, London: Allen Lane &The Penguin Press.

Foucault, Michel (2001 [1977]): "Le jeu de Michel Foucault", in: *Dits et écrits II, 1976–1988*, Paris: Gallimard, pp. 298–329.

Foucault, Michel (2003): *Society must be defended: Lectures at the Collège de France 1975–1976*, London: Allen Lane.

Foucault, Michel (2004 [1976]): "Society must be defended", in Mauro Bertani/Alessandro Fontana (eds), *Lectures at the College de France, 1975–76*, London: Penguin Books, pp. 239–265.

Francis, Elisabeth (1995): "Migration and changing divisions of labour: gender relations and economic change in Koguta, western Kenya", in: *Africa* 65(2), 197–215.

Frenk, Julio (2010): "The global health system: Strengthening national health systems as the next step for global progress", in: *PLoS Med* 7(1), pp. 1–3.

Freyhold, Michaela von (1979): *Ujamaa villages in Tanzania: analysis of a social experiment*, New York: Monthly Review Press.

Froment, Alain (1988): "Le Docteur Jamot, sa vocation africaine, et l'épidémiologie", in: *Bulletin de liaison et de documentation de l'OCEAC* 85, pp. 23–25.

Frye, Phyllis R. / Meiselman, Alyson D. 2001: "Same-sex marriages have existed legally in the United States for a long time now", in: *Albany Law Review* 64(3), pp. 1031–1072.

Gaudillière, Jean-Paul (2002): *Inventer la biomédecine: La France, l'Amerique et la production des savoirs du vivant (1945–1965)*, Paris: La Découverte.

Geissbühler, Yvonne et al. (2009): "Microbial larvicide application by a large-scale, community based program reduces malaria infection prevalence in urban Dar Es Salaam, Tanzania", in: *PLoS One* 4(3): e5107.

Geissbühler, Yvonne et al. 2007: "Interdependence of domestic malaria prevention measures and mosquito-human interactions in urban Dar es Salaam, Tanzania", in: *Malaria Journal* 6: pp. e126

Geissler, P. Wenzel (2011): "Studying Trial Communities: Anthropological and Historical Inquiries into Ethos, Politics and Economy of Medical Research in Africa", in: Paul W. Geissler/Catherine Molyneux (eds), *Evidence, ethos and experiment: The anthropology and history of medical research in Africa*, Oxford: Berghahn Books, pp.1–28.

Geissler, P. Wenzel (2012): "Introduction: Life-science in its African para-state", in: P. Wenzel Geissler (ed.), *Para-states of science: Ethnographic and historical perspectives on the life-sciences in 21st century Africa*, Durham: Duke University Press: in press.

Geissler, P. Wenzel et al. (2008): "'He is now like a brother, I can even give him some blood'—relational ethics and material exchanges in a malaria vaccine 'trial community' in The Gambia", *Social Science and Medicine* 67(5), pp. 698–707.

Geissler, P. Wenzel / Molyneux, Catherine (eds) (2011): *Evidence, ethos and experiment: the anthropology and history of medical research in Africa*, Oxford: Berghahn Publishers.

Geissler, P. Wenzel / Prince, Ruth J. (2010a): *The land is dying. Contingency, creativity and conflict in Western Kenya*, Oxford: Berghahn Books

Geissler, P. Wenzel / Prince, Ruth J. (2010b): "Order and decomposition: challenges of touch in a time of death", in: Ute Luig/Hansjörg Dilger (eds), *Morality, hope and grief: Anthropologies of AIDS in Africa*, Oxford: Berghahn.

Geissler, P. Wenzel / Pool, Robert (2006): "Popular concerns with medical research projects in Africa—a critical voice in debates about overseas research ethics", in: *Tropical Medicine and International Health* 11(7), pp. 975–982.

Gerrets, Rene (2010): *Globalizing international health: The cultural politics of 'partnership' in Tanzanian malaria control*, New York: New York University.

Gerstl, Sibylle, et al. (2010): "Successful introduction of artesunate combination therapy is not enough to fight malaria: results from an adherence study in Sierra Leone", in: *Trans R Soc Trop Med Hyg* 104(5), pp. 328–335.

Geschière, Peter (1982): *Village communities and the state: Changing relations among the Maka of southeastern Cameroon since the colonial conquest*, London/Boston: Kegan Paul International.

Geschière, Peter (1983): "European planters, African peasants and the colonial state: Alternatives in the mise en valeur of Makaland, Southeast Cameroun, during the Interbellum", in: *African Economic History* 12, pp. 83–108.

Geschière, Peter (forthcoming): "'Tournaments' of value in the forest area of Cameroon. 'Multiple self-realization' versus colonial coercion during the rubber-boom (1900–1913)", in: Wim Van Binsbergen/Peter Geschière (eds), *Commodifications and identities*, Durham, NC: Duke University Press.

Gessler, M. C., et al. (1995): "Traditional healers in Tanzania: the treatment of malaria with plant remedies", in: *J Ethnopharmacol* 48(3), pp. 131–144.

Gibson, Clark, Margaret A. McKean, and Elinor Ostrom (eds) (2000): *People and forests: Communities, institutions and governance*, Cambridge, MA: MIT Press.

Gieyrn, Thomas F. (2006): "City as Truth-Spot", in: *Social Studies of Science* 36(1), pp. 5–38.

Giles-Vernick, Tamara (2002): *Cutting the vines of the past: Environmental histories of the Central African rain forest*, Charlottesville, VA: University Press of Virginia.

GNP+ (2000): Positive Development, http://www.gnpplus.net/images/stories/Empowerment/PosDev/Positive_Development_English.pdf

Good, Byron (1994): *Medicine, rationality, and experience: an anthropological perspective*, New York: Cambridge University Press.

Gooldin, Sigal (2008): "Being anorexic: hunger, subjectivity, and embodied morality", in: *Med Anthropol Q* 22(3), pp. 274–296.

Government Gazette No. 26148 (2004): Alteration of Sex Description and Sex Status Act, 2003. Vol. 465, Cape Town, 15 March 2004. http://www.info.gov.za/gazette/acts/2003/a49-03.pdf last accessed 17.10.2010.

Graboyes, Melissa (2010): "Fines, orders fear... and consent? Medical research in East Africa, ca. 1950s", in: *Developing World Bioethics* 10(1), pp. 34–41.

Grebe, Eduard (2009): *Leaders, networks and coalitions in the AIDS response: a comparison of Uganda and South Africa*. Research paper 03, Leaders, Elites and Coalitions Research Program.

Green, Maia (2003): "Globalizing development in Tanzania: Policy franchising through participatory project management", in: *Critique of Anthropology*, 23(2), pp. 123–143.

Green, Maia (2010): "Making development agents: Participation as boundary object in international development", in: *Journal of Development Studies* 46, pp. 1240–1263.

Green, Richard (1992): *Sexual science and the law*, Cambridge, MA: Harvard University Press.

Greenberg, Julie A. (1999): "Defining male and female: Intersexuality and the collision between law and biology", in: *Arizona Law Review* 41, pp. 265–328.

Greenberg, Julie A. (2000): "When is a man a man and when is a woman a woman?", in: *Florida Law Review* 52, pp. 745–768.

Gremillion, Helen (2003): *Feeding anorexia: Gender and power at a treatment center*, Durham: Duke University Press.

Guyatt, Helen L. / Snow, Robert W. (2004): "The management of fevers in Kenyan children and adults in an area of seasonal malaria transmission", in: *Trans R Soc Trop Med Hyg* 98(2), pp. 111–115.

Guyer, Jane (2004): *Marginal gains: Monetary transactions in Atlantic Africa*, University of Chicago Press.

Hall, Budd L. (1974): "Revolution in rural education: Health education in Tanzania", in: *Community Development Journal* 9(2), pp. 133–139.

Hamers, Raph et al. (2011): "HIV-1 drug resistance in antiretroviral-naive individuals in sub-Saharan Africa after rollout of antiretroviral therapy: a multicentre observational study", in: *Lancet Infectious Diseases* 11(10), pp. 750–759.

Hardon, Anita (2006): "Confronting the HIV/AIDS epidemic in Sub-Saharan Africa: policy versus practice", in: *International Social Science Journal* 57(186), pp. 601–605.

Hardon, Anita / Daniels, Colleen (2006): *Universal access by 2010: 10 challenges on the way*, Amsterdam: Health Action International.

Hardon, Anita / Dilger, Hansjörg (2011): "Global AIDS medicines in East African health institutions" in: *Medical Anthropology* 30(2), pp. 136–157.

Hardon, Anita / Akurut, Dorothy. / Comoro, Christopher. / Ekezie, Cosmas. / Irunde, Henry. / Gerrits, Trudie. / Kglatwane, Joyce et al. (2007): "Hunger, waiting time and transport costs: time to confront challenges to ART adherence in Africa", in: *AIDS Care* 19(5), pp. 658–665.

Harms, Robert (1975): "The end of red rubber: A reassessment", in: *Journal of African history* 16(1), pp. 73–88.

Harper, Ian (2005): "Interconnected and Inter-infected: DOTS and the stabilization of the tuberculosis control programme in Nepal", in: David Mosse/David Lewis (eds), *The aid effect: giving and governing in international development*, London; Ann Arbor: Pluto, pp. 126–149.

Harrison, Graham (2008): "From the global to the local? Governance and development at the local level: Reflections from Tanzania", in: *The Journal of Modern African Studies* 46, pp. 169–189.

Harrison, Mark (1996): "Medicine and the culture of command: The case of malaria control in the British Army during the two World Wars", in: *Medical History* 40(4), pp. 437–452.

Harrison, Mark (2004): *Medicine and victory: British military medicine in the Second World War*, Oxford: Oxford University Press.

Harrison, Simon (1992): "Ritual as intellectual property", in: *Man*, New Series 27(2), pp. 225–244.

Hartwig, Kari A., et al. (2005): "AIDS and 'shared sovereignty' in Tanzania from 1987 to 2000: a case study", in: *Social Science & Medicine* 60(7), pp. 1613–1624.

Harvey, David W. (2006): *A brief history of neoliberalism*, Oxford: Oxford University Press.

Haugerud, Angelique (1993): *The culture of politics in modern Kenya*, Cambridge: Cambridge University Press.

Hausmann-Muela, Susanna, et al. (2002): "Medical syncretism with reference to malaria in a Tanzanian community", in: *Soc Sci Med* 55(3), pp. 403–413.

Hay, Margaret J. (1976): "Luo women and economic change during the colonial period", in: Nancy J.B. Hafkin/Edna G. Bay (eds), *Women in Africa: studies in social and economic change Stanford*, Stanford University Press, pp. 87–109.

Hayden, Cory (2007): "Taking as giving: bioscience, exchange, and the politics of benefit-sharing", in: *Social Studies of Science* 37, pp. 729–758.

Headrick, Rita (1994): *Colonialism, health and illness in French Equatorial Africa, 1885–1935*, Atlanta, GA: African Studies Association Press.

Hearn, Julie (1998): "The NGO-isation of Kenyan society: USAID and the restructuring of Health Care", in: *Review of African Political Economy* 25(1995): 89–100.

Heller, Kevin J. (1996): "Power, subjectification and resistance in Foucault", in: *SubStance: a Review of Theory and Literary Criticism* 25(1), pp. 78–110.

Henson, Graham E. (1914): "Man, the principal etiological factor, in the perpetuation of malaria, with special references to the endemicity of the disease in the temperate zone", in: *Journal of American Medical Association* 62, pp. 1374–1377.

Hetzel, Manuel W., et al. (2007): "Understanding and improving access to prompt and effective malaria treatment and care in rural Tanzania: the ACCESS Programme", in: *Malar J* 6: pp. 83.

Hickey, Sam / Mohan, Giles (eds) (2004): *Participation: From tyranny to transformation? Exploring new approaches to participation in development*, London: Zed Books.

Hines, Sally (2009): "A pathway to diversity?: Human rights, citizenship and the politics of transgender", in: *Contemporary Politics* 15(1), pp. 87–102.

Hodd, Michael (1988): *Tanzania after Nyerere*, New York: Pinter Publishers.

Hong, Kari (2002): "Categorical exclusions: Exploring legal resoinse to health care discrimination against transsexuals", in: *Columbia Journal of Gender and Law*

11 http://www.trans-health.com/hong_categorical_exclusion.pdf, last accessed 02.10.2011.

Hoppe, Kirk A. (2003): *Lords of the fly: Sleeping sickness control in British East Africa, 1900–1960*, Westport, CT: Praeger.

Hubbard, Ruth (1998): "Gender and genitals: Constructs of sex and gender", in: Dallas Denny (ed.), *Current concepts in transgender identity*, New York: Garland Press, pp. 45–54.

Hucker, Stephen J. (1985): "Medical-legal issues", in: Betty W. Steiner (ed.), *Gender Dysphoria: Development, Research, Management*, New York: Plenum Press, pp. 393–410.

Hugon, Anne (2005): "L'historiographie de la maternité en Afrique subsaharienne", posted on Clio http://clio.revues.org/document1466.html accessed 15 July 2008.

Hunt, Nancy Rose (1999): *A colonial lexicon of birth ritual, medicalization and mobility in the Congo*, Durham, NC: Duke University Press.

Iliffe, John (1979): *A modern history of Tanganyika*, New York: Cambridge University Press.

Iliffe, John (1998): *East African doctors: A history of the modern profession*, New York: Cambridge University Press.

Illife, John (2006): *The African AIDS epidemic: A history*, Oxford: James Currey Ltd.

Illich, Ivan (1976): *Limits to medicine. Medical nemesis: The expropriation of health*, Harmondsworth: Penguin.

Imperato, Pascal James (2005): "Review: Lords of the fly: Sleeping sickness control in British East Africa, 1900–1960", in: *African Studies Review* 48(1), pp. 166–169.

IMTSSA-Institut de Médecine Tropicale du Service de Santé des Armées, Marseille (1944): Instruction du commissaire aux colonies, Comité français de Libération Nationale, n°1283 Colslg/88.4, 18 juin 1944, "recommandation de la Conférence Africaine Française de Brazzaville". Arch. IMTSSA: 115.

Isin, Engin F. / Turner, Bryan S. (2008): "Citizenship studies: An introduction", in: Idem (eds.) *Handbook of citizenship studies*, London: Sage, pp. 1–9.

ITPC (2005): Missing the target: A report on HIV/AIDS treatment access from the frontlines, www.aidstreatmentaccess.org.

ITPC (2006): Off-Target for 2010: How to avoid breaking the promise of universal access.

Jacques, Juliet (2010): "They are the gatekeepers of my physical transition" in: http://www.guardian.co.uk/lifeandstyle/2010/sep/22/transgender-charing-cross#start-of-comments, last accessed 18.09.2011.

Janes, Craig R. / Corbett, Kitty K. (2009): "Anthropology and global health", in: *Annual Review of Anthropology* 38, pp. 167–183.

Jasanoff, Sheila (ed.) (2004): *States of knowledge. The co-production of science and social order*, New York: Routledge.

Jennings, Eric Thomas (2001): *Vichy in the tropics: Pétain's national revolution in Madagascar, Guadeloupe and Indochina, 1940–1944*, Stanford, CA: Stanford University Press.

Jennings, Eric Thomas (2006): *Curing the colonizers: Hydrotherapy, climatology and French colonial spas*, Durham, NC: Duke University Press.

Jennings, Michael (2007): "'A very real war': Popular participation in development in Tanzania during the 1950s & 1960s", in: *International Journal of African Historical Studies* 40(1), pp. 71–95.

Jitta, Jessica / Whyte, Susan Reynolds / Nshakira, Nathan (2002): "The availability of drugs: what does it mean in Ugandan primary care", in: *Health Policy* 65, pp. 167–179.

Johnston Hank / Larana, Enrique / Gusfield, Joseph. R. (1994): "Identities, grievances, and new social movements", in: Enrique Larana/Hank Joseph./Joseph. R Gusfield (eds), *New social movements: From ideology to identity*, Philadelphia: Temple University Press, pp. 3–35.

Jones, James H. (1981): *Bad blood: the Tuskegee syphilis experiment*, New York & London: Free Press.

Joseph, Richard (1986): *Le mouvement nationaliste au Cameroun: les origines sociales de l'UPC*, Paris: Karthala.

Juma, Calestous (1989): *The gene hunters: Biotechnology and the scramble for seeds*, Princeton: Princeton University Press.

Jurisprudential Annotations to the Yogyakarta Principles (2007) http://www.yogyakartaprinciples.org/yogyakarta-principles-jurisprudential-annotations.pdf, last accessed 27.11.2009.

Kachur, Stephen P., et al. (2004): "Adherence to antimalarial combination therapy with sulfadoxine-pyrimethamine and artesunate in rural Tanzania", in: *Am J Trop Med Hyg* 71(6), pp. 715–722.

Kamat, Vinay R. (2006): "'I thought it was only ordinary fever!' cultural knowledge and the micropolitics of therapy seeking for childhood febrile illness in Tanzania", in: *Soc Sci Med* 62(12), pp. 2945–2959.

Kaplan, Robert M. (2004): "Treatment of homosexuality during apartheid", in: *BMJ* (18 December) 329, pp. 1415–1416.

Kasper, Toby / Coetzee, David / Louis, Francoise / Boulle, Andrew / Hilderbrand, Katherine (2003): "Demystifying antiretroviral therapy in resource-poor settings", in: *Essential Drug Monitor* 32, pp. 20–21.

Keck, Margaret .E. / Sikkink, Kathryn (1998): *Activists beyond borders: Advocacy networks in international politics*, Ithaca: Cornell University Press.

Keller, Richard (2007): *Colonial madness: Psychiatry in French North Africa*, Chicago, IL: University of Chicago Press.

Kelly, Ann H. (2011): "Will he be there? A meditation on immobility and scientific labour", in: *Journal of Cultural Economy* 4(1), pp. 65–79.

Kelly, Ann H. / Beisel, Uli (2011): "Neglected malarias: Debugging the link between eradication and development", in: *Biosocieties* 4, pp. 71–87.

Kelly, Ann H. et al. (2010): "Like sugar and honey. The embedded ethics of a larval control project in the Gambia", in: *Social Science and Medicine* 70, pp. 1912–1919.

Kengeya-Kayondo, Jane F., et al. (1994): "Recognition, treatment seeking behaviour and perception of cause of malaria among rural women in Uganda", in: *Acta Trop* 58(3–4), pp. 267–273.

Khagram, Sanjeev / Riker, James.V. / Sikkink, Kathryn (eds) (2002): *Restructuring world politics: Transnational social movements, networks and norms*, Minneapolis: University of Minnesota Press.

Khantikul, Nardlada, et al. (2009): "Adherence to antimalarial drug therapy among vivax malaria patients in northern Thailand", in: *J Health Popul Nutr* 27(1), pp. 4–13.

Kidson, Chev (1992): "Global malaria challenge: the Amsterdam summit", in: *Southeast Asian J Trop Med Public Health* 23(4), pp. 635–640.

Killeen Gerry F. et al. (2003): "Taking malaria transmission out of the bottle: implications of mosquito dispersal for vector-control interventions", in: *Lancet Infectious Diseases* 3(5), pp. 297–303.

Killeen Gerry F. et al. (2006): "Habitat targeting for controlling aquatic stages of malaria vectors in Africa", in: *American Journal of Tropical Medicine & Hygiene* 74, pp. 517–518.

Kinung'hi, Safari M., et al. (2007): "Knowledge, attitudes and practices about malaria among communities: comparing epidemic and non-epidemic prone communities of Muleba district, North-western Tanzania", in: *BMC Public Health* 10, pp. 395.

Kironde, J.M. Lusugga (1995): "Access to land by the urban poor in Tanzania: Some findings from Dar es Salaam", in: *Environment and Urbanization* 7, pp. 77–96.

Kiunsi, Robert et al. (2009): "Building disaster-resilient communities: Dar es Salaam, Tanzania", in: Mark Pelling/Ben Winser (eds), *Disaster risk reduction: Cases from urban Africa*, London: Earthscan, pp. 127–145.

Klein, Thamar (2009): "Intersex and transgender activism in South Africa". Liminalis 3. http://www.liminalis.de/2009_03/Liminalis-2009-Klein.pdf, last accessed 17.10.2010.

Koch, Henri (1949): "Aperçu démographique des territoires de l'AOF", in: *Bulletin Médical de l'AOF* 6, pp. 161–173.

Koch, Henri (1967): *La médecine de l'espérance*, Paris: Maloine.

Koch, Henri (1968): *Magie et chasse dans la forêt camerounaise*, Paris: Éditions Berger Levrault.

Kohler, Robert E. (2002): *Labscapes and landscapes*, Chicago: University of Chicago Press.

Kombe, Wilbard J. / Kreibich, Volker (2001): "Informal land management in Tanzania and the misconception about its illegality." Paper presented at the ESF/N-Aerus Annual Workshop "Coping with informality and illegality in human settlements in developing countries" in Leuven and Brussels, May 23–26.

Krause, Monika (2010): "Organized need. Humanitarian relief, NGOs and the market for projects." Unpublished manuscript.

Kuhn, Philalethes (1914): "Die Schlafenkrankheit in Kamerun", in: *Medizinische Klinik* 27, pp. 1131–1135.

Kyakuwa, Margaret (2009): "Ethnographic experiences of HIV-positive nurses in managing stigma at a clinic in rural Uganda", in: *African Journal of AIDS Research* 8(3), pp. 381–392.

Kyakuwa, Margaret (2010): *Going the extra mile: An ethnography of care giving and care designing among nurses in Uganda*. Unpublished PhD thesis, Amsterdam.

Kyessi, Alphonce G. (2005): "Community-based urban water management in fringe neighbourhoods: the case of Dar es Salaam, Tanzania", in: *Habitat International* 29, pp. 1–25.

Laborit, Henri / Grenié, Claude (1997): *Une vie: Derniers entretiens avec Claude Grenié*, Paris: Éditions du Félin.

Laburthe-Tolra, Philippe (1999): *Vers la lumière? ou, Le désir d'Ariel: À propos des Beti du Cameroun: sociologie de la conversion*, Paris: Karthala.

Lachenal, Guillaume (2006): *Biomédecine et décolonisation au Cameroun, 1944–1994. Technologies, figures et institutions médicales à l'épreuve*, Dissertation, Paris: Denis-Diderot.

Lachenal, Guillaume / Taithe, Bertrand (2009): "Une généalogie missionaire et coloniale de l'humanitaire: Le cas Aujoulat au Cameroun, 1935–1973", in: *Le Mouvement Social* 227(2), pp. 45–63.

Laing, Richard / Hodgekin, Catherine (2006): "Overview of antiretroviral therapy, adherence and drug-resistance", in: Anita Hardon et al. (eds), *From access to adherence: The challenges of antiretroviral treatment*, Geneva: WHO, pp. 21–31.

Lairumbi, Godfrey M. / Parker, Michael et al. (2011): "Stakeholders understanding of the concept of benefit sharing in health research in Kenya: a qualitative study", in: *BMC Medical Ethics* 12, pp. 20.

Lakoff, Andrew (2010): "Two regimes of global health", in: *Humanity: An International Journal of Human Rights, Humanitarianism, and Development* 1, pp. 59–79.

Langwick, Stacey A. (2007): "Devils, parasites, and fierce needles: Healing and the politics of translation in Southern Tanzania", in: *Science Technology Human Values* 32(1), pp. 88–117.

Lapeyssonnie, Léon (1982): *Toubib des tropiques*, Paris: Laffont.

Larkin, Brian (2008): *Signal and noise: Media, infrastructure, and urban culture in Nigeria*, Durhan, NC: Duke University Press.

Last, Murray (2012): The peculiarly political problem behind Nigeria's primary health care provision, in: Ruth J. Prince (ed.), *Shifting regimes of care: Anthropological perspectives on trajectories of public health in Africa*, Athens: Ohio University Press: in press.

Latour, Bruno (1984): *Les microbes guerre et paix suivi de Irréductions*, Paris: A.M. Métailié.

Latour, Bruno (2005): "From Realpolitik to Dingpolitik or How to make things public", in Bruno Latour/Peter Weibel (eds), *Making things public*, Cambridge, MA: MIT Press.

le Grand, Amanda, H. V. Hogerzeil / Haaijer-Ruskamp, F. M. (1999): "Intervention research in rational use of drugs: a review", in: *Health Policy Plan* 14(2), pp. 89–102.

Le Rouzic, Dr. Colonel / Koch Henri, Dr., Captain (1949): "Le SGHMP en AOF. Étude historique et statistique", in: *Bulletin Médical de l'AOF* 6, pp. 9–35.

Leach, James (2000): "Situated connections. Rights and intellectual resources in a Rai Coast society", in: *Social Anthropology* 8(2), pp. 163–179.

Leach, Melisse / Fairhead, James (2007): *Vaccine Anxieties: Global Science, Child Health and Society*, London, Earth Scan.

Lemmens, Trudo / Elliott, Carl (1999): "Guinea Pigs on the payroll: The ethics of paying research subjects", in: *Accountability in Research: Policies and Quality Assurance* 7(1), pp. 3–20.

Lewinson, Anne S. (2007): "Viewing postcolonial Dar es Salaam, Tanzania through civic spaces: a question of class", in: *African Identities* 5(2), pp. 199–215.

Lewis, Joanna (2000): *Empire State-building: War and welfare in Kenya 1925–52*, Oxford: James Currey.

Lezaun, Javier (2011): "Bees, beekeepers, and bureaucrats: Parasitism and the politics of transgenic life", in: *Environment and Planning D: Society and Space* 29(4), pp. 738 – 756.

Li, Tania M. (2005): "Beyond 'the State' and failed schemes, in: *American Anthropologist* 107(3), pp. 383–394.

Li, Tania M. (2007): *The will to improve. Governmentality, development and the practice of politics*, Durham and London: Duke University Press.

Linklater, Andrew (2008): "Cosmopolitan citizenship", in: Engin F. Isin/Bryan S. Turner (eds.), Handbook of citizenship studies, London: Sage, pp. 317–332.

Lister, Ruth (1997): Citizenship: Feminist perspectives, Basingstoke: Macmillan.

Lister, Ruth (2008): "Sexual citizenship", in: Engin F. Isin/Bryan S. Turner (eds.), Handbook of citizenship studies, London: Sage, pp. 191–207.

Livingstone, Julie (2012): *Improvising Medicine: An African Oncology Ward in an Emerging Cancer Epidemic*, Durham: Duke UP.

LNHO: League of Nations Health Organization (1925): Minutes of the international conference on sleeping sickness, held in London at the Colonial Office from May 19th to 22nd, 1925, Geneva: League of Nations.

Locke, John (1689): Second Treatise of Government. http://www.gutenberg.org/files/7370/7370-h/7370-h.htm, last accessed 02.10.2011.

Louet, Sabine (2003): "Public-private partnerships boost research on neglected diseases", in: *Nat Biotechnol* 21(11), pp. 1254–1255.

Lugalla, Joe L. (1995): "The impact of structural adjustment policies on women's and children's health in Tanzania", in: *Rev Afr Polit Econ* 22(63), pp. 43–53.

Lwoba, Albred / Ombongi, Kenneth / Geissler, Wenzel P. / Malowany, Maureen (2011): "'Take up the land!': Negotiating space, framing governmentality in Lambwe Valley, 1954–1975." Unpublished paper.

Lyons, Maryinez (1992): *The colonial disease: A social history of sleeping sickness in northern Zaire, 1900–1940*, Cambridge, UK: Cambridge University Press.

Madiega, Philister (2011): *Challenges faced by community-health workers in HIV/AIDS support and treatment: Patient support centers in western Kenya 2010–11.* Unpublished M.A. thesis, London School of Hygiene and Tropical Medicine.

Makemba, Ahmed M., et al. (1996): "Treatment practices for degedege, a locally recognized febrile illness, and implications for strategies to decrease mortality from severe malaria in Bagamoyo District, Tanzania", in: *Trop Med Int Health* 1(3), pp. 305–313.

Makundi, Emmanuel A., et al. (2006): "Role of traditional healers in the management of severe malaria among children below five years of age: the case of Kilosa and Handeni Districts, Tanzania", in: *Malar J* 5, pp. 58.

Malinowski, Bronislav (1922): *Argonauts of the Western Pacific*, London: Routeledge

Mamdani, Mahmood (1996): *Citizen and subject: Contemporary Africa and the legacy of late colonialism*, Princeton: Princeton University Press.

Marks, Shula (1997): "South Africa's early experiment in social medicine: Its pioneers and politics", in: *American Journal of Public Health* 87(3), pp. 452–459.

Marsland, Rebecca (2006): "'Community participation the Tanzanian way: Conceptual contiguity or power struggle?'", in: *Oxford Development Studies* 34(1), pp. 65–79.

Martin, Gustave (1921): *L'existence au Cameroun. Études sociales, études médicales, études d'hygiène et de prophylaxie*, Paris: Émile Larose.

Martin, Gustave (1931): "La collaboration administrative et médicale dans l'hygiène coloniale appliquée", in: *Les grandes endémies tropicales. Études de pathogénie et de prophylaxie* 2, pp. 63–81.

Martin, Gustave (1932): "L'influence du climat tropical sur le psychisme de l'Européen", in: *Les grandes endémies tropicales. Études de pathogénie et de prophylaxie* 3, pp. 101–116

Martinez-Jones, Astrid / Anyama, Norbert (2002): *Access to Antiretroviral Therapy in Uganda*, OXFAM GB.
Martonne, Édouard Guillaume de (1930): *Le savant colonial*, Paris: Larose.
Massey, Doreen (1999): *Power-geometries and the politics of space-time*, 2nd Hettner-Lecture, Stuttgart: Franz Steiner Verlag.
Mattes, Dominik (2011): "We are just supposed to be quiet: patient adherence to antiretroviral treatment in urban Tanzania", in: *Medical Anthropology* 30(2), pp. 158–183.
Maurer, Bill (2006): "The anthropology of money", in: *Annual Review of Anthropology* 35, pp. 15–36.
Mauss, Marcel (1990 [1923]): *The gift. The form and reason for exchange in archaic societies*, London, Routledge.
Mazenot, Georges (1996): *Carnets du Haut-Congo, 1959–1963*, Paris: L'Harmattan.
Mbembe, Achille (1996): *La naissance du maquis dans le Sud-Cameroun, 1920–1960*, Paris: Karthala.
Mbembe, Achille (2000): *On the postcolony*, Berkeley: University of California Press.
Mburu, F.M. (1985): "Evaluation of government rural health centers and UNICEF essential drug inputs", in: Dodge, Cole D./Wiebe, Paul D. (eds), *Crisis in Uganda: the breakdown of health services*, Oxford; New York: Pergamon Press, pp. 87–96.
McCombie, Susan C. (1996): "Treatment seeking for malaria: a review of recent research", in: *Soc Sci Med* 43(6), pp. 933–945.
McGoey, Linsey / Reiss, Julian / Wahlberg, Ayo (2011): "The global health complex", in: *BioSocieties* 6(1), pp. 1–9.
McKelvey, John (1975): *Man against tsetse, struggle for Africa*, Ithaca, NY: Cornell University Press.
McNeely, Ian (2002): *Medicine on a grand scale: Rudolf Virchow, liberalism and the public health*, London: Wellcome Trust.
Meagher, Kate (2007): "Manufacturing disorder: Liberalization, informal enterprise and economic 'ungovernance' in African small firm clusters", in: *Development and Change* 38(3), pp. 473–503.
Médecin-Chef de Région (1944): Étude sur l'administration médicale directe d'une région démographique éprouvée, 18 January 1944. Arch. IMTSSA: 115.
Medecines Sans Frontieres (2001): *Fatal imbalance: The crisis in research and development for drugs for neglected diseases*, Geneva: MSF.
Médecins Sans Frontières (MSF) (2006): "Human African Trypanosomiasis: Facing the Challenges Caused by Neglect, the Need for New Treatment and Diagnostics", in: Francesco Checchi/Graciela Diap/Unni Karunakara, *Campaign for Access to Essential Medicines*, Geneva: MSF.
Meinert, Lotte (forthcoming, 2012): "Regimes of homework in AIDS care. Questions of responsibility and imagination of lives in Uganda", in: Ruth

Prince/Rebecca Marsland, *The changing order of public health in Africa: Anthropological perspectives*, Athens: Ohio University Press.

Meinert, Lotte / Mogensen, Hanne O. / Twebaze, Jennifer (2009): "'Tests for life chances: CD4 miracles and obstacles in Uganda", in: *Anthropology & Medicine* 16(2), pp. 195–209.

Melucci, Alberto (1989): *Nomads of the present: Social movements and individual needs in contemporary society*, Philadelphia: Temple University Press.

Mfecane, Sakhumzi (2010): *Exploring masculinities in the context of ARV use: A study of men living with HIV in a South African village.* Unpublished PhD thesis, Witwatersrand.

Minja, Happiness, et al. (2001): "Introducing insecticide-treated nets in the Kilombero Valley, Tanzania: The relevance of local knowledge and practice for an information, education and communication (IEC) campaign", in: *Trop Med Int Health* 6(8), pp. 614–623.

Mission de Doumé (1941): Résumé du journal (no date). Arch.CSE: 2D54 A, Résumé de journaux de communautés, Fascicule 1 (Doumé).

Mission de Doumé (1944): Résumé du journal (no date). Arch.CSE: 2D54 A, Résumé de journaux de communautés, Fascicule 12.

Mission de Lomié (1941a): Journal (21 Décember 1941). Arch.CSE: 2D54 A, Résumé de journaux de communautés, Fascicule 11 (Lomié).

Mission de Lomié (1941b): Résumé du journal, (28 Novembre 1941). Arch.CSE: 2D54 A, Résumé de journaux de communautés, Fascicule 1 (Doumé).

Mission de Lomié (1942a): Journal (26 September 1942). Arch.CSE: 2D54 A, Résumé de journaux de communautés, Fascicule 11 (Lomié).

Mission de Lomié (1942b): Journal (no date). Arch.CSE: 2D54 A, Résumé de journaux de communautés, Fascicule 11 (Lomié).

Mission de Lomié (1942c): Résumé du journal (no date). Arch.CSE: 2D54 A, Résumé de journaux de communautés, Fascicule 1 (Doumé).

Mission de Lomié (1943): Journal (no date). Arch.CSE: 2D54 A, Résumé de journaux de communautés, Fascicule 11 (Lomié).

Mission de Lomié (1944): Journal (no date). Arch.CSE: 2D54 A, Résumé de journaux de communautés, Fascicule 11 (Lomié).

Mission de Messamena (1943): Résumé du journal (no date). Arch.CSE: 2D54 A, Résumé de journaux de communautés, Fascicule 9 (Messamena).

Mitchell, Timothy (2002): *Rule of experts: Egypt, techno-politics, modernity*, Berkeley: University of California Press.

Mkandawire, Thandika (2001): "Thinking about developmental states in Africa", in: *Cambridge Journal of Economics* 25(3), pp 289–314.

Mogensen, Hanne Overgaard (1995): *AIDS is a kind of Kahungo that kills: The challenge of using local narratives when exploring AIDS among the Tonga of Southern Zambia*, Oslo: Scandinavian University Press.

Molyneux, Catherine. S. / Mutemi, Wilfred et al. (2005): "Trust and informed consent: insights from community members on the Kenyan Coast", in: *Social Science & Medicine* 61, pp. 1463–1473.

Montgomery, Catherine M., et al. (2006): "'To help them is to educate them': power and pedagogy in the prevention and treatment of malaria in Tanzania", in: *Trop Med Int Health* 11(11), pp. 1661–1669.

Moran, Mary (2005): "A breakthrough in R&D for neglected diseases: new ways to get the drugs we need", in: *PLoS Med* 2(9), pp. e302.

Morolake, Odetoyinbo / Stephens, David / Welbourn, Alice (2009): "Greater involvement of people living with HIV in health care", in: *Journal of the International AIDS Society* 12(4).

Morris, Rosalind C. (2008): "Rush/panic/rush: Speculations on the value of life and death in South Africa's age of AIDS", *Public Culture* 20(2), pp. 199–231.

Mosse, David (2005): *Cultivating development. An ethnography of aid policy and practice*, London: Pluto Press.

Mukabana, W. Richard et al. (2006): "Ecologists can enable communities to implement malaria vector control in Africa", in: *Malaria Journal*, 5.

Murard, Lion (1996): *L'hygiène dans la République: la santé publique en France, ou l'utopie contrariée: 1870–1918*, Paris: Fayard.

Murard, Lion / Zylberman, Patrick (1984): "De l'hygiène comme introduction à la politique expérimentale (1875–1925)" in: *Revue de Synthèse* 105(115), pp. 313–341.

Mushita, Andrew / Thompson, Carol (2007): *Biopiracy of biodiversity: Global exchange as enclosure*, Trenton, NJ: Africa World Press.

Mwabu, Godfrey / Mwanzia, J. et al. (1995): "User charges in government health facilities in Kenya: effect on attendance and revenue" in: *Health Policy Plan* 10(2), pp. 164–170.

Mwenesi, Halima A. (2005): "Social science research in malaria prevention, management and control in the last two decades: An overview", in: *Acta Trop* 95(3), pp. 292–297.

Najera, Jose A. (2001): "Malaria control: Achievements, problems and strategies", in: *Parassitologia* 43(1–2), pp. 1–89.

Nash, T.A.M. (1948): *The Anchau rural development and settlement scheme*, London: Colonial Office.

Nguyen, Vin Kim (2004): "Antiretroviral globalism, biopolitics, and therapeutic citizenship", in: Aihwa Ong/Steve J. Collier (eds), *Global assemblages: Technology, politics and ethics as anthropological problems*, London: Blackwells, pp. 124–144.

Nguyen, Vinh-Kim (2009): "Government-by-Exception: Enrolment and experimentality in mass HIV treatment programs in Africa", in: *Social Theory and Health* 7(3), pp. 196–218.

Nguyen, Vinh-Kim (2010): *The republic of therapy: Triage and sovereignty in West Africa's time of AIDS*, Durham, NC, Duke University Press.

Nicolle, Charles (1934): *L'expérimentation en médecine*, Paris: Alcan.

Nnadozie, Kent / Lettington, Robert / Bruch, Carl / Bass, Susan (eds.) (2003): *African perspectives on genetic resources: A handbook on laws, policies and institutions*, Washington DC: Environmental Law Institute.

Nsungwa-Sabiiti, Jesca, et al. (2007): "Home-based management of fever and malaria treatment practices in Uganda", in: *Trans R Soc Trop Med Hyg* 101(12), pp. 1199–1207.

Ntozi, James P.M. / Zirimenya, Samuel (1999): "Change in household composition and family structure during the AIDS epidemic in Uganda", in: Israel O. Orubuloye/John C. Caldwell/James P.M. Ntozi (eds.), *The continuing HIV/AIDS epidemic in Africa: Responses and coping strategies*, Canberra: Health Transition Centre, pp. 193–209.

Nwaka, Solomon (2005): "Drug discovery and beyond: The role of public-private partnerships in improving access to new malaria medicines", in: *Trans R Soc Trop Med Hyg* 99(Suppl 1): pp. S20–S29.

Nyambedha, Erik O. (2008): "Ethical dilemmas of social science research on AIDS and orphanhood in western Kenya", in: *Social Science and Medicine* 67(5), pp. 771–779.

Nyambedha, Erik O. / Wandibba, Simiyu / Aagaard-Hansen, Jens (2003): "Changing patterns of orphan care due to the HIV epidemic in western Kenya", in: *Social Science and Medicine* 57, pp. 301–311.

Nyerere, Julius K. (1962 [1975]): "Ujamaa: the basis of African Socialism", in: Gideon-Cyrus Makau Mutiso/S.W. Rohio (eds), *Readings in African political thought*, London: Heinemann, pp. 512–515.

Nyerere, Julius K. (1967): "The Arusha declaration: socialism and self-reliance", in: J. K. Nyerere (ed.), *Freedom and development (Uhuru na Maendeleo): A selection from writings and speeches 1968–1973*, Open University Press, Dar es Salaam.

Oakley, Ann / Barker, Jonathan (2004): *Private complaints and public health. Richard Titmuss on the National Health Service*, Bristol: Policy Press.

Oberlander, Lars / Elverdan, Beth (2000): "Malaria in the United Republic of Tanzania: Cultural considerations and health-seeking behavior", in: *Bull World Health Organ* 78(11), pp. 1352–1357.

Odell, John S. (2006): *Negotiating trade: Developing countries in the WTO and NAFTA*, Cambridge: Cambridge University Press.

O'Farrell, Clare (2010): Frequently Asked Questions. http://www.michel-foucault.com/info/faq.html, last accessed 02.10.2011.

Ogot, Bethwell A. (2004): *Politics and the AIDS epidemic in Kenya 1983–2003*, Kisumu: Anyange Press.

Okonta, Ike / Douglass, Oronto (2003): *Where vultures feast: Shell, human rights, and oil in the Niger Delta*, London: Verso.

Ollwig, H. (1903): "Die Bekaempfung der Malaria", in: *Zeitschrift für Hygiene und Infektionskrankheiten* 43, pp. 133–155.

Ong, Aihwa (2005): "(Re)Articulations of citizenship", in: PSOnline, pp. 697-699. http://journals.cambridge.org/download.php?file=%2FPSC%2FPSC38_04%2FS1049096505050377a.pdf&code=a124352d121409a067d2aaa56a4c8e16, last accessed 17.10.2010.

Ong, Aihwa (2006): *Neoliberalism as exception: Mutations in citizenship and sovereignty*, Durham, Duke UP.

Ooms, Gorik, et al. (2010): "Financing the millennium development goals for health and beyond: sustaining the 'Big Push'", in: *Globalization and Health* 6(1), pp. 17.

Ordinioha, B. (2007): "The use of insecticide-treated bed net in a semi-urban community in south-south, Nigeria", in: *Niger J Med* 16(3), pp. 223–226.

Orenstein, Alexander J. (1914): "Contribution to the study of the value of quininization in the eradication of malaria", in: *Journal of the American Medical Association* 63, pp. 1931–1933.

Oster, Candice / Cheek, Julianne (2008): "Governing the contagious body: Genital herpes, contagion and technologies of the self", in: *Health* 12(2), pp. 215–232.

Oudart, J.L. (2005): "Les pharmaciens coloniaux", in: *Médecine tropicale* 65(3), pp. 263–272.

Oyebade, Adebayo (1998): "Feeding America's war machine: The United States and economic expansion in West Africa during World War II", in: *African Economic History* 26, pp. 119–140.

Packard, Randall M. (1984): "Maize, cattle and mosquitoes: The political economy of malaria epidemics in colonial Swaziland", in: *J Afr Hist* 25(2), pp. 189–212.

Packard, Randall M. (1989): *White plague, black labour: Tuberculosis and the political economy of health and disease in South Africa*, Berkeley: University of California Press.

Packard, Randall M. (1990): *White Plague, Black Labour: Tuberculosis and the political economy of health and disease in South Africa*, Oxford: James Currey.

Packard, Randall M. (1998): "'No other logical choice': Global malaria eradication and the politics of international health in the post-war era", in: *Parassitologia* 40(1–2), pp. 217–229.

Packard, Randall M. (2007): *The making of a tropical disease: A short history of malaria*, Balimore, MD: Johns Hopkins University Press.

Packard, Randall M. / Peter J Brown (1997): "Rethinking health, development, and malaria: Historicizing a cultural model in international health", in: *Med Anthropol* 17: 181–194.

Pallotti, Arrigo (2008): "Tanzania: Decentralising power or spreading poverty?" in: *Review of African Political Economy* 116, pp. 221–235.

Parry, Jonathan / Bloch, Maurice (1989): *Money and the morality of exchange*, Cambridge: Cambridge University Press.

Pecoul, Bernard / Chirac, Pierre / Trouiller, Patrice / Pinel, Jacques (1999): "Access to essential drugs in poor countries: A lost battle?" in: *JAMA* 281, pp. 361–362.

Pelis, Kimberly Ann (1995): *Pasteur's imperial missionary: Charles Nicolle (1866–1936) and the Pasteur Institute of Tunis.* Unpublished dissertation, Baltimore, MD.

PEPFAR (2009): Celebrating life: *The president's emergency plan for AIDS relief*, Annual report to Congress.

Pestre, Dominique (2004): "Le nouvel univers des sciences et des techniques: une proposition générale", in: Amy Dahan/Dominique Pestre (eds.), *Les sciences pour la guerre, 1940–1960*, Paris: Éditions de l'ÉHÉSS, pp. 11–47.

Petersen, Alan / Lupton, Deborah (1996): The new public health: Health and self in the age of risk, London: Sage.

Peterson, Kristin (2001): "Benefit sharing for all?—Bioprospecting NGOs, intellectual property rights, new governmentalities" in *PoLAR: Political and Legal Anthropology Review* 24(1), pp. 78–91.

Peterson, Kristin (2012): "AIDS policies for markets and warriors: Dispossession, capital, and pharmaceuticals in Nigeria", in: Kaushik Sunder Rajan (ed.), *Lively Capital*, Durham, NC: Duke University Press.

Petryna, Adriana (2002): *Life exposed: Biological citizens after chernobyl*, Princeton: Princeton University Press.

Petryna, Adriana (2005): "Ethical variability: Drug development and globalizing clinical trials", in: *American Ethnologist* 32(2), pp. 183–197.

Petryna, Adriana / Lakoff, Andrew / Kleinman, Arthur (2006): *Global pharmaceuticals: Ethics, markets, practices*, Durham: Duke University Press.

Pfeiffer, James / Nichter, Mark (2008): "What can critical medical anthropology contribute to global health?" in: *Medical Anthropology Quarterly* 22(4), pp. 410–415.

Pfeiffer, James / Chapman, Rachel (2010): "Anthropological perspectives on structural adjustment and public health", in: *Annual Review of Anthropology* 39(1): 149–165.

Picard, Louis A. (1980): "Socialism and the field administrator: Decentralization in Tanzania", in: *Comparative Politics* 12(4), pp. 439–457.

Plummer, Ken (2001): "The square of intimate citizenship: Some preliminary proposals", in: *Citizenship Studies* 5(3), pp. 237–53.

Pratt, Cranford (1976): *The critical phase in Tanzania, 1945–1968: Nyerere and the emergence of a socialist strategy*, Cambridge: Cambridge University Press.

Pratt, Cranford (1999): "Julius Nyerere: Reflections on the legacy of his socialism", in: *Canadian Journal of African Studies* 33(1), pp. 137–152.

Prince, Ruth J. (2011): "Public debates about 'Luo widow inheritance' in relation to Christianity, tradition and AIDS in western Kenya", in Harri Englund (ed.), *Christianity and public culture in Africa*, Athens: Ohio University Press.

Prince, Ruth Jane / Geissler, Paul Wenzel (2010): *"The land is dying": Contingency, creativity and conflict in Western Kenya*, Oxford: Berghahn Books.

Priotto, Gerardo / Kaboyo, Winyi (2002): Final evaluation of the MSF-France trypanosomiasis control program in West Nile, Uganda, from 1987 to 2002, Epicentre.

Pschyrembel (1994): *Klinisches Wörterbuch*, Berlin, New York: de Gruyter.

Rabinow, Paul (1996): "Artificiality and enlightenment: from sociobiology to biosociality", in: Paul Rabinow (ed.), *Essays on the anthropology of reason*, Princeton: Princeton University Press, pp. 91–111.

Rabinow, Paul (1999): *French DNA: Trouble in purgatory*, Chicago, IL: University of Chicago Press.

Rabinow, Paul (2005 [1996]): "Artificiality and enlightenment: from sociobiology to biosociality", in: J. Xavier Inda (ed.), *Anthropologies of modernity. Foucault, government, and life politics*, Malden, Oxford, Victoria: Blackwell Publishing, pp. 179–193.

Rabinow, Paul (2005): *Une France si moderne. Naissance du social, 1800–1950*, Paris: Buchet-Chastel.

Rabinow, Paul / Rose, Nikolas (2006): "Biopower today", in: *BioSocieties* 1, pp. 195–217.

Rajan, Kaushik Sunder (2006): *Biocapital: The constitution of postgenomic life*, Durham: Duke University Press.

Raman, Sujatha / Tutton, Richard (2010): "Life, science, and biopower", in: *Science, Technology & Human Values* 35(5), pp. 711–734.

Rankin, F. Harrison (1836): *The white man's grave: a visit to Sierra Leone, in 1834*, London: R. Bentley.

Rankin, Johanna (2005): "A new frontier for humanitarianism? Médecins Sans Frontiers responds to neglected diseases", UNC-Chapel Hill.

Ravishankar, Nirmala, et al. (2009): "Financing of global health: tracking development assistance for health from 1990 to 2007", in: *Lancet* 373(9681): pp. 2113–2124.

Redfield, Peter (2005): "Doctors, borders, and life in crisis", in: *Cultural Anthropology* 20(3), pp. 328–361.

Redfield, Peter (2006): "A less modest witness: Collective advocacy and motivated truth in a medical humanitarian movement", in: *American Ethnologist* 33(1), pp. 3–26.

Redfield, Peter (2008): "Vital mobility and the humanitarian kit", in: Andrew Lakoff/Stephen Collier (eds), *Biosecurity interventions: Global health and security in question*, New York: Columbia University Press, pp. 147–71.

Redfield, Peter (2012). "The unbearable lightness of ex-pats: Double binds of humanitarian mobility", in: *Cultural Anthropology* 27(2), pp. 358–382.

Redfield, Peter / Bornstein, Erica (eds) (forthcoming): *Forces of compassion: Humanitarianism between ethics and politics*, Santa Fe, NM: School of Advanced Research Press.

Reubi, David (2010): "The will to modernize: A genealogy of biomedical research ethics in Singapore", in: *International Political Sociology* 4(2), pp. 142–158.

Richardson, Diane (1998): "Sexuality and citizenship", in: *Sociology* 32(1), pp. 83–100.

Richter, Judith (2004): "Public-private partnerships for health: A trend with no alternatives?", in: *Development* 47(2): pp. 43–48.

Riles, Annelise (2008): "The anti-network: Private global governance, legal knowledge, and the legitimacy of the state", in: *American Journal of Comparative Law* 56, pp. 605–630.

Robins, Steven (2004): "'Long live Zackie, long live': AIDS activism, science and citizenship after apartheid", in: *Journal of Southern African Studies* 30(3), pp. 651–672.

Robins, Steven (2006): "From 'rights' to 'ritual': AIDS activism in South Africa", *American Anthropologist* 108(2): pp. 312–323.

Roitman, Janet (2005): *Fiscal disobedience: An anthropology of economic regulation in Central Africa*, Princeton: Princeton University Press.

Rose, Dale / Blume, Stuart (2003): "Citizens as users of technology: An exploratory study of vaccines and vaccination", in: Nelly Oudshorn/Trevor Pinch (eds), *How users matter. The co-construction of users and technologies*, Cambridge, MA: MIT Press, pp. 103–131.

Rose, Nikolas (1996): "The death of the social? Reconfiguring the territory of government", in: *Economy and Society* 25, pp. 327–356.

Rose, Nikolas (2007): The Politics of Life Itself: Biomedicine, Power, and Subjectivity in the Twenty-First Century, Princeton: Princeton University Press.

Rose, Nikolas / Miller, Peter (1992): "Political Power beyond the State: Problematics of Government", in: British Journal of Sociology 43(2): pp. 172–205.

Rose, Nikolas / Novas, Carlos (2005): "Biological citizenship", in: Aihwa Ong and Steven J. Collier. (eds), *Global assemblages. Technology, politics, and ethics as anthropological problems*, Oxford: Blackwell, pp. 439–463.

Ross, R. (1902 [2009]) *Mosquito brigades and how to organize them.* Milton Keynes, UK: General Books.

Ross, Robert (1898): "The role of the mosquito in the evolution of the malarial parasite", in: *Lancet* 152(3912): pp. 488–490.

Rottenburg, Richard (2009): "Social and public experiments and new figurations of science and politics in postcolonial Africa", in: *Postcolonial Studies* 12(4), pp. 423–440.

Rottenburg, Richard (2009): *Far-fetched facts: A parable of development aid*, Cambridge, MA: The MIT Press.

Roussin, Philippe (2005): *Misère de la littérature, terreur de l'histoire: Céline et la littérature contemporaine*, Paris: Gallimard.

Sabatello, Maya (2009): Transgendered parenthood: Science and family life. Draft—Work in Progress. http://www.fondazionefeltrinelli.it/dm_0/FF/FeltrinelliCmsPortale/0388.pdf, last accessed 17.10.2010.

Samelius, Lotta / Wagberg, Erik (2005): Sexual orientation and gender identity issues in development. A study of policy and administration. http://www.sida.se/shared/jsp/download.jsp?f=SIDA4948en_Sexual+Orientation+web.pdf&a=4855, last accessed 02.10.2011.

Samoff, Joel. (1974): *Tanzania: Local politics and the structure of power*, Madison: The University of Wisconsin Press.

Sartre, Jean-Paul (2007): *Typhus* (unpublished scenario, c. 1944), Paris: Gallimard.

Sattler, Michael A. et al. (2005): "Habitat characterization and spatial distribution of Anopheles sp. mosquito larvae in Dar es Salaam (Tanzania) during an extended dry period", in: *Malaria Journal* 4(4).

Schellenberg, Joanna R., et al. (1999): "KINET: A social marketing programme of treated nets and net treatment for malaria control in Tanzania, with evaluation of child health and long-term survival", in: *Trans R Soc Trop Med Hyg* 93(3), pp. 225–231.

Schinkel, Willem (2010): "From zoepolitics to biopolitics: Citizenship and the construction of 'society'", in: *European Journal of Social Theory* 13(2), pp. 155–172.

Schneider, William H. / Drucker, Ernest (2006): "Blood transfusions in the early years of AIDS in sub-Saharan Africa"; in: *American Journal of Public Health* 96(6), pp. 984–994.

Semboja, Joseph / Therkildsen, Ole (1995): *Service provision under stress in East Africa: The state, NGOs & people's organizations in Kenya, Tanzania & Uganda*, Portsmouth, NH: Heinemann.

Serdobova, Irina / Kieny, Marie-Paule (2006): "Assembling a global vaccine development pipeline for infectious diseases in the developing world", in: *Am J Public Health* 96(9): pp. 1554–1559.

Service, Mike W. (1993): "Community participation in vector-borne disease control", in: *Ann Trop Med Par* 87(3), pp. 223–234.

Shah, Sonia (2006): *The body hunters: Testing new drugs on the world's poorest patients*, New York: New Press.

Shapiro, Eve (2010): *Gender circuits. Bodies and identities in a technological age*, New York NY: Routledge (Contemporary sociological perspectives).

Sharpe, Andrew N. (2007): "Endless Sex: The gender recognition act and the persistence of a legal category", in: *Feminist Legal Studies* 15(1), pp. 57–84.

Shiffman, Jeremy (2006): "Donor funding priorities for communicable disease control in the developing world", in: *Health Policy Plan* 21(6), pp. 411–420.

Shipton, Parker (1989): *Bitter money: Cultural economy and some African meanings of forbidden commodities*, Washington, DC: American Anthropological Association.

Shipton, Parker (2007): *The nature of entrustment: Intimacy, exchange and the sacred in Africa*, New Haven: Yale University Press.

Shivji, Issa G. (2004): "Reflections on NGOs in Tanzania: What we are, what we are not, and what we ought to be", in: *Development in Practice* 14(5), pp. 689–695.

Sibeud, Emmanuelle (2002): *Une science impériale pour l'Afrique? La construction des savoirs africanistes en France, 1878–1930*, Paris: Éditions de l'ÉHÉSS.

Sicé, A (1946): *L'AEF et le Cameroun au service de la France*, Paris: Presses Universitaires de France.

Sicé, A. (1943): 'L'Assistance medicale en Afrique Noire Francaise. *Africa* 14(1), pp. 27–34.

Silva, Kalinga Tudor (1997): "'Public health' for whose benefit? Multiple discourses on malaria in Sri Lanka", in: *Med Anthropol* 17(3), pp. 195–214.

Simone, Abdul Maliq (2006): "Pirate towns. Reworking social and symbolic infrastructures in Johannesburg and Douala", in: *Urban Studies* 43(2). pp. 357–370.

Simons, Jon (2006): "Michel Foucault (1926–84)", in: idem (Hg.), *Contemporary critical theorists. From Lacan to Said*, Edinburgh: Edinburgh Univ. Press, pp. 185–200.

Sodipo, Bankole (1997): *Piracy and counterfeiting: GATT, TRIPS, and developing countries*, London, Boston: Kluwer Law International.

Sonné, Wang (1998): "Approche historique de la gestion de la Région médicale du Haut-Nyong (Cameroun), 1939–1948", in: A. Guerci (ed.), *Treating illness, historical routes*, Genoa: Erga Edizione, pp. 371–383.

Souares, Aurelia, et al. (2008): "Adherence and effectiveness of drug combination in curative treatment among children suffering uncomplicated malaria in rural Senegal", in: *Trans R Soc Trop Med Hyg* 102(8), pp. 751–758.

South African Law Commission (1995): Report on the investigation into the legal consequences of sexual realignment and related matters. Project 52.

Ssewaya, Achilles (2010): *Sustaining adherence to antiretroviral therapy among HIV/AIDS patients in Uganda*. Unpublished PhD thesis, Amsterdam.

Stambach, Amy (2000): *Lessons from Mount Kilimanjaro: Schooling, community, and gender in East Africa*, New York: Routledge.

Stapleton, Darwin H. (2009): "Historical perspectives on malaria: The Rockefeller antimalaria strategy in the 20th century", in: *Mt Sinai J Med* 76(5), pp. 468–73.

Stoler, Ann Laura / Cooper, Frederick (1997): "Between métropole and colony: Rethinking a research agenda", in: ead. (eds), *Tensions of empire: Colonial cultures in a bourgeois world*, Berkeley/London: University of California Press. pp. 1–56.

Strathern, Marilyn (1988): *The gender of the gift. Problems with women and problems with society in Melanesia*, Berkeley, Los Angeles, London, California UP.

Strathern, Marilyn (1999): *Property, substance, and effect: Anthropological essays on persons and things*, New Brunswick, NJ: Athlone Press.

Sufian, Sandra M. (2007): *Healing the land and the nation: Malaria and the Zionist Project in Palestine, 1920–1947*, Chicago: University of Chicago Press.

Sullivan, Noelle (2011): "Mediating abundance and scarcity: Implementing and HIV/AIDS targeted project within a government hospital" in: *Medical Anthropology* 30(2), pp. 202–221.

Sunder Rajan, Kaushik (2006): *Biocapital: The constitution of post-genomic life*, Durham: Duke University Press.

Sutter, Paul (2007): "Nature's agents or agents of empire? Entomological workers and environmental change during the construction of the Panama Canal", in: *Isis* 98(4), pp. 724–754.

't Hoen, Ellen (2002): "TRIPS, pharmaceutical patents, and access to essential medicines: A long way from Seattle to Doha", in: *Chicago Journal of International Law* 3(1), pp. 27–46.

't Hoen, Ellen (2009): *The global politics of pharmaceutical monopoly power*, Amsterdam: Amb.

Taithe, Bertrand (2009): *The killer trail: A colonial scandal in the heart of Africa*, Oxford: Oxford University Press.

Tanner, Marcel, et al. (1987): Longitudinal study on the health status of children in a rural Tanzanian community: Parasitoses and nutrition following control measures against intestinal parasites", in: *Acta Trop* 44(2), pp. 137–74.

Tanner, Marcel / Kitua, Andrew / Degremont, A. A. (1994): "Developing health research capability in Tanzania: From a Swiss Tropical Institute field laboratory to the Ifakara Centre of the Tanzanian National Institute of Medical Research", in: *Acta Trop* 57(2–3), pp. 153–173.

Tanon, Louis (1930): "Préface", in: *Les grandes endémies tropicales.* Études de pathogénie et de prophylaxie I, pp. ii.

Tantchou, Josiane (2007): *Epidémie et politique en Afrique. Maladie du sommeil et tuberculose au Cameroun*, Paris: L'Harmattan.

Tarimo, Donath S., et al. (2000): "Mothers' perceptions and knowledge on childhood malaria in the holendemic Kibaha district, Tanzania: Implications for malaria control and the IMCI strategy", in: *Trop Med Int Health* 5(3), pp. 179–184.

Taylor, Verta / Whittier, Nancy E. (1992): "Collective identity in social movement communities: Lesbian feminist mobilization", in Aldon D. Morris/Carol McClurg Mueller (eds), *Frontiers of social movement theory*, New Haven: Yale University Press, pp. 104–129.

The Advisory Committee of the People with AIDS (1983): The Denver Principles. http://www.actupny.org/documents/Denver.html (accessed 14.10.2010).

Thomas, T., R. Masaba, et al. (2008): PMTCT of HIV-1 among breastfeeding mothers using HAART: the Kisumu Breastfeeding Study, Kisumu, Kenya,

2003–2007. 15th Conference on Retroviruses and Opportunistic Infections (CROI). Boston, Massachusetts.

Tilley, Helen (2001): *Africa as a "living laboratory"—The African Research Survey and the British colonial empire: Consolidating environmental, medical, and anthropological debates, 1920–1940*. Unpublished dissertation, Oxford, UK.

Tilley, Helen (2004): "Ecologies of complexity: Tropical environments, African trypanosomiasis, and the science of disease control strategies in British colonial Africa, 1900–1940", in: *Osiris* 19, pp. 21–38.

Tilley, Helen (2011): *Africa as a living laboratory: Empire, development, and the problem of scientific knowledge*, Chicago: University of Chicago Press.

Titmuss, Richard M. (1964): *The health services of Tanganyika: A report to the government*, London: Pitman Medical Pub. Co.

Titmuss, Richard M. (1970): *The gift relationship: From human blood to social policy*, London: Allen and Unwin.

Trigg, Peter I. / Kondrachine, Anatoli V. (1998): "Commentary: Malaria control in the 1990s", in: *Bull World Health Organ* 76(1), pp. 11–16.

Tripp, Aili Mari (1997): *Changing the rules: The politics of liberalization and the urban informal economy in Tanzania*, Berkeley: University of California Press.

Trouiller, Patrice, et al. (2001): "Drugs for neglected diseases: A failure of the market and a public health failure?" in: *Trop Med Int Health* 6(11), pp. 945–951.

Turnbull, David (2003): "Making malaria curable: Extending a knowledge space to create a vaccine", in: David Turnbull, *Masons, tricksters and cartographers*, London, Routledge, pp. 161–181.

Turshen, Meredeth (1999): *Privatizing health services in Africa*, New Brunswick, N.J.: Rutgers University Press.

UNAIDS (1999): "From principle to practice: Greater involvement of people living with or affected by HIV/AIDS", in: *UNAIDS* 99.43E.

UNAIDS (2000): AIDS becoming Africa's top human security issue, UN warns, Press Release, 10 January.

UNECA (1996): Africa and the multilateral trading system and the World Trade Organization (WTO): Seattle and Beyond, Addis Ababa: UNECA.

Vanek, Michael J. et al. (2006): "Community based surveillance of malaria vector larval habitats A baseline study in urban Dar es Salaam, Tanzania", in: *BMC Public Health* 6, pp. 154.

Vaucel Marcel (1952): *Médecine Tropicale*, Paris: Flammarion.

Vaucel, Marcel (1940): Rapport Annuel. Année 1939. Service de Santé. Cameroun Français. B.—Partie Médicale. Arch. IMTSSA: Boite 107.

Vaughan, Megan (1991): *Curing their ills. Colonial power and African illness*, Cambridge: Polity Press.

Vincent, Louise / Camminga, Bianca (2009): "Putting the 'T' into South African human rights: Transsexuality in the post-Apartheid order", in: *Sexualities* 12(6), pp. 678–700.

Virchow, Rudolf (1848): *Medicinische Reform*, n°18", 3 November 1848, Rudolf Virchow, Gesammelte Abhandlungen aus dem Gebiete der öffentlichn Medicine und der Seuchenlere (2 vols.), Berlin, Hirschwald, 1879.

Wadman, Meredith (2006): "London's disastrous drug trial has serious side effects for research", in: *Nature* 440, pp. 388–389.

Walker, Kristen (2001): "Moving gaily forward? Lesbian, gay and transgender human rights in Europe", in: *Melbourne Journal of International Law* 2(1), http://www.austlii.edu.au/au/journals/MelbJIL/2001/4.html, last accessed 02.10.2011.

Watts, Michael (ed.) (2010): *Curse of the black gold: 50 years of oil in the Niger Delta*, Brooklyn, NY: PowerHouse Books.

Weindling, Paul (1995): "Social medicine at the League of Nations Health Organization and the International Labour Office compared", in: Paul Weindling (ed.), *International health organizations and movements, 1918–1939*, Cambridge, UK: Cambridge University Press, pp. 134–153.

Wendland, Claire L. (2010): *A heart for the work: Journeys through an African medical school*, Chicago: Chicago University Press.

Wendt, Paul (1947): "The control of rubber in World War II", in: *Southern Economic Journal* 13(3), pp. 203–227.

White, Luise (2000): *Speaking with vampires: Rumor and history in colonial Africa*, Berkeley, University of California Press.

Whiteside, Alan / Smith, Julia (2009): "Exceptional epidemics: AIDS still deserves a global response", in: *Globalization and Health* 5(1), pp. 1–6.

Whittle, Stephen et al. (2008): "Transgender Eurostudy: legal survey and focus on the transgender experience of health care. ILGA-Europe." http://www.ilga-europe.org/europe/publications/non_periodical/transgender_eurostudy_legal_survey_and_focus_on_the_transgender_experience_of_health_care_april_2008, last accessed 27.11.2009

WHO (2003): Scaling Up Antiretroviral Therapy: Experience in Uganda, in: *Perspectives and practice in antiretroviral treatment*, WHO.

WHO (2006): Evaluation of WHO's Contribution to '3 by 5', Main Report, Geneva: WHO.

WHO (2010): Towards universal access: scaling up priority HIV/AIDS interventions in the health sector: progress report 2010, WHO.

WHO / UNAIDS (2008): Towards Universal Access: Scaling Up Priority HIV/AIDS Interventions in the Health Sector, Progress Report 2008, Geneva: WHO.

Whyte, Susan Reynolds (1992): "Pharmaceuticals as folk medicine: Transformations in the social relations of health care in Uganda", in: *Cult Med Psychiatry* 16(2), pp. 163–186.

Whyte, Susan Reynolds (1997): *Questioning misfortune. The pragmatics of uncertainty in eastern Uganda*, Cambridge: Cambridge University Press.

Whyte, Susan Reynolds (2009): "Health identities and subjectivities: The ethnographic challenge", in: *Medical Anthropology Quarterly* 23(1), pp. 6–15.

Whyte, Susan Reynolds (2012): "The publics of the new public health: Life conditions and 'lifestyle diseases' in Uganda", in: Ruth J. Prince (ed.), *Shifting regimes of care: Anthropological perspectives on trajectories of public health in Africa*, Athens: Ohio University Press: in press.

Whyte, Susan Reynolds / van der Geest, Sjaak / Hardon, Anita (2002): *Social lives of medicines*, Cambridge: Cambridge University Press.

Whyte, Susan Reynolds / Whyte, Michael [forthcoming]: "Therapeutic clientship: Belonging in Uganda's mosaic of AIDS projects", in: *When people come first: Anthropology and social innovation in global health*, Joao Biehl/Adriana Petryna (eds), Princeton: Princeton University Press.

Whyte, Susan Reynolds / Whyte, Michael / Meinert, Lotte / Kyaddondo, Betty (2006): "Treating AIDS: Dilemmas of unequal access in Uganda", in: Adriana Petryna/ Andrew Lakoff/Arthur Kleinman (eds), *Global pharmaceuticals: Ethics, markets, practices*, Durham: Duke University Press, pp. 240–290.

Wilder, Gary (2005): *The French imperial nation-state: Négritude and colonial humanism between the two World Wars*, Chicago, IL: University of Chicago Press.

Winch, Peter J., et al. (1996): "Local terminology for febrile illnesses in Bagamoyo District, Tanzania and its impact on the design of a community-based malaria control programme", in: *Soc Sci Med* 42(7), pp. 1057–1067.

Wolf, Angelika. (2001): "AIDS, morality and indigenous concepts of sexually transmitted diseases in Southern Africa", in: *Africa Spectrum* 36(1), pp. 97–107.

Worboys, Michael (1994): "The comparative history of sleeping sickness in East and Central Africa, 1900–1914", in: *History of Science* 32, pp. 89–102.

World Bank. 2001. *World Development Report 2002: Building institutions for markets*, New York: Oxford University Press.

World Health Organization (2003): *Scaling up antiretroviral therapy in resource-limited settings: Treatment guidelines for a public health*, Geneva: WHO.

World Health Organization (2006): *The world health report 2006: Working together for health*, Geneva: WHO

World Health Organization (2009): *Rapid advice: Antiretroviral therapy for HIV Infection in Adults and Adolescents*, Geneva: WHO.

WTO (No date): The GATT years: from Havana to Marrakesh. http://www.wto.org/English/thewto_e/whatis_e/tif_e/fact4_e.htm. Accessed October 1, 2009.

Yamagata, Yoshi (1996): Review of Tanzania-Japan urban malaria control project (UMCP) in Dar es Salaam and Tanga (1988–1996), Dar es Salaam, Tanzania: Japan International Cooperation Agency, pp. 46.

Yamba, Bawa C. (1997):"Cosmologies in turmoil: Witchfinding and AIDS in Chiawa, Zambia", in: *Africa* 67(2); pp. 200–222.

Yaoundé / Divers (1942): Correspondances des Pères de Messamena, 1935–1953. Arch.CSE: 2J1 11b.

Yarrow, Thomas / Venkatasan, Soumhya (eds) (2012): *Differentiating development: Beyond an anthropology of critique*, Kumerian Press: Bloomfield, CT

Yeatman, Anna (1990): "Voice and representation in the politics of difference", in: Anna Yeatman and Sneija Gunew (eds), *Feminism and the politics of difference*, St.Leonards, Australia: Allen and Unwin, pp. 228–245.

Yhdego, Michael / Majura, Paul (1988): "Malaria control in Tanzania", in: *Environment International* 14, pp. 479–483.

Young, Iris M. (1990): *Justice and the politics of difference*, Princeton: Princeton University Press.

Zerbe, Noah (2007): "Contesting privatization: NGOs and farmers' rights in the African model law", in: *Global Environmental Politics* 7(1), pp. 97–119.

Contributors

Paul Wenzel Geissler teaches social anthropology at the Institute of Social Anthropology, University of Oslo and the London School of Hygiene and Tropical Medicine, where he founded the research group 'Anthropologies and Histories of African Biosciences'. He was an associate member of the LOST project at the Max Planck Institute for Social Anthropology. He studied zoology in Hamburg and Copenhagen (Ph.D. 1998) and social anthropology in Copenhagen and Cambridge (Ph.D. 2003). He wrote the monograph (with Ruth Prince) *The Land is Dying* (2010, Amaury Albot Price), and co-edited *Aids and Religious Practice in Africa* (2007) and *Evidence, Ethos and Experiment—the anthropology and history of medical research in Africa* (2010).

Rene Gerrets currently holds a postdoc position at the University of Amsterdam. His research uses malaria as a lens to investigate expertise and governance in East Africa. His current project examines how biomedical institutions dating back to the colonial era generate memory in African settings.

Ann Kelly is a Lecturer with the Anthropologies of African Biosciences (AAB) group at the London School of Hygiene and Tropical Medicine. Her work focused on international public health interventions. Her ethnographic fieldwork in Tanzania and The Gambia explores the production of scientific facts in Africa, with special attention to the built-environments, material artefacts and practical labours of experimentation. A second focus is on malaria control interventions, how rural and urban spaces are configured to manage the flow of human, parasite and mosquito populations. She is currently developing a project exploring the forms, mobilities and genres of memory among municipal health-workers in African cities.

Thamar Klein is research associate at the Somatechnics Research Centre, Macquarie University in Sydney, Australia. Ze serves on the editorial board of Liminalis and the advisory board of TvT: Transrespect Versus Transphobia Worldwide. From 2009—2010 ze has been elected vice-chair of the Work Group

Anthropological Gender Studies and since 2010 elected vice-chair of the Work Group Medical Anthropology of the German Anthropological Association. Hir current research interests include Queer Studies, Medical Anthropology as well as Science and Technology Studies. Hir major publication is *Alafia: Globale und lokale Medizinen in Benin* (Lit Verlag, 2009).

Guillaume Lachenal is a lecturer in the department of history and philosophy of science at Université Paris Diderot Sorbonne Paris Cité. His current research interest is the history of colonial and post-colonial medical research in Africa, especially in the (former) French colonies. He has published articles in the Lancet and Annales, and he is finishing a book manuscript for the publisher Karthala on the biography of Pentamidine, a colonial wonder drug that was used for the prevention of sleeping sickness and provoked major accidents in late colonial Africa.

Kristin Peterson is a cultural anthropologist based at the University of California, Irvine. Her research interests include science and technology studies, theories of property and capital, pharmaceuticals, AIDS policies, clinical research and humanitarianism in Africa. She is currently completing a book on pharmaceutical markets in Lagos, entitled *Speculative Markets: Drug Circuits and Derivative Life in Nigeria.*

Ruth Prince is Mellon Fellow in Science, Medicine and Society in Africa at the Department of History and Philosophy of Science and the Centre of African Studies, University of Cambridge. Her research interests include the history and ethnography of medicine, health and healing in Africa; public health, development and the African city; memory and material culture; Christianity, subjectivity and personhood, with a focus on East Africa. Her current research explores the intersections between biomedical technologies, moral economies of care, survival and hope, governance and political economy in the city of Kisumu, Kenya. Her publications include *The Land is Dying: Contingency, Creativity and Conflict in Kenya* (Oxford: Berghahn, 2010), which received the 2010 Amaury Talbot prize for African Anthropology.

Peter Redfield is associate professor of anthropology at the University of North Carolina at Chapel Hill. Trained as a cultural anthropologist sympathetic to history, he concentrates on circulations of science and technology in colonial and postcolonial contexts, and currently focuses on humanitarian inspired design. The author of *Space in the Tropics: From Convicts to Rockets in French Guiana* (University of California Press, 2000) and *Life in Crisis: The Ethical Journey of Doctors Without Borders* (University of California Press, forthcoming), he is also the coeditor, with Erica Bornstein, of *Forces of Compassion: Humanitarianism Between Ethics and Politics* (School for Advanced Research Press, 2011).

Richard Rottenburg holds a chair in Social and Cultural Anthropology at the University of Halle (Germany). His research focuses on the anthropology of law, organization, science and technology (LOST). He has written and edited books on economic anthropology, networks of formal organizations, the transcultural production of objectivity, biomedicine and society, and on theorizing post-neoliberal governance (2009 *Far-fetched facts. A parable of development aid*, Cambridge, Mass.: MIT; 2009 Social and public experiments and new figurations of science and politics in postcolonial Africa. *Postcolonial Studies* 12 (4): 423-440).

Julia Zenker currently teaches medical anthropology at the University of Bern (Switzerland). She is an associate member of the LOST Research Group at the Max Planck Institute for Social Anthropology. She is currently turning her PhD thesis *The modernization of traditional healing in South Africa: Healers, biomedicine and the state*, which focuses on processes of standardization and professionalization in the course of a juridification of so-called traditional healing, into a book. Her publications include *Traditionelle Medizin und Afrikanische Renaissance in Südafrika*, in: Hansjörg Dilger, Bernhard Hadolt (eds.), Medizin im Kontext. Frankfurt a.m., Peter Lang: pp. 223-244